The Prevention of Eating Problems and Eating Disorders

Theory, Research, and Practice

Michael P. Levine
Linda Smolak
Kenyon College

LAWRENCE ERLBAUM ASSOCIATES, PUBLISHERS
2006   Mahwah, New Jersey   London

Copyright © 2006 by Lawrence Erlbaum Associates, Inc.
All rights reserved. No part of this book may be reproduced in
any form, by photostat, microform, retrieval system, or any other
means, without the prior written permission of the publisher.

Lawrence Erlbaum Associates, Inc., Publishers
10 Industrial Avenue
Mahwah, New Jersey 07430
www.erlbaum.com

Cover art by Samuel A. Malone
Cover design by Kathryn Houghtaling Lacey

Library of Congress Cataloging-in-Publication Data

Levine, Michael P.
  The prevention of eating problems and eating disorders : theory,
research, and practice / Michael P. Levine & Linda Smolak.
      p. cm.
  Includes bibliographical references and indexes.
  ISBN 0-8058-3925-9 (cloth)
  ISBN 0-8058-3926-7 (paper)
  1. Eating disorders—Prevention.
  [DNLM: 1. Eating Disorders—prevention & control. 2. Body Image.
3. Community Health Planning. 4. Preventive Health Services. 5. Risk Factors.
WM 175 L665p 2005] I. Smolak, Linda, 1951– II. Title.

RC552.E18L487 2005
616.85'2605—dc22   2005040028
                                                                         CIP

Books published by Lawrence Erlbaum Associates are printed on acid-free paper,
and their bindings are chosen for strength and durability.

Printed in the United States of America
10 9 8 7 6 5 4 3 2 1

The Prevention of Eating Problems and Eating Disorders

Theory, Research, and Practice

We dedicate this to the memory of Lori M. Irving (1962–2001) and to the future of Sabrina Lynn and the girls of her generation, that they might not struggle so mightily with these problems.

Contents

Preface ix

PART I: INTRODUCTION

1 Introduction to Prevention 3

2 Defining Eating Disorders 19

3 Important Controversies 42

PART II: GUIDES TO PREVENTION: MODELS AND RISK FACTORS

4 Developmental Psychopathology 73

5 Risk Factors as Guides to Prevention Program Design 95

6 Social Cognitive Approaches 108

7 The Non-Specific Vulnerability-Stressor Model 134

8 The Feminist-Empowerment-Relational Model: A Critical Social Perspective 149

PART III: REVIEW OF PREVENTION RESEARCH

9 Prevention of Body Image Disturbances and Disordered Eating: A Review of the Research — 179

PART IV: PREVENTION RESEARCH: LESSONS FROM THE FIELD

10 Lessons From the Field I: Curriculum and Program Development — 227

11 Lessons From the Field II: Practical Issues in Program Evaluation and Delivery — 264

12 Changing the Ecology — 282

13 Media Literacy as Prevention — 306

14 Deciding the Level of Prevention: Universal, Selective, or Targeted? — 335

PART V: CONCLUSIONS AND FUTURE DIRECTIONS

15 Conclusions and Future Directions — 361

Appendices A–E — 393

References — 409

Author Index — 445

Subject Index — 463

Preface

In the past 10 years the prevention of eating disorders and eating problems has been a burgeoning field of research and theory in a number of countries across the world. Since 1995 over 70 empirical studies evaluating universal-selective prevention programs have been published or made available as dissertations, theses, and conference papers. As documented by the numerous literature reviews that have also appeared, there has been considerable progress in this field. However, the research has often been marked by ambiguity of purpose, methodology, and outcomes. The result has been controversy—about the meaning of prevention, what can be prevented, the groups most likely to be helped, and the risk of well-intentioned efforts resulting in harm instead of prevention. As recently as the spring of 2000, the Academy of Eating Disorders' International Conference included a featured debate as to whether prevention is even possible.

This book was conceived within these strong cross-currents of progress and controversy. Whether one approaches the topic of prevention as a beginner or as an "expert," a thorough reading of the prevention literature in our field makes one key point very clear: Efforts to prevent eating problems and disorders typically have not been well rooted in general prevention theories and established prevention methodologies. With some notable exceptions, our field has not made good use of the models, theories, research strategies, data, and hard-earned wisdom of prevention science, health education, and community psychology. This has often led to a lack of precision as to what types of programs or techniques are most likely to be effective in achieving particular short-term and long-term outcomes. Research design problems have further limited the interpretation of findings. Yet, despite these problems, there are many reasons to believe that it is indeed possible to prevent body image and eating problems. In fact, the evidence concerning the continued spread of these problems internationally, as well as the limited access to and limited success of treatments, makes it evident that prevention efforts are essential.

In this book we adopt the perspective that not only *can* prevention work, but a broad coalition of people must try to find ways to *make* it work. We also believe that the best way to facilitate prevention is by mixing knowledge from the field of eating disorders with research, theory, and experience from other fields such as community psychology, public health, health education, developmental psychology, dietetics, and social work. Thus, this book is intended to be (a) an introduction to the prevention of eating problems and eating disorders, (b) a thorough review and critique of this topic in light of empirical studies within the fields of eating problems and substance abuse, and (c) a multidimensional guide for further development of the field, whether one is new to it or a veteran looking for new ideas. We hope the broad scope of this approach, coupled with detailed reviews of exemplary studies in the field, will be of use to prevention researchers in the aforementioned disciplines, health educators in schools, nonprofit eating disorder organizations, community activists, and students.

This is the first volume on the prevention of eating problems and disorders that is not an edited collection of chapters. To provide the depth, breadth, and integration that are unique features of this book, we have divided it into four major sections plus a final chapter. In Part I (*Introduction*) we discuss the definitions and necessity of prevention (chapter 1), the spectrum of eating problems and eating disorders that are the focus of prevention programs (chapter 2), and important but controversial issues such as the challenges posed by biopyschiatry, the role of males in prevention, and the significance of public concerns about obesity in children and adolescents (chapter 3).

Part II (*Models and Risk Factors*) considers the risk and protective factors that need to be decreased and increased, respectively, in order to prevent eating problems and disorders (chapter 5). Part II also presents in detail four models that have guided prevention efforts to date:

developmental psychopathology (chapter 4), social cognitive and cognitive-behavioral theories (chapter 6), the nonspecific vulnerability-stressor model (chapter 7), and feminist approaches (chapter 8). Part III (*Review of Prevention Research*) describes published and unpublished studies of prevention, characterizing them in terms of target audience, outcome, and the model or models that shaped the program (chapter 9). Part IV (*Lessons from the Field*) offers suggestions for curriculum and program development (chapter 10) and program evaluation (chapter 11) in light of both the extensive review in chapter 9 and research on the prevention of cigarette smoking and alcohol use by adolescents. The *Lessons* section also addresses three other very important topics for the development of our field: an ecological model of prevention (chapter 12), media literacy (chapter 13), and the question of whether prevention programs should be universal, selective, or targeted (chapter 14). Part V offers our major conclusions, that is, our answers to the major questions posed in chapter 1, and then integrates them into a detailed example of a feminist-ecological-developmental approach to community-based prevention.

ACKNOWLEDGMENTS

Collaboration is a cornerstone of prevention and professional development, and in our fields this is an international process. We wish to thank the following professionals for providing supplemental materials and constructive feedback to sharpen our analyses: Niva Piran (Canada), Dianne Neumark-Sztainer (USA), Jennifer O'Dea (Australia), Gail McVey (Canada), S. Bryn Austin (USA), Susan Paxton and Eleanor Wertheim (Australia), J. Kevin Thompson and Susan Stormer (USA), Riccardo Dalle Grave (Italy), Eric Stice (USA), and Linn Goldberg and Diane Elliot (USA). We single out Professors Austin, McVey, and Neumark-Sztainer for additional special thanks because they also served as reviewers for the first four chapters. In addition to Linda (his co-author, colleague, good friend, and astute critic), Michael would like to thank the following people for their abiding support during the writing of this book: Mary Suydam, Zeva Levine, Jim Keeler, Camille Collett, Michael Brint, Margo Maine, Carolyn Costin, Jane Martindell, Robin Cash, and Craig Johnson.

Linda wishes to first acknowledge that Michael is the guiding force of this book. Prevention is Michael's passion and this book represents his vision. She is grateful for his collegiality, great friendship, good humor, and hard work. As always, Linda is grateful to her family, particularly to her husband, Jim Keeler, for their support and patience, as well as to her friends and colleagues at Kenyon, especially Mary Suydam, Sarah Murnen, and Dana Krieg, for their support and good humor.

I

INTRODUCTION

1

Introduction to Prevention

Eating disorders constitute an array of problems that create a substantial amount of misery and dysfunction for sufferers and their families. As such, disordered eating is a significant social and economic issue for industrialized societies around the world. Testimonies from patients and their families, as well as reflections from sensitive clinicians, often include the statement "if only"—if only she had developed a stronger sense of self, if only something like a sexual assault had never happened, if only something could have been done at an earlier point in the child's life—then it is likely that the eating disorder would have been prevented.

Theorists in other areas of health psychology and psychosomatic medicine have long argued for a shift of emphasis away from the "detect it–treat it" medical model to a more behavioral, integrated model focusing on personal and environmental changes, broadly conceived, that contribute to health and prevention of illness (Kaplan, 2000; see Albee & Gullotta, 1997, for a succinct historical review). The success of public health programs to innoculate children against diseases such as polio, mumps, and measles suggests that prevention is potentially a straightforward solution to health promotion on a mass scale. However, the field of mental health prevention in general and the specific application of prevention ideals and practices to the phenomena of eating disorders and eating problems are both so dense that controversy regarding models, methodology, economics, and politics seems to arise at every turn

(Albee, 1996; Heller, 1996). In the area of the prevention of eating disorders, the ratio of programming, speculation, and controversy to solid research remains disconcertingly high (see Cowen, 1973). This book carefully examines theories, programs, empirical data, and important, unresolved issues pertaining to the prevention of the continuum of disordered eating and eating disorders in children, adolescents, and young adults.

MAJOR QUESTIONS

Price (1983) divides the prevention process into four interlocking components (see Bloom, 1996, for an overlapping but alternative theory of the steps involved). The first component is a full *description of the problem*, including precise definitions, prevalence and incidence, correlates, and risk factors. This phase requires a variety of methods, ranging from epidemiology to ethnography (Nichter, 2000), so as to get a description that is complete as well as sensitive to the needs and perspectives of those whom one is trying to help. Risk factors that are modifiable determine the nature of the second component, *design innovation*. During this phase, theories of change are integrated with evidence from previous research to select or create policies and programs for influencing the factors in question. In the third phase these policies and programs are linked to two types of *field research*: (a) collaboration with people (e.g., school staff or community leaders) who serve as facilitators and supporters of the "intervention"; and (b) program evaluation, which involves assessing the context, implementing the innovative program, and measuring the effects of the innovation. The final component in Price's scheme is *diffusion* of the innovative development, for example, a curriculum or set of community-based changes. This special type of marketing involves not only outreach to potential users, but the challenging task of continually refining the program to foster adjustment to the particular needs of those populations. This set of phases becomes a cycle as new applications clarify both the problem and the expected trade-offs between the general principles and practices of the program and the challenges posed by specific contexts.

Guided in part by Price's (1983) model, this book is designed to answer, or at least clarify, a number of basic questions:

1. What is prevention and how is it distinct from treatment?

INTRODUCTION TO PREVENTION 5

2. What is the rationale for an emphasis on prevention?
3. What exactly are we trying to prevent?
4. What is the role of models of problem etiology and preventive change in the development of prevention programs?
5. What is the status of evidence for the effectiveness of prevention programs?
6. What specifically have we learned about program development, evaluation, and refinement?

We believe that progress in the prevention of eating disorders and disordered eating has been severely hampered by lack of attention to the larger, more well-established field of community psychology, which has been working on prevention and mental health promotion for well over 40 years (Albee & Gullotta, 1997; Bloom, 1996; Cowen, 1983; Perry, 1999). Therefore, in this book we try to address these additional questions:

7. What can eating disorder prevention specialists learn from current theory and research regarding the prevention of health problems, such as cigarette smoking? What theories of health education, attitude change, and social change have informed these areas, and are they relevant to the prevention of eating disorders and disordered eating?

8. What are the implications, for prevention, of recent developments in neuroscience?

9. Are prevention programs, however well-meaning, potentially dangerous? What are the risks of transmitting unhealthy knowledge and motivation to impressionable youth? Do programs that "target" high-risk participants create a potentially stigmatizing situation for those people?

This is a daunting list of questions, but it is necessary to add two more that we feel are extremely significant:

10. What is the relationship between efforts to prevent disordered eating and public health concerns about obesity in children and adolescents? Are efforts to reduce risk factors for disordered eating (e.g., drive for thinness and intense fear of fat) necessarily at odds with the goals of people committed to the prevention of obesity?

11. Eating disorders and disordered eating affect many more females than males (van Hoeken, Lucas, & Hoek, 1998). Moreover, there is substantial evidence that disordered eating thrives in the soil of prejudices such as sexism and weightism that disproportionately affect females within patriarchal societies (Fallon, Katzman, & Wooley, 1994; Smolak & Murnen, 2001, 2004). This raises two questions: (a) What is it about the experience of growing up female that contributes to the development of eating problems and disorders? (b) What is the position of males as target audiences for change, as agents of prevention, and as obstacles to prevention?

PREVENTION: KEY DEFINITIONS AND CONCEPTS

General Considerations

As noted previously, the logic of prevention seems straightforward on the surface: If you know what factors and processes cause an illness or problem, if you know the factors whose presence make the illness or problem less likely, and if you know the prototypical age(s) of onset, then presumably you could create well-timed changes in people and their environments so as to reduce the number of new "cases" of the illness or problem, or delay onset (Muñoz, Mrazek, & Haggerty, 1996). Analogous to the concept of psychotherapy, prevention is both a goal and a broad set of methods for achieving that goal.

"Prevention" is derived from the Latin *praevenire*, meaning to come before, anticipate, and/or forestall. However, the semantics of prevention are more confusing than they first appear, and they have remained in a state of constant flux for over 50 years (Bloom, 1996; Cowen, 1983; Kessler & Albee, 1975). Most definitions of prevention focus on three interrelated goals: (a) evading or forestalling the development of psychological disorder or unhealthy behavior; (b) protecting current states of health and effective functioning; and (c) promoting greater well-being so as to strengthen resilience in the event of predictable or unforeseen stressors (Albee, 1996; Bloom, 1996). This perspective links prevention of disease and disability with a variety of multidisciplinary and interdisciplinary theories, goals, and strategies subsumed under the rubric of *health promotion*. According to the World Health Oganization, "health" is both the absence of illness and the presence of psychological, physical, and social resources that enable one to meet one's needs, cope with change, and contribute to society (Macrina, 1999).

Given the long-standing confusion about the definition of prevention, it is necessary to try to clarify what prevention does and does not mean. Consequently, we next consider several important approaches to articulating the types and goals of prevention. Important nomenclature is summarized in Table 1.1.

Caplan's (1964) Model

The familiar terms *primary prevention* and *secondary prevention* were first proposed in a 1957 report by the Commonwealth Fund's Commission on Chronic Illness (Mrazek & Haggerty, 1994). Then in 1964 Caplan published the scheme that for 30 years served as the standard in the prevention of eating disorders and other mental health problems: Prevention is designed to reduce "(1) the incidence of mental disorders of all types in a community (primary prevention), (2) the duration of a significant number of those disorders which do occur (secondary prevention), and (3) the impairment which may result from those disorders (tertiary prevention)" (pp. 16–17). According to Caplan (1964), primary prevention reduces the rate of new cases (i.e., the incidence) of mental disorder in a population of people by eliminating or modulating the negative circumstances that produce disorder in the first place. Secondary prevention reduces the prevalence or number of established cases in the population at risk. This is accomplished primarily by combining detection in the early phases of the disorder with effective referral and treatment. Interestingly, Caplan (1964) maintained that good secondary prevention programs should (a) have a widespread reach; (b) target

TABLE 1.1
Semantics of Prevention

Focus	Mrazek & Haggerty's (1994) IOM Terminology	Caplan (1964)
Populations or large groups of healthy people	Universal or Public Health	Primary
Smaller groups of nonsymptomatic people at high risk	Selective	Primary
Smaller groups of people at very high risk for the disorder because of clear precursors	Indicated or Targeted	Secondary
People clearly suffering from the disorder	[Treatment]	Tertiary

patients who will not recover on their own; and (c) target patients who have a favorable prognosis and thus are likely to recover without enormous expenditure of time and energy. Based on this definition of secondary prevention, Caplan (1964) reserved the term *tertiary prevention* for therapeutic programs that help people who have been treated for mental disorders to avoid chronic debilitation and return to being productive.

Cowen's Critique

Cowen (1973, 1983) feels that confusion would be reduced by no longer using the word *prevention* to refer to the important activities subsumed under Caplan's secondary and tertiary categories. Cowen (1983) maintains that both categories encompass attempts to detect and treat, in individuals, signs of dysfunction that are already in place to a lesser (secondary) or greater (tertiary) degree. Thus, he argues vehemently for dropping the amorphous phrases *prevention* and *prevention in mental health* for the more definitive *primary prevention in mental health*, which seeks to "strengthen *psychological* wellness and to prevent *psychological* dysfunction (i.e., 'maladjustment')" (p. 12; italics in the original). Ultimately, Cowen's (1973, 1983) perspective focuses on Caplan's (1964) broad concept of primary prevention and elaborates it to emphasize four quintessential components, including health promotion. Primary prevention (a) targets a group, not individuals; (b) targets those who are well, although they may be at risk by virtue of life circumstances; (c) has a more impersonal focus on changing groups, institutions, and communities; and (d) is an "intentional" intervention that applies a knowledge base to strengthening psychological health and forestalling maladjustment.

The IOM Nomenclature

In 1992 the Institute of Medicine (IOM), a subsidiary of the United States' National Academy of Sciences, joined the National Institute of Mental Health and several other Department of Health and Human Service agencies to form the IOM Committee on Prevention of Mental Disorders. This committee produced a 605-page report, released as a book edited by Mrazek and Haggerty (1994; see also Muñoz et al., 1996). Acknowledging that prevention is fundamentally designed to head off the emergence of disorder (Cowen, 1983; Kessler & Albee, 1975), the IOM agreed that treatment should no longer be labeled *tertiary prevention*. Furthermore, building on the work of Robert Gordon (1983; cited in Mrazek & Haggerty, 1994), the IOM recommended that "primary prevention" should now be divided into two subcategories. *Universal prevention*, sometimes known as "public health prevention," tries to implement changes seen as desirable for the population at large, including all members of specific groups at risk, such as girls making the early adolescent transition (Smolak & Levine, 1996). Presumably both the cost per individual and the threat posed by the intervention to the population are low. Examples would be childhood immunization and changing the laws that regulate advertising practices of the over-the-counter diet industry. The second type of primary prevention is *selective prevention*. This characterizes programs that focus on nonsymptomatic people who are considered high risk due to biological, psychological, and/or sociocultural factors. Examples are home visitation and infant day care for low-birthweight children (Mrazek & Haggerty, 1994) and programs for children ages 8 to 11 who are entering an environment that is competitive, perfectionist, and focused on weight and shape, such as an elite ballet company (Piran, 1999a). Note that the IOM categorizes selective prevention as a type of "primary" prevention, whereas many scholars in the eating disorders field have tended to think of programs for either "high risk" *or* "mildly symptomatic" as "secondary" prevention. In this book we use the IOM terminology because it is slightly more descriptive than Caplan's categories of primary and secondary prevention.

The third category along the IOM's continuum of prevention and mental health intervention is *indicated* or *targeted prevention* (Mrazek & Haggerty, 1994). This clearly corresponds to Caplan's (1964) category of secondary prevention. The target audience does not "have" the disease or disorder (yet), but is at very high risk because of the presence of clear precursors to the condition in question. An eating disorders prevention program for girls ages 13 to 14 selected on the basis of a high degree of weight concerns (Killen, 1996) would be an example of targeted prevention. These interventions require a good deal of effort on the part of the individuals involved, and they are more costly to the professionals and to society.

Before proceeding, we want to acknowledge that the distinctions between selective prevention, targeted prevention, and treatment remain in need of substantial clarification. Stating that prevention refers to interventions that take place before the onset of a disorder (Mrazek & Haggerty, 1994; Muñoz et al., 1996) runs the risk of becoming a slick tautology unless one can tease apart risk factors from prodromal manifestations of disorder and, ultimately, from the early signs and symptoms that define the clear onset of an eating disorder. This challenge means that we will often revisit the issue of what constitutes universal, selective, and/or targeted prevention.

Risk and Resilience

Relative to the definition of prevention, there is greater agreement among experts that prevention programs have multiple goals (Cowen, 1983; Prevention Research Steering Committee, 1993; Price, 1983). The *proximal* goal is to reduce risk and/or increase resilience. The *distal* goal is to avoid or head off the onset of disorder. Where this is not possible, an alternative distal goal is to delay the onset of the disorder so as to increase the time and opportunities for nonpathological development and to reduce stress on families, professionals, and society in general.

A *risk factor* is "a characteristic, experience, or event that, if present, is associated with an increase in the *probability* (risk) of a particular outcome over the base rate of the outcome in the general (unexposed) population" (Kazdin, Kraemer, Kessler, Kupfer, & Offord, 1997, p. 377). Risk factors are, by definition, probabilistic. In some instances the risk factor is necessary but not sufficient for the disease or disorder. For example, the organic psychosis called general paresis is "caused" by syphilitic infection, but only a small minority of those infected go on to develop this devastating disorder (Albee & Gullotta, 1997). In other instances a risk factor is neither necessary nor sufficient. Internalization of the slender beauty ideal increases the probability of an eating disorder in young women (Thompson & Stice, 2001), but eating disorders can occur in the absence of this factor, and many young women who endorse this ideal do not have an eating disorder.

Some risk factors are *fixed* insofar as it is impossible or nearly impossible to change one's gender, genotype, race, or in the case of children, socioeconomic status. These factors may signify increased risk as a function of their connection with other factors, for example, increased exposure to beliefs about the centrality of slender beauty for the definition of self. Some risk factors are *variable* or malleable, but they should be considered warning signs of risk until their status as a causal risk factor has been demonstrated. Examples of such variable markers for bulimia nervosa for British females ages 16 to 35 are childhood obesity and parents' critical comments about weight and shape (Shisslak & Crago, 2001). A risk factor plays a *causal* role (but should not be considered *the* cause) when it can be demonstrated that altering the risk factor changes the probability of the outcome. This proposition means that prevention research, which seeks this very demonstration, is therefore a critical aspect of basic risk factor research (Kazdin et al., 1997; Stice, 2001b).

Conversely, *resilience* or *protective* factors decrease the probability of disorder or increase the probability of health (Kazdin et al., 1997, p. 377). Some experts think of protective factors as the dimensional opposite of a risk factor. For example, if negative body image is a risk factor for eating disorders, then a positive body image might be a protective factor. Other experts tie this concept to the modulation of risk factors, arguing that protective factors contribute to relatively more healthy and adaptive outcomes for groups that are at risk because of significant adversity (Kazdin et al., 1997; Luthar, Cicchetti, & Becker, 2000). For example, even girls who have internalized the slender beauty ideal and are thus at risk for disorder eating (Thompson & Stice, 2001) may be protected from the development of eating problems by the presence of multiple interests and competencies in areas unrelated to appearance (Smolak & Murnen, 2001).

Some protective factors may be personality characteristics, but resilience refers to a set of processes, not to resiliency as a relatively fixed disposition (Luthar et al., 2000). Resilience, like risk, is not a static state. Understanding risk and resilience as dynamic processes operating in the transaction between individuals and environments reinforces the synergistic connection between prevention and health promotion (Albee, 1996; Cowen, 1997). Chapter 4 demonstrates that the principles of developmental psychopathology are very useful for organizing research on risk and resilience to guide prevention programming.

RATIONALE FOR PREVENTION

Prevention is vitally important. As discussed more fully in chapter 2, full-blown eating disorders and clinically significant subthreshold variants probably affect at least 10% of girls and women between the ages of 10 and 30. In addition, a large number of elementary school children and many adolescents—the overwhelming majority of whom are girls—embrace cultural values about the glories of thinness and the horrors of fat in ways that leave them dissatisfied with their weight, shape, and self, and therefore inclined to engage in unhealthy forms of eating and weight management (Berg, 2001; Neumark-Sztainer, 1995; Smolak & Levine, 1996, 2001b; Smolak, Levine, & Schermer, 1998b).

Full-blown eating disorders such as anorexia nervosa and bulimia nervosa are debilitating, life-threatening conditions (Andersen, 1985). Thus, preventing eating disorders would spare many people and their families years of suffering and the specter of death from starvation or suicide. In general, eating disorders are very difficult and time-consuming to treat, even with multidisciplinary and expert intervention, and all too often they deteriorate into chronic and even fatal conditions (Herzog, Deter, & Vandereycken, 1992; Richards et al., 2000). *The Statistical Abstracts of the United States* (U.S. Bureau of the Census, 1999) estimates that in 1998 there were approximately 27.5 million girls and women ages 15 to 30. This means that a conservative estimate of the number afflicted with clinically significant eating disorders (AN, BN, binge-eating disorder, and eating disorders not otherwise specified; American Psychiatric Association, 2000; see Table 2.1) in the United States is (.10 × 27.5 million =) 2.75 million. Even if these were not complex disorders shrouded in anxiety, secrecy, rigidity, and shame, there simply are nowhere near enough mental health professionals to meet this challenge, let alone provide treatment for other prominent disorders such as depression (Albee & Gullotta, 1997; Levine, 1996). Moreover, a recent report by the United States Surgeon General indicates that only about 50% of those who need mental health treatment get it, and that many women, children, minority groups, and people living in rural areas are not being well-served by private or community-based mental health specialists (United States Office of the Surgeon General, 1999; see also Cowen, 1983).

Traditional medical and psychological approaches to one-on-one and small group treatment of established disorders remain a sometimes viable and sometimes lifesaving intervention for a fairly large number of people in need. However, these approaches are far from capable of stemming the tide of eating disorders and other significant psychiatric problems (e.g., mood disorders, substance abuse) that face the United States and other countries (Gordon, 2000). This is but one aspect of a more general mental health crisis that was poignantly described by Cowen (1973) some 30 years ago. Today, in an era of spiraling health care costs and continued widespread health problems despite large expenditures on health care, prevention is not only a reasonable approach, it is a necessary approach to problems of this magnitude (Albee & Gullotta, 1997; Cowen, 1973, 1983; Holden & Black, 1999).

Another reason to emphasize prevention derives from the connection between universal prevention and social change (Albee, 1996; Albee & Gullotta, 1997; Mrazek & Haggerty, 1994). Over the past 25 years there has been growing concern with the ways in which our culture(s) is/are contributing to the high rates of eating disorders, depression, anxiety disorders, and psychosomatic problems among females and with the pronounced increase in risk that occurs in early adolescence (Petersen, Sargiani, & Kennedy, 1991; Silverstein & Perlick, 1995; Smolak & Levine, 1996). In fact, as discussed in chapters 4 through 8, there is substantial evidence that modifiable sociocultural factors—embodied in economic enterprises such as the multibillion diet industry, and in mass media, families, schools, and peer interactions—help eating disorders and eating problems among girls to flourish (Groesz, Levine, & Murnen, 2002; Stice, 1994; Thompson, Heinberg, Altabe, & Tantleff-Dunn, 1999). Increased risk for eating disorders in particular has been connected directly to natural phenomena (pubertal development), normative psychosocial development (dating and the intensification of sexual interest during early adolescence), and various nonnormative but all too frequent stressors such as sexual abuse and sexual harassment (Smolak & Levine, 1996; Smolak & Murnen, 2001, 2004). Strong evidence for the influence of sociocultural factors in the creation of risk for eating disorders and eating problems has motivated many people to embrace the possibility of prevention through changes in the cultural contexts for girls and young women. Social changes that have led to, for example, increased female participation in athletics, increased use of seat belts, and reductions in the percentage of adult males who smoke cigarettes demonstrate the viability of such massive sociocultural change.

GUIDING PRINCIPLES AND ASSUMPTIONS

The structure and substance of this book reflects not only a list of basic questions, but also a set of five principles that have emerged from our work over the past 20 years (see e.g., Levine, 1999; Smolak, 1999; Smolak, Levine, & Striegel-Moore, 1996).

Principle 1: Beware of the Distance Created by Medicalization and the "-ics"

It is convenient and vaguely authoritative to use medical nouns like *anorexics* and *bulimics*. Nevertheless, whenever possible we refer to those suffering, as, for example, "girls suffering from anorexia nervosa." People with eating disorders and eating problems are, like those committed to prevention, *people*, not "ics." They are people struggling with fantasies, motives, anxieties, and coping mechanisms established and vigorously reinforced by our culture (Gordon, 2000; Silverstein & Perlick, 1995). At a basic level, individuals suffer. In equally significant ways, however, eating disorders and eating problems express (embody) issues (e.g., the meaning of femininity and of power) and processes (e.g., the construction of body image, engagement with mass media) embedded in the culture(s) we all live in and create (Gordon, 2000; Thompson et al., 1999). *Prevention needs to acknowledge the context as much, if not more so, than individuals* (Cowen, 1973, 1983). In thinking about universal prevention of eating disorders and eating problems, the issue is "us" and the cultural contexts that we create, not a small group of distant others ("them").

Principle 2: Prevention Requires an Integrated, Ecological Approach

The symptoms and causes of eating disorders and eating problems are biopsychosocial and multidimensional. Therefore, prevention requires an ecological approach that integrates intervention at personal, group (e.g., family or team), organizational, community, and cultural levels. This means that prevention programming, including risk factor and evaluation research, should unfold on multiple and, hopefully, integrated levels (Perry, 1999; Winett, 1998). As this perspective emphasizes the multiple environments that influence and are influenced by individual behavior, we refer to it as an "ecological" principle (Bronfenbrenner, 1979; see chapter 4). Prevention work will necessarily affect children and youth, so the family, school, peers, and mass media are some of the major systems that must be evaluated and changed (Cowen, 1973; Smolak, 1999).

Felner and Felner (1989) propose a model for guiding prevention that argues for the importance of nonspecific environmental and individual factors early in development, followed by more specific developmental person–environment transactions (pathways) that shape the nature of the disorder or comorbid disorders that emerge. This "transactional–ecological" (p. 18) perspective reinforces a shift in the focus of theory and preventive actions from the individual child or adolescent to the contexts of the child's life and her attempts to adapt to the normative and nonnormative challenges in those environments (Felner & Felner, 1989; Smolak & Levine, 1996; see chapter 4). This has two significant implications for designing prevention programs (Smolak, 1999). First, one must acknowledge the ways in which eating disorders and eating problems are *adaptive* within the sociocultural ecology of the child. Second, prevention efforts with young children in particular must work to change the various limiting settings (e.g., family, school) in which they are immersed.

Principle 3: Prevention Is Necessarily and Essentially Collaborative

Price's (1983) cycle of prevention, operating within an ecological framework, points to the need for collaboration among a wide variety of professionals and lay people, including psychologists, epidemiologists, physicians, social workers, dietitians, parents, coaches, media consultants, educators and students, lay volunteers, etc. (see also Neumark-Sztainer, 1996). At a minimum, prevention research needs to be informed by developmental psychology, epidemiology, clinical psychology, and a broad-based community psychology that draws heavily from sociology and anthropology (Prevention Research Steering Committee, 1993). Epidemiology, the science of determining the presentation, distribution, correlates, and control of disease, is an especially important discipline for prevention specialists (Antoniadis & Lubker, 1997). Statistics concerning prevalence and incidence are the basis for the fiscal support of research and for other social changes requiring public acknowledgment of problems. Data regarding distribution according to type, gender, age, social class, geography, and so forth, point to theories of risk and therefore to programs for prevention. Data pointing to varying levels of risk and resilience among ethnic groups in the United States (such as African Americans, Hispanics, and Native Americans) also point to the importance of sociology and anthropology in understanding the interplay between context, risk, and prevention. And, of course, the ultimate proof of the effectiveness of population-based, universal prevention efforts requires a set of epidemiological studies demonstrating a reduction over time in the incidence of the problems in question.

Implementation of prevention programs, complete with solid evaluation research, requires consideration of what Reiss and Price (1996) call the "scientist–community fit." This means there is a need for substantial dialogue, collaboration, and understanding between researchers and the people (e.g., teachers), institutions (e.g., school systems), and communities who will be participating in prevention programming (Heller, 1996; Perry, 1999; Piran, 1999b). This collaboration should be an ongoing part of the development and evaluation of prevention programs, not the marketing endpoint of programming to be "disseminated" by privileged experts (Heller, 1996; Price, 1983). An important aspect of collaboration is egalitarian and respectful relationships between men and women, because this provides young people with models for healthy development through mutual empowerment of males and females.

Principle 4: Prevention Is an Important Aspect of Science

Prevention research is a critical part of the effort to prevent eating problems. Experimental demonstrations of a prevention effect are also a crucial final step in establishing a variable as a causal risk factor (Kraemer et al., 1997; Stice, 2001b). Thus, for those professionals "whose primary commitment is to research, preventive trials offer the possibility of new insights into developmental processes, causal mechanisms, and the role of social and community context in shaping life trajectories and well-being" (Reiss & Price, 1996, p. 114). As noted by Rosenvinge and Børresen (1999), research on the prevention of disordered eating has often lacked a strong, clear connection to prominent models of psychological, behavioral, and social change (see Kohler, Grimley, & Reynolds, 1999, for an introductory review). Unfortunately, research on the prevention of disordered eating has also lacked a strong, clear connection to bedrock issues of research design such as sampling and recruitment strategies, reliable and valid measurement, monitoring of the strength and fidelity of program implementation, and longitudinal analysis of prevention effects (Levine & Smolak, 2001; Perry, 1999; Prevention Research Steering Committee, 1993). Practitioners in the field of eating disorders must follow the lead of Killen, Taylor, and colleagues (Killen, 1996) and O'Dea and Abraham (2000) in clearly formulating theoretical models of prevention (and health promotion) and then subjecting model-based programs to rigorous scientific and ethical scrutiny (Prevention Research Steering Committee, 1993).

Principle 5: Prevention Is a Social Justice Issue

Eating disorders thrive in the "soil" of prejudice against women, fat people, and ethnic minorities (Fallon et al., 1994; Smolak & Murnen, 2001, 2004; Smolak & Striegel-Moore, 2001). It is unlikely that significant progress in prevention will be made without addressing emotionally and politically charged topics such as fear of women's desires and hungers; sexual harassment and sexual abuse; limitations in women's avenues for success apart from beauty and sexual objectification; and the role of big businesses that profit from female anxieties about weight and shape (Piran, 1995, 2001). People committed to prevention must consider carefully the implications of the facts that (a) at least eight or nine times as many females as males develop eating disorders; (b) the high-risk periods of early and late adolescence are those that highlight the meanings of femininity in terms of body shape, sexuality, and achievement; and (c) eating disorders have proliferated during historical periods like the present in which there is marked tension between expanding opportunities for females and continued reactionary emphasis on domesticity and subservience to males (Silverstein & Perlick, 1995; Smolak & Levine, 1996; Smolak & Murnen, 2001, 2004).

We agree with Winett's (1998) contention that prevention in mental health must be proactive in two ways. First, prevention specialists build systems that reduce stressors and increase access to resources and opportunities. This enables a very wide variety of people, including those who have been traditionally disenfranchised, to increase their competencies, self-esteem, and positive relationships. Prevention work, perhaps like all scientific endeavors, unavoidably combines political activism with professional and personal development (Albee, 1996; Irving, 1999; Maine, 2000). Second, those involved in prevention are necessarily engaged in social marketing and media advocacy. To achieve specific health goals, they use existing systems of power (e.g., school, mass media, government) to distribute information, programs, and/or other products in places and ways that engage the intended audience (Winett, 1998).

We close this introduction with an assumption that represents the hope of this book and of those who seek to prevent eating disorders and eating problems: "It is more sensible, humane, pragmatic, and cost-effective to build psychological health and prevent maladjustment than to struggle valiantly and compassionately to stay its awesome tide" (Cowen, 1983, p. 14).

2

Defining Eating Disorders

There is probably very little that prevention program designers and researchers all agree on. One point of agreement is that the first step in developing and evaluating a prevention program is to carefully and clearly define the goals. Thus, defining what problem behaviors or risk factors are to be prevented (or changed) and which protective factors or health enhancing behaviors are to be strengthened is the starting point. The prevention of problem behavior is typically a distal goal, whereas changing risk or protective factors may represent more proximal or immediate goals of prevention programs.

In the field of eating disorders prevention the task of identifying the distal goal seems fairly straightforward: prevention of eating disorders, their symptoms, or their subclinical forms. There are widely accepted definitions of the major eating disorders, anorexia nervosa (AN) and bulimia nervosa (BN), namely those in the *Diagnostic and Statistical Manual of Mental Disorders* (4th edition, Text Revision; *DSM-IV-TR*; American Psychiatric Association, 2000). These definitions are commonly used by both clinicians and researchers. The current definition of a third well-known eating disorder, binge eating disorder (BED), is considered provisional in *DSM-IV-TR* (2000, see pp. 785–787) and hence is a bit less broadly accepted. Nonetheless, there is substantial agreement concerning BED also.

These *DSM-IV-TR* definitions provide a reasonable starting point for defining the aims of prevention programs. Yet, there are two important issues that demand our attention before we can simply use these definitions. First, there are questions about the validity of the definitions of AN, BN, and BED, particularly in terms of their application to children and to people from American ethnic minority groups or from other cultures. Second, for a variety of reasons, prevention programs are often directed toward behaviors, such as calorie-restrictive dieting, or toward attitudes, such as body dissatisfaction, that are considered elements of or precursors to eating disorders. These approaches rely on the validity of the concept of a continuum (or spectrum) of eating disorders (Shisslak, Crago, & Estes, 1995). The examination of these two issues is the focus of this chapter.

DSM-IV-TR AND EATING DISORDERS

The *DSM-IV-TR* (2000) definitions of eating disorders are important for several reasons. They may be used to define the goals of prevention programs and thus the measurement instruments commonly used to evaluate the long-term success of these interventions. Many prevention efforts, including grassroots organizations and Web sites (see Appendix A), also use *DSM-IV-TR* (2000) criteria to describe the disorders to parents, students, and teachers.

Relative to many other public health problems, such as diabetes or alcohol abuse, full-syndrome eating disorders are fairly rare. Within a 6- to-12-month period, AN probably affects less than 1% of postpubertal females while BN affects approximately 1% to 3% (Hoek & van Hoeken, 2003). Using the higher estimates, these may add up to nearly 4% of adolescent and adult females. However, perhaps an additional 5% to 15% of girls and women exhibit some symptoms of eating disorders that are severe enough to warrant a diagnosis of Eating Disorder Not Otherwise Specified (EDNOS; Herzog & Delinsky, 2001). The diagnosis of EDNOS is given if a person presenting for clinical assistance is clearly suffering but does not meet all of the criteria for AN or BN. This category includes BED, which may affect 2% to 3% of adolescent and adult females. If we put the percentage of females suffering from EDNOS at 10% and those suffering from BN and AN at a total of 4%, then we would estimate that around 4 million girls and women ages 15 to 30 are affected by eating disorders. A substantially smaller number of males suffer from eating disorders (Hoek & van Hoeken, 2003). Probably no more than 10% of diagnosed victims of AN or BN are male (*DSM-IV-TR*, 2000). The percentage of BED sufferers who are male is probably higher, perhaps as many as 40% to 50% (Striegel-Moore, 1993). Numbers for male cases of EDNOS are not available, but several large-scale survey studies of adolescents suggest a point prevalence of roughly 2% to 3% (see chapter 3). Assuming prevalence figures of 0.2% for AN or BN, and 2.5% for EDNOS, and assuming that there are approximately 27.5 million males ages 15 to 30 in the United States (U.S. Bureau of the Census, 1999), a rough estimate of males with clinically significant eating disorders is 740,000.

Four to five million or more people suffering from eating disorders is not a negligible problem. Furthermore, the psychological and physical costs of eating disorders are extraordinarily high (Hill & Pomeroy, 2001), with particularly serious consequences among children (Garvin & Striegel-Moore, 2001). Most dramatically, over 10% of AN sufferers admitted to university hospitals eventually die from the disorder (*DSM-IV-TR*, 2000). These disorders, then, are clearly worthy of prevention efforts.

Anorexia Nervosa

Definition. Table 2.1 shows the *DSM-IV-TR* definition of AN. We begin with AN because it is considered the most basic of the eating disorders in that a diagnosis of AN "trumps" a diagnosis of BN. This probably reflects the greater seriousness of AN, in terms of sequelae and intractability. There are two subtypes of AN: restricting type and binge-eating/purging type. AN is a heavily gendered disordered, with about 90% of the diagnosed and population cases involving females (*DSM-IV-TR*, 2000; Hoek & van Hoeken, 2003). This is reflected in *DSM-IV-TR*'s inclusion of amenorrhea in the diagnostic criteria. There may also be substantial ethnic group differences in rates of AN; specifically, it may be considerably more rare among African Americans than among Whites (Smolak & Striegel-Moore, 2001). The lack of epidemiological data, however, leaves this an open question.

AN most commonly onsets during adolescence, with peaks at ages 14 and 18 (*DSM-IV-TR*, 2000). However, it has long been evident that AN can and does begin prepubertally (e.g., Atkins & Silber, 1993). This makes the applicability of AN's diagnostic criteria to children an important issue.

Weight Criterion. Extremely low weight is certainly the feature most likely to result in entry into treatment or into the hospital. It is arguably the hallmark feature of AN, but its precise definition has proven

TABLE 2.1
DSM-IV-TR (American Psychiatric Association, 2000)
Diagnostic Criteria for Anorexia Nervosa, Bulimia Nervosa,
and Eating Disorders Not Otherwise Specified
(Including Binge-Eating Disorder)

Anorexia Nervosa
- Refusal to maintain body weight at or above a minimally normal weight for age and height (e.g., weight loss leading to maintenance of body weight less than 85% of that expected; or failure to make expected weight gain during period of growth, leading to body weight less than 85% of that expected).
- Intense fear of gaining weight or becoming fat, even though underweight.
- Disturbance in the way in which one's body weight or shape is experienced, undue influence of body weight or shape on self-evaluation, or denial of the seriousness of the current low weight.
- In postmenarcheal females, amenorrhea, i.e., the absence of at least three consecutive menstrual cycles. (A woman is considered to have amenorrhea if her periods occur only following hormone, e.g., estrogen, administration.)
- **Restricting Type**: During the current episode of Anorexia Nervosa, the person has not regularly engaged in binge-eating or purging behavior (i.e., self-induced vomiting or the misuse of laxative, diuretics, or enemas).
- **Binge-eating/Purging Type**: During the current episode of Anorexia Nervosa, the person has regularly engaged in binge-eating or purging behavior (i.e., self-induced vomiting or the misuse of laxatives, diuretics, or enemas).

Bulimia Nervosa
- Recurrent episodes of binge eating. An episode of binge eating is characterized by both of the following:
  (1) eating, in a discrete period of time (e.g., within any 2-hour period), an amount of food that is definitely larger than most people would eat during a similar period of time and under similar circumstances.
  (2) a sense of lack of control over eating during the episode (e.g., a feeling that one cannot stop eating or control what or how much one is eating).
- Recurrent inappropriate compensatory behavior in order to prevent weight gain, such as self-induced vomiting; misuse of laxatives, diuretics, enemas, or other medications; fasting; or excessive exercise.
- The binge-eating and inappropriate compensatory behaviors both occur, on average, at least twice a week for 3 months.
- Self-evaluation is unduly influenced by body shape and weight.
- The disturbance does not occur exclusively during episodes of Anorexia Nervosa.
- **Purging Type**: During the current episode of Bulimia Nervosa, the person has regularly engaged in self-induced vomiting or the misuse of laxatives, diuretics, or enemas.
- **Nonpurging Type**: During the current episode of Bulimia Nervosa, the person has used other inappropriate compensatory behaviors, such as fasting or excessive exercise, but has not regularly engaged in self-induced vomiting or the misuse of laxatives, diuretics, or enemas.

(Continued)

TABLE 2.1
(Continued)

Eating Disorder Not Otherwise Specified
The Eating Disorder Not Otherwise Specified category is for disorders of eating that do not meet the criteria for any specific Eating Disorder. Examples include:
- For females, all of the criteria for Anorexia Nervosa are met except that the individual has regular menses.
- All of the criteria for Anorexia Nervosa are met except that, despite significant weight loss, the individual's current weight is in the normal range.
- All of the criteria for Bulimia Nervosa are met except that the binge eating and inappropriate compensatory mechanisms occur at a frequency of less than twice a week or for a duration of less than 3 months.
- The regular use of inappropriate compensatory behavior by an individual of normal body weight after eating small amounts of food (e.g., self-induced vomiting after the consumption of two cookies).
- Repeatedly chewing and spitting out, but not swallowing, large amounts of food.
- **Binge-eating disorder** (for which the research criteria are:)
  A. Recurrent episodes of binge eating. An episode of binge eating is characterized by both of the following:
     (1) eating, in a discrete period of time (e.g., within any 2-hour period), an amount of food that is definitely larger than most people would eat in a similar period of time under similar circumstances.
     (2) a sense of lack of control over eating during the episode (e.g., a feeling that one cannot stop eating or control what or how much one is eating).
  B. The binge-eating episodes are associated with three (or more) of the following:
     (1) eating much more rapidly than normal
     (2) eating until feeling uncomfortably full
     (3) eating large amounts of food when not feeling physically hungry
     (4) eating alone because of being embarrassed by how much one is eating
     (5) feeling disgusted with oneself, depressed, or very guilty after overeating
  C. Marked distress regarding binge eating is present.
  D. The binge eating occurs, on average, at least 2 days a week for 6 months.
  E. The binge eating is not associated with the regular use of inappropriate compensatory behaviors (e.g., purging, fasting, excessive exercise) and does not occur exclusively during the course of Anorexia Nervosa or Bulimia Nervosa.

Note. Reprinted with permission from the *Diagnostic and Statistical Manual of Mental Disorders* (4th ed., Text Revision). Copyright 2000, American Psychiatric Association.

elusive. *DSM-IV-TR* provides an example of severe underweight at 85% of expected weight. Some researchers have suggested that a Body Mass Index (BMI) of 17.5 (e.g., 5'5" and 105 pounds) be used as a marker of severe underweight. These criteria, however, are all somewhat arbitrary inasmuch as it remains unclear exactly when the physiological effects of severe weight loss or extreme underweight become evident (Herzog & Delinsky, 2001).

These questions are even more complicated with children. The National Center for Health Statistics of the Centers for Disease Control (2000) recently issued new height and weight growth charts. These charts include BMI percentiles for girls and boys ages 2 to 20. These CDC data provide researchers with a relatively easy way to identify an epidemiologically low BMI at any given age. Even with these standards, however, differences in growth rates and patterns, particularly around the high-risk period of puberty, may make it difficult to identify a level of underweight that can be consistently applied to diagnose prepubertal AN, particularly in its early stages. This underscores the difficulty of using the current diagnostic criterion of some percentage (in *DSM-IV-TR*, 85%) of "expected" growth and weight. It is difficult to know what is "expected" in an individual child. Hence, providing information to, for example, teachers to help them quickly identify girls who might be in some danger is very difficult.

Amenorrhea. A similar statement can be made about amenorrhea. It is rarely clear precisely when to expect an individual girl to begin menstruating. The first "peak" age of onset of AN, 14, occurs before a girl would be obviously late had she not begun to menstruate. In the rare cases of AN among boys, the comparable criteria of reduced fertility and hormonal levels are even more difficult to identify prepubertally.

Intense Fear of Weight Gain and Disturbance in Experience of One's Body. Intense body image problems, including unrealistic fears about being or becoming fat, and distortion in bodily self-perception, were at the core of early descriptions of AN (Bruch, 1973; Crisp, 1980). More recent theorists have also posited that extreme fear of weight gain is at the heart of the disorder. On the other hand, Lee and colleagues (Lee, Ho, & Hsu, 1993; Lee, Lee, Ngai, Lee, & Wing, 2001) have suggested that women suffering from AN in Hong Kong do not always show this intense fear of fat, inciting a debate as to whether or not AN without the fear of fat is really AN or a different disorder (Herzog & Delinsky, 2001). Rieger, Touyz, Swain, and Beumont (2001) have suggested that the criterion might be altered to be positive valuation of weight loss rather than fear of fat. This change, they claim, will effectively encompass all of the currently available reports as well as some of the historical descriptions of religion-affiliated anorexia (Brumberg, 1988).

The question is what this extreme fear of fat or positive valuation of both weight loss and low body weight might look like in young children;

indeed, there is some question as to whether young children are cognitively capable of the type of fear of fat and disturbance in bodily experience seen in adults with AN (Bryant-Waugh, 2000; Netemeyer & Williamson, 2001). There are a variety of techniques available to measure perceptual size estimates in children. Using these techniques, children as young as 6, and possibly as young as 4, show considerable accuracy and consistency in estimating their body size (Gardner, 2001). There may be a small tendency for young children to overestimate their body size, however (Gardner, Sorter, & Friedman, 1997). When simply observing a child in a classroom setting, it is important to keep in mind that beginning in late elementary school, many girls engage in "fat talk" (Nichter, 2000) during which they complain about being fat more to communicate distress and to connect with peers than as a reflection of real weight concerns. Again, this may make it difficult for program designers to advise elementary school and even middle school educators what to look for in terms of poor body estimation.

Bulimia Nervosa

Definition. The *DSM-IV-TR* definition is also shown in Table 2.1. In the popular press, BN is often depicted as the "binge–purge" syndrome in which young girls eat huge amounts of food and then, to compensate, induce vomiting. Consistent with this image, *DSM-IV-TR* does require "recurrent" (≥ 2 times per week for at least 3 months) binge eating coupled with "inappropriate compensatory behavior." If the compensatory behavior involves vomiting or the abuse of laxatives, diuretics, or enemas, the diagnosis is "purging subtype." If instead the compensatory behaviors consist primarily of fasting or excessive exercise, the diagnosis is "nonpurging subtype."

BN is also a heavily gendered disorder with at least 90% of the diagnoses going to females (Hoek & van Hoeken, 2003). Both binge eating and purging appear to be at least as common among adolescent girls from several ethnic groups, especially Native Americans, as among Whites, although it is not yet clear whether these similarities extend to diagnosis of the full-blown syndrome (Crago, Shisslak, & Estes, 1996; Dounchis, Hayden, & Wilfley, 2001). Onset is most commonly in late adolescence or early adulthood. BN is rarely diagnosed among prepubertal children, although there is now evidence that it can occur in children (Bryant-Waugh, 2000; Stein, Chalhoub, & Hodes, 1998).

Binge Eating. There is broad agreement that a person must feel out-of-control when eating in order to consider an episode of overeating a binge (Fairburn & Wilson, 1993). What is more controversial is how to determine whether a person has overeaten enough to constitute a binge and, perhaps more important, whose impression of overeating is the one that matters. Should binge eating be "objectively" defined so that any two observers can agree reliably whether or not an episode of overeating constitutes a binge? Or should an incident be considered a binge if the person herself thinks she ate "an amount of food that is definitely larger than most people would eat under similar circumstances" (*DSM-IV-TR*, 2000, p. 589; see Table 2.1). It is not clear how much this distinction matters, as the amount of food consumed during a binge is not necessarily related to the level of psychopathology (Herzog & Delinsky, 2001).

Nonetheless, there is considerable room for error in recognizing a binge among children. Even among adults, binge eating is rarely observed directly by others. Particularly during periods of growth spurts, children, especially boys, may eat (and indeed require) more calories than most adults normally would. This might result in comments by adults that make some children wonder whether they are overeating. In line with this concern, more than 26% of the third-grade boys in one study reported that they binged (Maloney, McGuire, Daniels, & Specker, 1989). Such questionnaire self-reports by children, and even adolescents, do not appear to be remarkably reliable. For example, the McKnight Risk Factor Survey (MRF Survey; see Appendix E) included two binge-related questions, one concerning loss of control and the other focusing on amount eaten (Shisslak et al., 1999). Neither question showed adequate one-week test-retest stability. In the late elementary school sample, the stability coefficient was .41 for the control question and only .31 for the amount question.

Compensatory Behaviors. Although everyone agrees that vomiting and laxative or diuretic abuse following binge eating should be considered compensatory behavior, there is considerable debate as to whether to include fasting and excessive exercise in this category (Herzog & Delinsky, 2001). Even if we limit ourselves to the agreed-upon components, vomiting and laxative/diuretic abuse, children are unreliable reporters of purging behavior. Maloney et al. (1989) found that more fifth-grade boys than girls reported purging and that such purging occurred at a rate of almost 3% among those boys. This is an implausibly high level of true purging. In the same vein, the MRF Survey included questions about laxative/diuretic use and vomiting for weight loss. Among the elementary school sample, stability coefficients for these two questions were .43 and .48, respectively, whereas among middle school girls, the same coefficients were .45 and .34 (Shisslak et al., 1999).

This state of affairs raises two questions for prevention specialists. The first is: How can researchers identify the warning signs of disordered eating in order to conduct targeted interventions? The second is: How can prevention specialists help educators and parents to identify signs of binge eating and purging that are observable, are reliably correlated with BN, and do not rely on child self-report? These issues are addressed in detail in chapter 13.

Eating Disorder Not Otherwise Specified (EDNOS): Binge Eating Disorder

Definition. The provisional *DSM-IV-TR* (2000) criteria for Binge Eating Disorder (BED) as a prototypical form of EDNOS are presented in Table 2.1. The focus is on binge eating, which is defined similarly to BN, without regular use of any form of compensatory behavior. In fact, *DSM-IV-TR* (2000) criteria for BED expand the BN criteria for a pattern of binge eating to include (a) six months duration; and (b) a set of descriptive features that revolve around feeling embarrassed, disgusted, and otherwise distressed over the amount consumed and over the inability to stop eating even when uncomfortably full.

BN and BED are sufficiently similar that some people think that BED is simply an early form of BN. A recent community study does suggest that over a quarter of the BN sufferers had a history of BED. Only about 11% of women with symptoms of BED had a history of BN (Striegel-Moore et al., 2001). Despite such relationships, research indicates that these are two different disorders. So, for example, BED is more strongly associated with obesity but less strongly associated with AN than is BN (Striegel-Moore et al., 2001). The relationship of binge eating to dieting may differ in the two disorders, with BN typically being preceded by dieting, whereas dieting more frequently follows the onset of binge eating in BED (Spurrell, Wilfley, Tanofsky, & Brownell, 1997). BED also seems to resolve without treatment much more frequently than does BN

(Herzog & Delinsky, 2001), although data are mixed as to whether women suffering from BED exhibit less psychopathology than do women suffering from BN (Hay & Fairburn, 1998; Striegel-Moore et al., 2001). This state of affairs is complicated further by research showing that women who began binge eating before age 18 are not only likely to have binged before they began dieting, but that they are also at risk for BN and for mood disorders (Marcus, Moulton, & Greeno, 1995). In general, though, both the precursors and the outcomes of BN and BED seem to differ.

Given the provisional nature of the definition of BED, epidemiological research concerning this disorder is still very limited. The gender difference in BED does not appear to be as pronounced as in BN and AN, with women about 1.5 times more likely to demonstrate BED, at least among those involved in weight control behaviors. BED is associated with obesity. Although the majority of obese people are not binge eaters, BED occurs in about 30% of people enrolling in weight control programs (*DSM-IV-TR*, 2000). BED is probably as common among African American as White women (Striegel-Moore, Wilfley, Pike, Dohm, & Fairburn, 2000).

Age of onset of BED is not well established, although it may be similar to BN (Striegel-Moore et al., 2001). At this time, BED is not commonly diagnosed among children or young adolescents. This may reflect the relative newness of the category rather than the rarity of the disorder. Retrospective reports by women who engage in binge eating, particularly perhaps those who seem to eat as a source of comfort and to control stress, indicate that they began this pattern in childhood (Thompson, 1994; see also Marcus et al., 1995).

Other Forms of EDNOS

Definition. The *DSM-IV-TR* (2000) EDNOS criteria are presented in Table 2.1. Generally speaking, this category is used when an individual presents with symptoms that are similar to those of AN and BN but do not quite meet all the criteria for those disorders. Despite the facts that perhaps half of those presenting for treatment of eating disorders are assigned a diagnosis of EDNOS (Garvin & Striegel-Moore, 2001), and that adolescents with body image and eating problems are particularly likely to qualify for this diagnosis (Levine & Piran, in press), the demographics of EDNOS are poorly understood.

Food Avoidance Emotional Disorder. An important question is whether there are any serious childhood eating disorders that are not explicitly included in *DSM-IV-TR* and hence might only be picked up in EDNOS. Such disorders may be overlooked by professional as well as casual observers who are relying on the widely used *DSM-IV-TR* criteria for guidance. One candidate for this possibility is Food Avoidance Emotional Disorder (FAED; Bryant-Waugh, 2000; Lask, 2000; Nicholls, Chater, & Lask, 2000). This disorder shows some similarities to AN in that the child avoids food, has lost weight, is underweight, and is often dehydrated and sickly. Otherwise, however, the symptom patterns of the two disorders differ, in that the child with FAED does not have an intense interest in, or distorted view of, weight and shape.

The question of the applicability of *DSM-IV-TR* criteria and categories to young children has arisen several times during this discussion. Research suggests marginal validity for the categories when applied to a sample of children ages 7 through 16 who presented with eating problems at a London hospital (Nicholls et al., 2000). The Great Ormond Street Children's Hospital Criteria, which define several disturbed eating patterns among children, showed greater validity. These criteria (Bryant-Waugh, 2000, pp. 38–39) are shown in Table 2.2. Further research is needed to determine whether these criteria indeed define childhood eating disorders that ought to be included in the DSM system (Nicholls et al., 2000). In the meantime it is critically important for prevention designers and evaluators to recognize that the *DSM-IV-TR* eating disorders categories may be particularly inadequate when applied to children. This is true whether the *DSM-IV-TR* criteria are being used to define the distal prevention goals of reduced incidence of the disorders or the more proximal goals of reducing risk factors or increasing protective factors. After all, the *DSM-IV-TR* categories are commonly used in the research concerning the etiology and course of eating problems.

Summary

As a source of target behaviors for the definition of distal prevention goals, *DSM-IV-TR* appears to be of limited usefulness to prevention researchers. The disorders themselves are rather rare, a factor that may

TABLE 2.2
**Great Ormond Street Criteria: Working Definitions
of the Types of Eating Disorder and Eating Disturbance
Seen in Children Ages 8 through 14**

- *Anorexia Nervosa*
  (1) determined weight loss (e.g., through food avoidance, self-induced vomiting, excessive exercising, abuse of laxatives)
  (2) abnormal cognitions regarding weight and/or shape
  (3) morbid preoccupation with weight and/or shape, food and/or eating
- *Bulimia Nervosa*
  (1) recurrent binges and purges and/or food restriction
  (2) sense of lack of control
  (3) abnormal cognitions regarding weight and/or shape
- *Food Avoidance Emotional Disorder*
  (1) food avoidance
  (2) weight loss
  (3) mood disturbance
  (4) no abnormal cognitions regarding weight and/or shape
  (5) no pre-occupations regarding weight and/or shape
  (6) no organic brain disease, psychosis, illicit drug use, or prescribed drug related side-effects
- *Selective Eating*
  (1) narrow range of foods (for at least two years)
  (2) unwillingness to try new foods
  (3) no abnormal cognitions regarding weight and/or shape
  (4) no morbid pre-occupations regarding weight and/or shape
  (5) weight may be low, normal, or high
- *Restrictive Eating*
  (1) smaller than usual amounts for age eaten
  (2) diet is normal in terms of nutritional content, but not in amount
  (3) no abnormal cognitions regarding weight and/or shape
  (4) no morbid pre-occupations regarding weight and/or shape
  (5) weight and height tend to be low
- *Food Refusal*
  (1) food refusal tends to be episodic, intermittent, or situational
  (2) no abnormal cognition regarding weight and/or shape
  (3) no morbid pre-occupations with weight and/or shape
- *Functional Dysphagia*
  (1) food avoidance
  (2) fear of swallowing, choking or vomiting
  (3) no abnormal cognitions regarding weight and/or shape
  (4) no morbid pre-occupation with weight and/or shape
- *Pervasive Refusal Syndrome*
  (1) profound refusal to eat, drink, walk, talk or self care
  (2) determined resistance to efforts to help.

Note. From Bryant-Waugh (2000, pp. 38–39). Reprinted with permission of Psychology Press, a subsidiary of Taylor & Francis.

cause funding agencies to be reluctant to provide money for these over other public health problems. More important, perhaps, it is not clear how the *DSM-IV-TR* criteria apply to children and, sometimes, young adolescents. In regard to targeted prevention, it is difficult to know how to describe the disorders in a way that will enable teachers and parents, and perhaps even medical personnel, to accurately identify children who might be in the early phases of eating disorders.

These are some of the reasons that people rely on the continuum of eating problems to focus their eating disorders prevention programs.

THE CONTINUUM OF EATING DISORDERS

Theorists have long debated whether there is continuity between subthreshold eating problems and the clinical eating disorders, AN and BN. Some theorists, including several classic writers such as Bruch (1973) and Crisp (1980), have argued that AN and BN are *qualitatively* different from the subthreshold variants and, by extension, from the normative dieting and body dissatisfaction common among at least White and perhaps Hispanic girls and women. In statistical terms, opponents of the continuity theory (also called the continuum model) would predict that the extent and intensity of eating disorder symptoms would vary in a nonlinear fashion as one moves from nondieters to normative dieters to chronic dieters to subthreshold eating disorders to fullblown, clinical eating disorders. Specifically, there would be a sharp and abrupt rise in disturbed eating behaviors and attitudes, as well as in psychopathology, as one moved along the continuum from chronic dieters to subthreshold eating disorders and, in particular, from the subthreshold to the clinical groups.

More recently, several theorists have argued that there is a continuum, or at least a partial continuum, of eating problems and eating disorders (e.g., Gordon, 2000; Levine & Smolak, 1992; Shisslak et al., 1995; Striegel-Moore, Silberstein, & Rodin, 1986). These authors argue that AN and BN are the extreme end of a continuum that begins with body dissatisfaction, overconcern about weight and shape, and calorie-restrictive dieting. This particular continuum reflects the weight-and-shape-related symptoms of eating disorders. There may also be continua for some personality characteristics (e.g., negative emotionality or perfectionism) and for psychopathology. Certainly, continua proponents expect some differences between nondieters, dieters, and the subthreshold and clinical groups. However, such differences are assumed to be quantitative and gradually (linearly) incremental.

The issue of whether there is a continuum (or set of continua) of eating problems and disorders is an important one for prevention efforts. The existence of a continuum suggests that intervention any place along the path would result in a decrease in the incidence and/or prevalence of eating disorders. This argument would especially apply to preventing or decreasing the earliest steps in the continuum—body dissatisfaction, weight concerns, and dieting—because these may devolve into disordered eating and because they are associated with other health-compromising phenomena such as cigarette smoking and depression. Given the normative nature of body dissatisfaction, weight concerns, and dieting, particularly among White and Hispanic girls and women, universal prevention becomes a very reasonable approach (Levine & Smolak, 2001; Smolak, Levine, & Schermer, 1998b). If, however, there is substantial discontinuity, then prevention efforts aimed at body dissatisfaction and dieting are unlikely to prevent eating disorders. Indeed, a much more targeted approach, perhaps even one bordering on therapy rather than prevention, might be necessary (see chapter 14).

The question of whether there is a continuum of eating problems and disorders actually consists of several aspects:

1. Is there a continuum between subthreshold disorders, which might sometimes receive a diagnosis of EDNOS, and eating disorders?
2. Does this continuum extend back to more normative groups of dieters or restrained eaters or binge eaters?
3. Is there a continuum for disturbed eating attitudes and behaviors, including body dissatisfaction, weight and shape concerns, dieting, bingeing, and purging?
4. Is there a continuum or set of continua for personality characteristics associated with eating disorders, for example, perfectionism or problems with interoceptive awareness?
5. Do continua exist for all of the eating disorders? Or might there be a continuum for bulimic but not anorexic behaviors, attitudes, and symptomology?

Research to date probably does not permit an adequate answer to all of these questions, particularly the last one. We can, nevertheless, point to several types of evidence that address issues of continuity.

Definitional Issues

In some sense, a relationship between body dissatisfaction, weight concerns, dieting, and AN and BN is built in. For example, the *DSM-IV-TR* (2000) diagnostic criteria for AN include "an intense fear of gaining weight or becoming fat even though underweight" and a "refusal to maintain body weight" (p. 589), which can be accomplished through dietary restriction (see Table 2.1). It would not be surprising to find that weight concerns and dieting predated AN, worsening as the disorder consolidated. In other words, it seems unlikely that weight concerns and dieting would suddenly appear at a pathological level; instead they would gradually worsen to such levels (see Bruch, 1978).

The likelihood of a continuum between EDNOS and the eating disorders is even more clearly implied in the definitions of the disorders. EDNOS might be diagnosed, for example, if all symptoms of AN are present except for amenorrhea (see Table 2.1). This would appear to insure at least some continuity in the other symptoms. The point here is that, although the definitions probably do not require continuity, they do appear to facilitate findings supporting continuity. If the definitions were changed, for example, to de-emphasize concerns about weight in AN as per Lee et al.'s (1993) suggestion, discontinuity may be more evident.

Prospective Risk Factor Studies

If there is continuity between certain behaviors (e.g., dieting) and eating disorders, one would expect that (a) the behaviors would predate the disorders; and (b) the strength of the early forms of the behaviors would prospectively predict the onset of subthreshold and clinical eating disorders. There is substantial and converging prospective evidence from community samples to suggest that dieting, body dissatisfaction, and weight concerns predate and predict the onset of eating pathology (e.g., Attie & Brooks-Gunn, 1989; Field, Camargo, Taylor, Berkey, & Colditz, 1999; Killen et al., 1994, 1996; The McKnight Investigators, 2003; Stice & Agras, 1999; but see Leon, Fulkerson, Perry, & Early-Zald, 1995). Case studies also support the argument that dieting, body dissatisfaction and weight concerns are precursors of eating disorders (Bruch, 1978). Thus, we have a convergence between empirical studies using community samples and clinical experience. The predictive value of these attitudes and behaviors is evident by middle school.

Negative emotions such as anxiety, depression, and irritability are a well-established feature of the constellation of psychological problems associated with eating disorders (see, e.g., Johnson & Connors, 1987). Negative emotionality is a well-established psychological dimension that refers to an individual's characteristic tendency to become anxious, irritable, guilt-ridden, distressed, and, in general, dysphoric. Several theorists (e.g., Stice, 2001a; Striegel-Moore, 1993) have argued that negative emotionality may be at the root of some binge eating. Limited prospective research supports this relationship. It is noteworthy that depression does not appear to be as strong a predictor as negative emotionality is (Stice, 2002).

Thus, the empirical, longitudinal data seem to indicate that there is a continuum between unhealthy eating attitudes and behaviors, as well as negative emotionality, and later development of eating pathology. We offer this conclusion cautiously for several reasons. First, eating pathology has been defined in a variety of ways in these risk-factor studies (Stice, 2002). It is not always synonymous with diagnosed (or diagnosable) clinical cases. Second, the research focuses more on BN and its symptoms than on AN, so the data certainly do not demonstrate that there is a continuum for AN. Finally, the prospective data provide little evidence of continuity in the personality aspects of AN and BN, with the possible exception of negative emotionality. Perfectionism, self-esteem, interoceptive awareness, and impulsivity are among the personality characteristics that have not received consistent support (see Stice, 2002, for a review).

Thus, the prospective data suggest that there may be a partial continuum in which some eating attitudes and behaviors are continuous across the recognized categories of nondieters, normative dieters, chronic dieters, EDNOS, and AN and BN, whereas personality characteristics and psychopathology are discontinuous (Connors, 1996; Levine & Smolak, 1992).

Group Comparisons

Several cross-sectional studies have tried to address directly the question of continua in the eating and personality dimensions of eating disorders. In general, the findings are quite mixed. For example, Garner, Olmsted, Polivy, and Garfinkel (1984, p. 265) reported that whereas some weight-preoccupied women are "quite similar" to those with AN, others only "superficially resemble" AN clients. More specifically, AN clients scored higher on personality variables including ineffectiveness, interpersonal distrust, and lack of interoceptive awareness than did weight-preoccupied women. Research concerning BN seems to indicate more continuity although, again, there is some inconsistency. For example, Lowe et al. (1996) found general support for the continuity hypothesis, particularly in terms of restraint/weight concerns and psychopathology. However, they did find discontinuity in binge eating with very low binge eating scores among the unrestrained and restrained eaters, as well as the dieters, but a much higher rate among the bulimic sample. Stice, Killen, Hayward, and Taylor (1998) found that weight concerns and psychopathology loaded on a single factor that discriminated controls from subthreshold bulimic and bulimic women. In other words, there was not a factor that discriminated the bulimic women from the subthreshold women. Franko and Omori (1999) found an orderly, decreasing pattern in automatic "bulimic" thoughts and total scores on the EDI-2 across groups of EDNOS/probable bulimics, intensive dieters, casual dieters, and nondieting women college students. Thus, in the work of Franko and Omori (1999) and Stice et al. (1998) the continuity hypothesis was again supported.

Differences in findings are at least partly attributable to wide variation in methodology, including sample characteristics, measures, and statistical analyses. Garner et al.'s (1984) study focused on AN, whereas the others examined BN. Stice et al. (1998) used a variety of scales, but only one, the Drive for Thinness Scale to measure thin ideal internalization, was an EDI subscale. By contrast, all the measures used by Garner et al. (1984) were from the EDI. Lowe et al. (1996) used trend and regression analyses to evaluate their data; Stice et al. (1998) used ANOVA and discriminant function analyses.

Until there is more methodological consistency across studies, it is difficult to evaluate the continuum hypothesis. Some cross-sectional studies compare AN, BN, EDNOS, and non-eating-disordered samples, whereas other studies include normative dieters and chronic dieters. Williamson (2003) conducted a taxometric analysis and factor analysis of large groups of AN, BN, EDNOS, BED, and non-eating-disordered participants. Taxometric analysis, which is well-suited for determining continuity and/or discrete categories, indicated that the "anorexic" components of drive for thinness, fear of fat, and calorie-restrictive dieting appear to be on a continuum, whereas binge eating is more "categorical." Our review of prospective studies and studies including various types of dieters also supports the existence of a continuum of eating problems and disorders. However, these studies indicate that support is stronger for a continuum culminating in BN than for one ending in AN, though this may reflect the greater amount of research on the former. This continuum appears to run from "normative" body dissatisfaction and dieting to subthreshold cases to clinical cases. Despite the fact that questions about continuity and discontinuity have been raised for many years (see Levine & Smolak, 1992), much more research is needed to clarify the status of possible continua involving eating behaviors, personality characteristics, and psychopathology (Williamson, 2003).

These data, if they continue to be supported in future research, may be interpreted as supporting a sociocultural model of eating disorders. Indeed, it is probably impossible to argue for a sociocultural model without evidence of a continuum. Thus, Gordon (2000) has argued that a continuum between normative, highly valued attitudes and behaviors and pathological symptoms is one of the criteria defining a "cultural" or "ethnic" syndrome. The data supporting the existence of a continuum, including subthreshold disorders, provide part of the justification and rationale for using sociocultural models to design programs for the universal prevention of eating problems and eating disorders.

OVERWEIGHT AND OBESITY

Throughout this book, we grapple with complex but very important questions concerning the relationship of obesity to eating disorders (see, e.g., chapter 3). Indeed, it may well have been reasonable to include obesity as part of the continuum of eating disorders and disorders. But the relationship of obesity to eating disorders—and to "eating" and "disorder"—remains controversial (Cogan & Ernsberger, 1999; Irving & Neumark-Sztainer, 2002; Neumark-Sztainer, 1999, 2003). As discussed in chapter 3, there is some debate as to whether obesity is, for most overweight people, a serious health problem (e.g., see Ernsberger & Koletsky, 1999). Certainly, the vast majority of the medical and scientific community believes that obesity is a very serious and worsening problem. However, some authors view this position as part of an irrational and ultimately very unhealthy anti-fat bias that permeates our culture (Cogan & Ernsberger, 1999). This issue is argued even more intensely for children, as the long-term effects of childhood obesity are not completely clear. Moreover, even though the standards established by the Centers for Disease Control are now widely cited, there is a debate as to how to define obesity, especially among developing children (e.g., Barlow & Dietz, 1998; Wilfley & Saelens, 2002). That issue is the focus of this section.

Several things make it difficult to define obesity in childhood. First, children grow in different sequences and at different rates. For some children, a height spurt may precede a weight or fat spurt, leaving them seeming unusually thin for a period of time. For others, the two spurts coincide closely enough that the child has healthy-looking proportions most of the time. Still other children experience a weight or fat spurt prior to their height spurt. These children may appear to be too heavy.

Second, although being overweight as a child predisposes one to be overweight as an adult, the relationship is far from perfect. Generally, estimates indicate that 25% to 50% of overweight children will become overweight adults (Must, 1996). However, extremely overweight adolescents, that is, those who are in at least the 95th percentile for BMI, may run a greater risk of becoming overweight adults (Guo, Roche, Chumlea, Gardner, & Siervogel, 1994). This means it is unclear whether most overweight children are at risk for adult obesity and its attendant risks. In addition, data concerning the relationship between obesity in children and short- or long-term health risks are limited. Freedman, Dietz, Srinivasan, and Berenson (1999) did, however, recently report that children ages 5 to 10 who fell above the 85th percentile for BMI, and particularly those above the 95th percentile, have higher levels of cholesterol and higher blood pressure than do leaner children. The link between obesity and high blood pressure is better documented in late adolescence (Barlow & Dietz, 1998). The emerging emphasis on the unhealthy nature of relatively extreme BMI scores in children and adolescents is consistent with the CDC standards.

Body Mass Index (BMI) is a commonly used indicator of obesity in both children and adults. It is easy to measure BMI accurately because it requires only measurements of weight and height; BMI = (weight in kg)/(height in meters)^2. For both children and adults, BMI correlates fairly well with a variety of other measures of body fatness as well as with markers of the complications of obesity, but the strength of the relationship varies as a function of age and gender (Barlow & Dietz, 1998; National Task Force on the Prevention and Treatment of Obesity, 2000).

BMI must be interpreted within age and gender norms for children and adolescents.

Adult Standards

Although obesity refers to excessive body fat, the definition of overweight and obesity in adults is a controversial matter (Allison & Saunders, 2000; Cogan & Ernsberger, 1999). Based on their interpretation of the voluminous data on the health risks of increasing weight, the U.S. National Heart Lung and Blood Institute and the World Health Organization agree on the following categorization: BMI between 25 and 29.9 indicates "overweight," whereas BMIs from 30–34.9, 35–39.9, and over 40 constitute classes of increasing "obesity." If these are valid guidelines, then approximately 55% of adults in the United States are overweight and approximately 25% to 26% are obese (Devlin, Yanovski, & Wilson, 2000).

Some researchers believe these ranges are too narrow. For example, reviews by Troiano, Frongillo, and Levitsky (1996) and Ernsberger (1989) demonstrate that, for adult men, mortality is uncorrelated with BMIs between 22 and 28; for women, the relationship is even less clear, with a range perhaps of 22–32. In general, there seems to be more agreement in the scientific community about the health risks, that is, the predictive validity, of BMI > 30 for men than about the meaning of overweight in general or the meaning of BMI-defined obesity for females (Garner & Wooley, 1991). Nevertheless, there seems little doubt that a woman with a BMI > 35 is obese and at risk for significant health problems such as hypertension and diabetes, and 30 may indeed be too high for many women (Manson et al., 1995; National Task Force on the Prevention and Treatment of Obesity, 2000; Pi-Sunyer, 1999). An adult woman 5'4" tall would have a BMI of greater than 30 if she weighed 175 pounds, and greater than 35 if she weighed 204 pounds.

It should also be noted that BMI is a convenient but limited measure that many professionals consider a first step in screening for unhealthy levels and distribution of weight and fat. It does not distinguish between fat mass and fat-free mass, nor does it take into account the distribution of body fat. For example, it has been shown that central or upper body fat (stomach, chest), as opposed to lower body fat, is an independent predictor of health risk (Allison & Saunders, 2000; National Task Force on the Prevention and Treatment of Obesity, 2000). Chapter 3 discusses in more detail other significant limitations of using BMI as an indicator of health status.

Child Standards

The National Center for Health Statistics (2000) of the United States' Centers for Disease Control (CDC) has issued revised growth charts for children aged 2 to 20. As in the past, these charts included growth curves for height and for weight. What was new was the addition of gender-specific BMI growth charts that identify BMI percentiles at each age. Two things about these BMI growth charts are noteworthy. First, there is no correction for ethnicity. Clearly, the CDC believes that there is a "universal" healthy child. This approach might be criticized on the basis that the effects of obesity appear to vary across cultures (Kumanyika, 1995). In addition, there are considerable ethnic group differences in rates of obesity. These differences first appear around puberty (Rosner, Prineas, Loggie, & Daniels, 1998).

Second, the charts are based on corrected data from national surveys. These data are corrected in the sense that they do not simply reflect national norms. National demographic data would show the average child to be considerably heavier than the CDC growth curves recommend. These curves, then, are intended to represent what the CDC views as a healthy BMI for each age and gender. This distinguishes the BMI curves from the height curves, for example.

The CDC recommends that children who exceed the 95th percentile BMI for their age and gender be considered obese (National Center for Health Statistics, 2000; see also Barlow & Dietz, 1998). The CDC further recommends that children falling between the 85th and 95th percentiles be considered "at risk" for becoming obese. In both cases, but particularly in the former situation, the CDC suggests that the child undergo further evaluation as to the potential causes and effects of their weight status. Such an evaluation is deemed important to protect the child's health.

Barlow and Dietz (1998) contend that any child who shows rapid increases in BMI be considered for evaluation. "Rapid" increase would mean adding more than about 3 or 4 BMI units in one year. For example, a 13-year-old boy who grows from 4'10" and 90 pounds (BMI = 20.53) to 5'2" and 130 pounds (BMI = 23.82) would have undergone a "rapid increase," according to Barlow and Dietz. This level of increase has not clearly been associated with risk of obesity but, given its unusual nature, is seen as a potential warning sign. Additional research is needed to address this question.

Obesity and the Continuum of Eating Disorders

There are several potentially important links between eating disorders and obesity. First, at least some level of overweight is seen as a risk factor for the development of BN (e.g., Killen et al., 1994). However, not all prospective data support this relationship (e.g., Graber, Brooks-Gunn, Paikoff, & Warren, 1994; Stice & Agras, 1998). This suggests that the effect of BMI on the development of eating disorders is either inconsistent or is so small that it can only be picked up in some research projects (Stice, 2002). Second, BED is more common among obese people, or at least obese people who seek treatment for obesity, than among the general population. It is possible that the binge eating actually contributes to obesity. It should be noted, however, that the vast majority of obese people in the general population do not meet the diagnostic criteria for BED. Third, dieting appears to be a risk factor for both eating disorders and obesity (Field et al., 1999; Stice, Cameron, Hayward, Taylor, & Killen, 1999). This risk has been documented in prospective, longitudinal studies and so may constitute a causal risk factor. More research is needed before this claim can be considered definitive.

On the other hand, there are some important differences between eating disorders and obesity. Most notably, they differ on the dimension of psychological disturbance. Most victims of eating disorders manifest personality and psychological pathology that, by definition, interferes with normal functioning in social, academic, and vocational areas. Most obese people, although frequently victims of discrimination, are well-functioning members of society who work (or go to school) and have meaningful social relationships (Garner & Wooley, 1991; Lamertz, Jacobi, Yassouridis, Arnold, & Henkel, 2002; Yuker & Allison, 1994).

SUMMARY AND CONCLUSIONS

The long-term or distal goal of universal prevention programs is a reduction in the onset of new cases of eating disorders. In selective and targeted prevention programs, participants are chosen because they are at high risk and/or show the early symptoms of eating disorders. In these programs, the proximal goal is reduction of those risk factors or symptoms, while the distal goal continues to be a reduction in the incidence of eating disorders. In any case, the goals of the programs are rooted in definitions of eating disorders.

In this chapter we have examined the most commonly used definitions of eating disorders, those contained in *DSM-IV-TR* (2000). We have also considered the possibility that there are continua of disordered eating attitudes and behaviors and personality characteristics that might link nonpathological (but not necessarily healthy) practices and beliefs to eating disorders. Our analysis suggests that:

1. *DSM-IV* (1994, 2000) criteria have been immensely important in standardizing the definitions used in research concerning the identification of cases of and risk factors for eating disorders. The criteria reflect much of what clinicians and researchers have observed concerning, in particular, AN and BN.

2. However, there are serious shortcomings even in the AN and BN criteria. For example, the criteria concerning weight loss/low weight in AN are vague. This problem is exacerbated by the difficulty in determining an "expected" weight in children and young adolescents.

3. The EDNOS category is very troublesome, especially because 50% to 60% of the girls and women presenting with eating problems end up with this diagnosis. It remains to be determined whether these people are suffering at "subclinical" levels, are victims of syndromes that do not fit within the current nomenclature, or are presenting with variants of the currently defined syndromes. At present it would be very difficult to assess whether the incidence of EDNOS has been reduced by a prevention program because EDNOS is so poorly defined and understood.

4. There does appear to be a continuum of eating behaviors and attitudes. Normative discontent with weight and shape, accompanied by use of weight control techniques, appears to be quantitatively but not qualitatively different from its manifestation in women with eating disorders. Certain personality characteristics may also be continuous from disturbed eating to subthreshold to full-blown clinical cases, although support for this is more mixed.

5. Obesity may reflect a problem with eating, and obese people tend to have high levels of body dissatisfaction as well as a history of calorie-restrictive dieting. Obesity is, for example, associated with binge eating. Nonetheless, obesity is not an eating disorder. Obese children and adults do not routinely suffer from the levels of self and behavioral disturbances that are observed in people suffering from AN, BN, and BED.

3

Important Controversies

Research on the causes, treatment, and prevention of disorders such as depression and cancer is marked by controversies. The field of eating disorders and eating problems is no exception. This chapter considers three debates that are particularly relevant to our contentions about the fundamental importance of primary or universal prevention:

1. Shouldn't prevention acknowledge that eating disorders are neuropsychiatric illnesses and, therefore, concentrate, not on sociocultural factors, but on identifying individuals at high risk so special programs can be tailored to their unique needs?

2. The continuum of eating problems and eating disorders affects many girls and women, and certainly many more females than males. Should girls then be in the foreground of the target audiences for prevention efforts, with boys' behavior in the background as part of the sociocultural problems to be remedied? If girls are indeed seen as the appropriate target audience, does this perspective blame boys while ignoring body image and eating problems that they have too?

3. Isn't prevention of negative body image and disordered eating necessarily at odds with international concerns about the prevalence and incidence of obesity? Shouldn't there be *more* public concern about fat and a greater cultural drive for thinness, not less?

THE NEUROGENETIC PERSPECTIVE

Eating Disorders as Illnesses

Clinically, an eating disorder such as AN or BN appears as a powerful, self-contained, refractory, and chronic "illness" (Kaye & Strober, 1999). The relative rarity and severity of these illnesses, and their links to fundamental disturbances of hunger, feeding, and satiety, all suggest the operation of "neurogenetic factors" such as genetic vulnerability or dysregulation of neurotransmitters. Proponents of the neurogenetic model argue that cultural factors play a minimal causal role in the etiology of eating disorders (Kaye & Strober, 1999). According to these researchers, the important question is: Why are some individuals particularly vulnerable to assimilating toxic sociocultural messages or unhealthy family dynamics, while most girls and women are relatively immune?

The neurogenetic perspective raises important issues concerning the value of universal, in contrast to selective and targeted, prevention. The question of universal versus selected or targeted interventions remains an especially thorny one, so it is considered in detail in chapter 14. Nevertheless, there are serious limitations to the neurogenetic perspective.

Limitation 1: Behavior Genetics

Supporting Evidence. Advocates of the "new biology" of eating disorders offer several types of data as proof that risk is genetically transmitted (Bulik, 2001; Bulik, Sullivan, Wade, &, Kendler, 2000; Kaye & Strober, 1999; Strober, Freeman, Lampert, Diamond, & Kaye, 2000; see also the overview of theory, methodology, and research by Bulik, 2004). For example, the risk of a frank eating disorder (approximately 7%) or a partial syndrome in the first-degree female relatives (mother, sister, daughter) of women with an eating disorder is much greater than the comparable risk for first-degree relatives of matched comparison samples of non-ill women (approximately 1.5% for frank eating disorders; Lilenfeld & Kaye, 1998; Strober et al., 2000). Also, whether or not a person with AN also has Obsessive–Compulsive Personality Disorder (OCPD; *DSM-IV-TR*, 2000, pp. 725–729), the relative risk of OCPD in first-degree relatives is approximately double that of the general population (Kaye & Strober, 1999). Several cardinal features of OCPD (e.g., perfectionism, rigid thinking, and excessive concern with orderliness) overlap with key clinical aspects of AN and have been theorized to constitute aspects of vulnerability for that eating disorder.

Another source of data is the study of monozygotic (MZ) and dizygotic (DZ) twins (Bulik, 2001; Bulik et al., 2000; Klump, Wonderlich, Lehoux, Bulik, & Lilenfeld, 2002; Lilenfeld & Kaye, 1998). Reviews by Bulik (2001, 2004), Bulik et al. (2000), and Klump et al. (2002) conclude that individual differences in AN, BN, and components of disordered eating (measured using continuous scales such as the EDI) are best explained by an additive combination of heritability (multiple genes, each with a small effect) *plus* unique environments and experiences not shared by both twins in a set. Nonshared environments include experiences at school, with peers, and with the mass media. Estimates for the proportion of variance in liability across individuals accounted for by each of the two factors—genetic potential and nonshared environments—vary tremendously, but typically each is 20% to 50%. The contribution of environmental effects shared by both twins, such as exposure to similar family dynamics, appears to be negligible, especially for AN. Bulik does acknowledge that several studies of AN and BN could not rule out the effects of shared environments, given the small sample sizes involved (Bulik, 2001, 2004; Bulik et al., 2000).

Critique. Fairburn, Cowen, and Harrison (1999) caution against premature conclusions about the genetic "basis" of eating disorders. They note that even within groups of research collaborators there is disagreement and confusion about the role of genetic factors in AN and BN (Bulik et al., 2000; Kaye & Strober, 1999; cf. Klump et al., 2002). For example, different analyses of the same Virginia Twin studies by Kendler, Walters, Bulik, and colleagues (as reviewed in Fairburn et al., 1999) yield heritability estimates for BN that range from the negligible to 83%. The latter is an extraordinarily high estimate for a psychiatric disorder. Moreover, in three of the six major twin studies reviewed by Bulik (2001), the range of heritability estimates that can be postulated with 95% confidence includes zero, that is, no genetic contribution to individual variability in disordered eating.

Overall, the twin research has produced some inconsistent findings and troublesome methodological issues. Consequently, it is fair to say that our knowledge about the heritability of eating disorders, and thus the relative roles of shared and nonshared environments, is still in an early and unstable phase (Fairburn et al., 1999; Klump et al., 2002). Two points are particularly important in this regard. First, the three-factor model applied to date has limited or no power to detect the impact of either shared environments alone or the interaction between genetic vulnerability and shared environments. The second is a fundamental principle of behavior genetics: Heritability estimates for individual difference variables (e.g., body image) will necessarily be larger to the extent that environmental factors (e.g., the glorification of slenderness, the vilification of fat, the objectification of women) are relatively homogeneous and ubiquitously powerful.

Support for Fairburn et al.'s (1999) advocacy of a more open perspective concerning biological, psychological, and sociocultural factors is found in a set of studies by Klump, McGue, and Ianoco (2000, 2003) of eating attitudes and behaviors in 11- and 17-year-old twin pairs. Both shared and nonshared environmental effects explained virtually all the variance in total scores on the EDI and in weight preoccupation when the twins being studied were *pre*pubertal 11-year-old girls. In contrast, for 17-year-old twins and *post*pubertal 11-year-old twins, genetic and nonshared environmental influences each accounted for approximately half of the variance. Although the methodology of these studies renders the data open to alternate interpretations, the work of Klump et al. (2000, 2003) suggests that something about pubertal development, for example, ovarian hormones and/or new social experiences, activates a genetic vulnerability to the types of disordered eating measured by the EDI.

The behavioral genetic studies of Klump and colleagues also highlight the role of factors emphasized by prevention theorists who operate from a sociocultural model. Both members of prepubertal 11-year-old MZ and DZ twins appear to be influenced by differences in environments they share, which could include weight-and-shape teasing by peers, or family messages about the ideal beauty shape, including the types of magazines and other media that are prominent in the house (Thompson et al., 1999). And the eating pathology of one member of the 11- and 17-year-old twin pairs appears to be influenced by experiences that do not confront or affect the other, such as, perhaps, sexual harrassment or a coach intent on belittling athletes about being "fat and slow" (see Klump et al., 2002). The powerful effect of nonshared environments is entirely consistent with a sociocultural model, which does not require that all people in the "target" audience receive the same message or respond identically to it (Smolak & Levine, 1996; Thompson et al., 1999).

Limitation 2: Temperament, Personality, and Vulnerability

Lilenfeld and Kaye (1998) argue that personality traits, such as obsessional thinking and a neurogenetic tendency to avoid harm, are the most important heritable components of risk for eating disorders. Presumably, these genetic vulnerabilities are transformed into phenotypic eating disorders by a complex "trigger" such as the combination of pubertal development, dysphoria, and dieting (Klump et al., 2003; Stice, 2001b).

Kaye and Strober (1999) and other proponents of the neurogenetic perspective have argued that some girls have a "temperament" that puts them at risk for severe eating disorders. The concept of temperament refers to a genetically mediated set of tendencies toward emotions, preferences, behavioral styles, and so forth (see, e.g., Strober, 1990). One assumption underlying temperament theory is that characteristics that persist in samples of "recovered" ED patients provide clues to pathogenesis (Kaye & Strober, 1999). By "recovered" they mean weight restored and/or "free" of starvation, binge eating, and purging. Consistent with the data on familial cotransmission of AN and OCPD, Kaye and Strober (1999) reviewed four studies indicating that women who have recovered from AN continue to experience problems with rigid thinking, constricted emotional expression, obsessions, and over-control of impulses. These women also had continued difficulties with high levels of introversion, risk avoidance, and compliance, all of which suggest a narrowing of contact with the social world in order to minimize stimulation and potential harm. A review by Wonderlich (2002) supports this connection between obsessive–compulsive personality characteristics and AN.

Critique. In addition to the very generous definition of "recovered" that they adopt, there are four major problems with Kaye and Strober's (1999) conclusions about temperament, personality, and the presumed genetic bases of eating disorders. First, as acknowledged by Lilenfeld and Kaye (1998), no consistent residual characteristics have been reported for females who have recovered from BN. Second, although there is no doubt that AN and BN are associated with severe personality problems and disturbances in physiology (Johnson & Connors, 1987; Kaplan & Garfinkel, 1993; Kaye & Strober, 1999), the challenge for neuropsychiatric research is to distinguish pathogenic predispositions (risk factors) from the correlates or consequences of starvation, binge eating, purging, chronic stress, and comorbid substance abuse, depression, and anxiety. Kaye and Strober (1999) offer no data to disprove the contention that postmorbid personality characteristics reflect, not premorbid characteristics, but a combination of incomplete recovery and the "scarring" effects of a major psychiatric disorder with serious physical and neurological complications (Smolak & Murnen, 2001; Wonderlich & Mitchell, 2001). Statements like "Individuals who are long-term recovered from AN had continued core eating disorder symptoms, such as ineffectiveness, a drive for thinness, and significant psychopathology related to eating habits" (Kaye, Gendall, & Stroberg, 1998, p. 828) are perplexing. Are "recovered" and "correlates of recovery" applicable if such problems persist? As is the case for the behavior genetics of eating disorders, research on personality and disordered eating has yet to address many troubling conceptual and methodological problems, including a lack of prospective studies (Stice, 2001b; Wonderlich & Mitchell, 2001).

The third basic problem is Kaye and Strober's (1999) emphasis on Cloninger's theory that temperament consists of four heritable, neurogenetic dimensions: novelty seeking, harm avoidance, reward dependence, and persistence (see, e.g., Cloninger, Svrakic, & Przybek, 1993). The core of AN is thought to be extremely high harm avoidance, low novelty seeking, and, depending on whom one reads, high or low reward dependence (see, e.g., Fassino et al., 2002; Strober, 1990). This may be an appealing clinical proposition, but it has very little consistent empirical support. Except for the proposed associations between AN and obsessive–compulsive personality tendencies, and between BN and high novelty seeking and impulsivity, the differences between AN and BN are not at all clear, especially in regard to harm avoidance (the tendency to react to stressful situations with anxiety and behavioral inhibition). In general, the relationship between eating disorders and personality remains vague (Fassino et al., 2002; Raevuori, 2002; Wonderlich & Mitchell, 2001).

A brief review illustrates the shaky empirical foundation of the temperament hypothesis. Bulik, Sullivan, Weltzin, and Kaye (1995) compared the temperament characteristics of women with restricting AN, women with BN, and women with both diagnoses concurrently (AB) and found no evidence for the predicted differences between the AN and BN groups in harm avoidance, novelty seeking, and reward dependence. Fassino et al. (2002) compared women from four clinical groups: restricting AN, bulimic AN, BN, and no eating disorder. As predicted, the eating disordered groups were more harm avoidant than controls, whereas the two bulimic groups reported more novelty seeking. However, discriminant function analysis using temperament scores resulted in a correct overall categorization rate of only 60%. In another recent study, women receiving treatment for BN reported more harm avoidance than did nonpsychiatric controls, but there were no differences in novelty seeking and reward dependence (Berg, Crosby, Wonderlich, & Hawley, 2000). Finally, a longitudinal study of the relationship between temperament and scores on the EDI subscales of drive for thinness, body dissatisfaction, and bulimia indicated no prospective relationships between scores on withdrawal/approach (which overlaps with harm avoidance and novelty seeking) and those measures of psychopathology (Martin et al., 2000).

The fourth problem is also empirical. Developmental psychology has a long and active history of research concerning temperament. Developmental psychologists generally believe that there are temperament characteristics that are early appearing, relatively consistent across time, and genetically mediated. However, these characteristics do not include harm avoidance or reward dependence. The evidence does suggest that both negative and positive affect appear to be genetically mediated temperament characteristics (Bates, 1987; Fox, Henderson, Rubin, Calkins, & Schmidt, 2001). There is also evidence supporting behavioral inhibition, which might be a precursor of novelty seeking, as a temperament dimension, although recent evidence suggests that behavioral exuberance may show greater temporal consistency than does behavioral inhibition (Fox et al., 2001).

Furthermore, early appearing temperament differences do not generally show gender differences, much less gender differences of the magnitude found in eating disorders (Bates, 1987; Lemery, Goldsmith, Klinnert, & Mrazek, 1999). Proponents of the temperament-as-a-risk-factor argument need to explain how nongendered temperament differences become very gendered eating disorders (Smolak & Murnen, 2001). It is possible, of course, that the same temperament characteristic leads to different pathways depending on biopsychosocial aspects of gender, as developmental psychopathology models would suggest (see chapter 4). Although there is some research supporting this argument in terms of eating disorders, the predictive temperament characteristics involve negative affect, not the Cloninger triad (Martin et al., 2000).

Limitation 3: Disturbances of Serotonin Functioning

People suffering from eating disorders have profound disturbances in eating and satiety, in emotional functioning, and in coping with stressors. Therefore, it makes sense to investigate the relationship between eating disorders and the neurotransmitters involved in motivation and emotion. In general, the multiple neuroendocrine disturbances accompanying the eating disorders are reversed by effective therapy (Kaye & Strober, 1999). This strongly implies that dsyregulation of neurotransmitters is a concomitant of the illness and possibly a cause of chronicity, but not a predisposing factor, let alone a "genetic cause." Regardless, scientists seeking the causes of eating disorders have focused attention on the central nervous system neurotransmitter 5-Hydroxytryptophan (5-HT), better known as serotonin (Brewerton, 1995).

Serotonin activity helps inhibit many sets of behaviors, including feeding, exploration, stimulus reactivity, aggression, and sexuality (Kaye, 1995). In animals, increasing 5-HT activity reduces food consumption by affecting satiety mechanisms, whereas inhibiting 5-HT activity increases eating and weight gain. Serotonin probably plays an important role in other clinical features of eating disorders, including depression, obsessionality, and impulsivity (Brewerton, 1995). Serotonin activity is abnormally low during both AN and BN, but some measures are abnormally elevated during long-term "recovery" (Brewerton, 1995; Kaye, 1997; Kaye et al., 1998; Kaye & Strober, 1999).

Kaye theorizes that a high baseline level of serotonin activity is the foundation for personality characteristics (e.g., emotional restriction, harm avoidance, obsessionality) that constitute the risk for AN (see Kaye et al., 2003, for a recent review of the literature). When girls with this physiological vulnerability are confronted by the biological and psychosocial challenges of puberty, dieting helps to manage the resulting dysphoria. For females, dieting reduces the availability of plasma tryptophan and other nutrients (e.g., zinc) and thus reduces serotonin activity. This coping mechanism traps the girl in a downward spiral of starvation and restriction because reduced synaptic activity in the short run increases receptor sensitivity in long run, which increases the impact of 5-HT activity when the person does eat (Cowen, Clifford, Walsh, Williams, & Fairburn, 1996; Kaye, 2000; Kaye et al., 2003). According to Kaye, low levels of 5-HT activity are also associated with the illness phase of BN, but for various biological reasons this hypoactivity provides little relief. Instead, it is somehow related to dysphoria, impulsivity, mood instability, and a tendency to binge eat (Brewerton, 1995; Kaye et al., 1998; Kaye et al., 2003).

Critique. This is a provocative theory, and Kaye's contention that 5-HT dysregulation is a risk factor for AN is supported by at least five studies of molecular genetics indicating that people with AN have an abnormality in the gene that controls one type of serotonin receptor (Bergen & The Price Foundation Research Collaborative, 2003; Kaye & Strober, 1999). In addition, Kaye et al. (2003) found partial support for the 5-HT dysregulation theory in a double-blind, placebo-controlled study of responses to an amino acid mixture that produces an acute depletion of plasma tryptophan. As predicted, women with active AN and women who had recovered from AN reported a significant reduction in anxiety in the treatment versus control conditions, whereas healthy control women did not. However, contrary to prediction, the group × treatment interaction for anxiety was not statistically significant, and analysis of treatment versus control conditions using initial tryptophan levels as a covariate found a significant reduction in anxiety only in the actively ill women. Given the theory's reliance on the characteristics of recovered patients with AN, the fact that plasma tryptophan reduction has no distinguishing significant effect on the anxiety (or depression and irritability) of recovered patients is a troubling outcome. Furthermore, the fact remains that there is little evidence that a genetically mediated dysregulation of neurotransmitters such as 5-HT is a fundamental cause of eating disorders. Kaye and Strober (1999) themselves acknowledge that the multiple neuroendocrine abnormalities associated with eating disorders tend to normalize following clinical recovery. As noted before, the status of neurohormonal functioning in "recovered" patients is more parsimoniously explained as a scarring effect of the disorder or a correlate of incomplete recovery.

This does not mean that we see no causal role for serotonin or other neurotransmitters in the development of eating disorders. In both rats and humans, the females, as compared to the males, have higher levels of 5-HT and higher levels of 5-HT utilization. Females also have 5-HT systems that are less flexible in response to stress. And following even moderate dieting, women, but not men, demonstrate altered 5-HT neuroendocrine responses, probably as a function of decreased availability of plasma tryptophan (Anderson, Parry-Billings, Newsholme,

Fairburn, & Cowen, 1990; Brewerton, 1995). Together, these findings point to the likely impact of a variety of powerful sociocultural factors on neuronal functioning. Choosing to diet in order to achieve a narrow standard of ideal beauty and to manage stress is explained more effectively by sociocultural factors than by neurobiology, as is the fact that so many more females than males are affected by negative body image, dieting, and disordered eating (Gordon, 2000; Smolak & Murnen, 2001, 2004; Thompson et al., 1999). Research from various disciplines has shown that a variety of "environmental" effects, such as psychological trauma or disturbed mother–child interactions, shape long-term alterations in the functioning of serontonergic and other neurotransmitter systems (see Fishbein, 2000, for a review). Dysregulation of serotonin functioning could well be one mediator between many different environmental influences and the various physical and psychological disturbances that comprise an eating disorder.

Implications and Challenges for Prevention

It is indisputably humane and practical to treat full-blown eating disorders as serious, life-threatening, and potentially chronic illnesses. This clinical fact in no way establishes neurobiology as the dominant paradigm for thinking about risk factors for, and prevention of, the continuum of eating problems and eating disorders. Advocates of the neurogenetic perspective, in its current form, do not come anywhere close to doing what they argue has already been accomplished, that is, obliterating the sociocultural perspective and thereby undermining the basis for most universal prevention efforts (see, e.g., Kaye & Strober, 1999). Therefore, we are very uncomfortable with the prevailing sentiment among powerful people at the National Institute of Mental Health (see, e.g., Vitiello & Lederhendler, 2000) and the Academy for Eating Disorders that the neurogenetic paradigm is the scientific benchmark against which all other models of etiology and prevention should be measured. Indeed, it is impossible for the neurogenetic perspective, as currently formulated, to account for many of the compelling observations that form the basis of a sociocultural perspective (Gordon, 2000; Thompson et al., 1999; see chapters 5 through 8). In this respect, the neurogenetic perspective virtually ignores the critically important question of why females are at such greater risk than males for eating problems and eating disorders (Smolak & Murnen, 2001, 2004).

This is not to say to that the neurogenetic perspective is irrelevant to prevention. The need for universal prevention and health promotion rests in large part on the fact that eating disorders are indeed chronic and devastating illnesses for the person, her or his family, and society. Evidence for genetic transmission of liability to personality characteristics and to a spectrum of psychological disorders also forces us to think carefully about the interactions and transactions between social psychological experiences (e.g., family dynamics, sexual abuse, perfectionism in athletics) and vulnerability to long-term disturbances in central nervous system functioning (Fishbein, 2000). This point has two important implications, which are discussed further in chapter 14. First, demonstration of specific genetic or other neurogenetic markers would need to be incorporated into selective prevention programs for at-risk children and adolescents. Second, explication of reciprocal gene–environment interactions will require selective and targeted prevention programs whose content and processes will necessarily be quite distinct from universal prevention programs (Bulik, 2004; Fishbein, 2000).

MALES AND PREVENTION

AN and BN are much more prevalent in females than in males, particularly in adolescents and adults. The female-to-male ratio for well-defined cases is at least 10 to 1 and may be much greater for both AN and BN (Hoek & van Hoeken, 2003; van Hoeken et al., 1998). This is an extraordinarily pronounced disparity. The ratio for disorders ordinarily considered "gendered" is on the order of 2:1 (e.g., females to males for depression) or 3–4:1 (e.g., females to males for panic disorder with agoraphobia; males to females for antisocial personality disorder or alcohol dependence; *DSM-IV-TR*, 2000).

Compared to males, females in Western, urbanized cultures are more emotionally invested in appearance and in body image, and they have more problems related to body weight, body image, and disordered eating (Muth & Cash, 1997; Smolak & Murnen, 2004; see chapter 8). A meta-analysis of over 200 studies involving more than 140,000 participants indicated that (a) in general, females have a poorer body image than males; (b) body image is more variable among females than males; (c) this male–female difference is more pronounced in adolescence than in adulthood; and (d) the disparity *increased*, not declined, over the period 1970–1995 (Feingold & Mazzella, 1998). There is also considerable evidence that patriarchy, including heterosexual objectification of girls and women, contributes to negative body image, helplessness, dissociation from internal signals, and other components of disordered eating (Fallon et al., 1994; Smolak & Murnen, 2004; see chapter 8).

Advocates of prevention must continue working very hard to stimulate public awareness about weight and shape concerns, including eating disorders, as a topic with special relevance to women's health. We argue throughout this book that prevention programs need to increase the resistance of females to unhealthy cultural messages about food, weight, and shape, while changing the behaviors of males and females who objectify and disempower females (Levine, 1994; Maine, 2000; Piran, 1999b, 2001, 2002; Smolak & Murnen, 2001, 2004). To build female resistance and to promote cultural change, girls need special opportunities to speak candidly with each other and with adult women. These dialogues help females to articulate how intense private feelings (e.g., shame, anxiety, hopelessness), negative body image, appearance competition between women, and unhealthy weight management ideals and practices are encouraged by sociocultural factors (Friedman, 2003; Piran, 1999b, 2001, 2002).

During our prevention talks and workshops, we often hear how the presence of males inhibits or disrupts the ability of girls to work together in developing a critical perspective toward negative sociocultural influences. All too often boys and men, as products of gender role socialization within a patriarchal society, do not take girls or their concerns seriously. Presentations about physical development, body image concerns, and beauty may elicit a variety of inappropriate, defensive behaviors from boys, many of whom feel it is their masculine right or obligation to objectify females and deflect attention from their own bodies (Phelps, Dempsey, Sapia, & Nelson, 1999; Smolak & Murnen, 2001). Some boys and men who sincerely care about females still find it difficult to discuss body image and disordered eating. They feel that critical analyses of the origins of negative body image and disordered eating in females all too easily degenerate into the unfair implication that "males are to blame" for females' troubles.

Males as Part of the Cultural Context for Disordered Eating

We are strong advocates of the need to prevent negative body and disordered eating in females, and to create special opportunities for females to participate in this process. However, neither goal means that prevention is irrelevant for males, or that males are solely to blame for negative body image and disordered eating in females. Powerful cultural institutions and traditions guide the attitudes of both males and females about bodies, beauty, gender, health, and control (Bordo, 1993, 1999; Foucault, 1979; Piran, Carter, Thompson, & Pajouhandeh, 2002). Cultural forces are reinforced by, and embodied in, the behavior of both males and females as they live within families, friendships, schools, jobs, and other systems. In a very real sense, no one set of people (e.g., fashion designers, males) is solely to blame for cultural systems that encourage unhealthy behavior. But this diffusion of responsibility does not imply that no one has a responsibility to promote healthy changes. In a very real sense, it means that all individuals, males and females alike, share the obligation to improve health and well-being. In inextricably linking females and males, a systemic and sociocultural perspective reminds us that females play a role in sustaining their own unhealthy practices (Nichter, 2000; Rothblum, 1994).

That said, this state of affairs should in no way obscure the fact that males are a powerful, if not dominant, part of many cultural contexts for eating problems and eating disorders. As businessmen and as consumers, males figure prominently in the construction, marketing, and consumption of mass media that glorify slenderness, vilify fat, and transform the female body into a sexual commodity (Levine, 1994; Levine & Smolak, 1996; Thompson et al., 1999). Normative messages (e.g., "Fat women look silly and deserve ridicule for their lack of self-control") are translated and intensified by many males, including fathers and brothers operating within the close emotional quarters of a family, as well as physicians and coaches working with young people. Chapters 6 and 8 review some of the voluminous evidence linking negative body image and disordered eating specifically to teasing, criticism, harassment, assault, and other forms of objectification directed by males toward the female body (see Thompson et al., 1999; see also Piran et al., 2002). Chapter 7 explains how the continuum of eating problems and eating disorders is also sustained by general social conditions that subject many females to an unhealthy blend of stressors, inadequate coping skills, low levels of social support, and lack of opportunities to establish a multifaceted identity apart from appearance.

Boys and men as a social category are not solely responsible for these pathological influences; to reiterate, males are not "to blame" for eating disorders. Nevertheless, we are adamant in arguing that a large number of individual males need to be held accountable for their unhealthy attitudes and behaviors toward females; and that as fathers, brothers, physicians, teachers, coaches, and so forth, males have the opportunity and the responsibility to live in ways that prevent eating disorders and in general promote women's and men's health (Kelly, 2002a; Levine, 1994; Maine, 1991, 2000; Smolak & Murnen, 2001, 2004). As explained more fully in the final third of this book, adult men need to work with adult women in developing prevention programs that operate on multiple levels to change the attitudes and behaviors of boys as well as girls.

Males and Disordered Eating

The psychology of negative body image and disordered eating in females has been explored extensively (Cash & Pruzinsky, 2002). Much less is known about negative body image, dieting, and eating problems in males. Many boys and men report they are "dissatisfied" with their weight and shape (Cash, 1997; Pope, Phillips, & Olivardia, 2000), but it is clear that, relative to females, males are much less likely to see thinness, weight, and control of hunger as critically important aspects of self-concept. Consequently, beginning at least in early adolescence, males are much less inclined to engage in the weight management practices that may devolve into eating problems and eating disorders. For example, Field, Camargo, Taylor, Berkey, Frazier, and colleagues (1999; A. E. Field, personal communication, July 31, 2000) administered surveys to 8,591 girls and 7,523 boys ages 9 through 14. Between 15% and 19% of the girls ages 12 to 14 were "overweight" according to body mass, while 17% of those who were not objectively overweight thought that they were. The prevalence of girls trying to lose weight increased from 35% to 40% to 44% for ages 12, 13, and 14, respectively. By contrast, more of the boys (22% to 27%) were objectively overweight, but only 20% were trying to lose weight (a figure that declined from ages 12 through 14). In addition, only 1.2% of the boys (vs. 2.4% of the girls) reported they were "always on a diet to lose weight," and only 5% to 6% perceived themselves to be overweight when they were not.

Whitaker et al. (1989) and Neumark-Sztainer, Story, Falkner, Beuhring, and Resnick (1999) reported similar findings for older adolescents. In their large-scale study Whitaker et al. found that 38% of the boys (vs. 81% of the girls) indicated a desire to lose weight, but only 2% to 5% (vs. 16% to 27% of the girls) feared weight gain and looking fat, and only 9% (vs. 35% of the girls) worried about overeating. Furthermore, only 18% of the boys (vs. 63% of the girls) said they had dieted in the past year. Numerous studies of older adolescents have also found that heavier girls are much more likely than heavier boys to be concerned about their weight and to report more mild and more severe forms of weight control behavior (see, e.g., Centers for Disease Control, 1999; Steen, Wadden, Foster, & Andersen, 1996; Whitaker et al., 1989).

At present there are insufficient data to determine whether a continuum of eating problems, eating disorders, or weight and shape concerns exists among males. The evidence does suggest that, although full-blown AN and BN are exceedingly rare in the general population of males (Hoek & van Hoeken, 2003), prevention specialists need to be concerned about a minority of boys and men who have significant problems with partial syndrome eating disorders and with the components of disordered eating (see Muse, Stein, & Abbess, 2003). Leichner, Arnett, Rallo, Srikameswaran, and Vulcano (1986) surveyed a nonrandom sample of 4,659 adolescents (most of whom were ages 13 to 18), living in the Canadian province of Manitoba. Based on an Eating Attitudes Test (EAT) score ≥ 30, approximately 22% of the females and 5% of males fell into this high-risk, eating-disordered category (Leichner, et al., 1986). Whitaker et al. (1989) also administered the EAT and a measure of eating disorder symptoms to 2,564 males ages 14 to 18 attending high school in a semirural New York county. No boys met the *DSM-III* criteria for AN and only 0.4% met the criteria for BN. However, 1% of the boys met the criteria for partial syndrome. More recently, in a 3-year longitudinal study of approximately 1,000 Minnesota boys ages 13 through 18, Leon et al. (1995) found that 5.5% were consistently in the moderate risk category, which was defined as 2 to 6 risk factors derived from a symptom checklist, high scores on EDI drive for thinness and bulimia, and low or high body weight. This is consistent with a study of over 3,500 Norwegian boys ages 12 through 19, in which approximately 3% reported disordered eating as measured by an abbreviated form of the EAT (Wichstrøm, 1999).

Research also indicates that a more substantial minority of boys reports the components of disordered eating such as very unhealthy weight control techniques (e.g., fasting, smoking cigarettes, using diet pills) or binge eating. An analysis of surveys from over 39,000 boys ages 14 to 15 and 17 to 18 in Minnesota found that approximately 12.5% reported binge eating, and nearly 30% reported either binge eating or use of at least one form of unhealthy weight management. The greatest prevalence of these eating problems occurred in Hispanic and American Indian boys (Croll, Neumark-Sztainer, Story, & Ireland, 2002). In a study of a nationally representative sample of over 3,400 boys ages 12 through 18, approximately 7% answered "yes" to the question: "Have you ever binged and purged (which is when you eat a lot of food and then make yourself throw up, or vomit, or take something that makes you have diarrhea) or not?" (Ackard, Neumark-Sztainer, Hannan, French, & Story, 2001).

As is the case for females, negative body image and eating disorders tend to flourish where weight, size, and appearance are critical to success, where people are competing with each other for success, and where the competitive edge is measured in small increments. Such contexts include wrestling, jockeys, light-weight rowing, and the gay community for males (Mickalide, 1990). For example, Williamson and Hartley (1998) found that gay males are more likely than males with a heterosexual orientation to have a slender ideal, to be dissatisfied with their bodies, and to report disordered eating. As another example, Johnson, Powers, and Dick (1999) surveyed 562 female and 883 male athletes from universities in Division I of the National Collegiate Athletic Association (USA). Approximately 43% of the male athletes were football players. Although this sample of male athletes was very unlikely to have a full-blown (0%) or subthreshold eating disorder (<0.5%), 38% were considered "at risk" based on high levels of body dissatisfaction and a high drive for thinness, or on multiple episodes of binge eating, vomiting, or purging during the past 3 months.

Coupled with the epidemiological studies of eating problems in general among adolescent boys, research on at-risk subcultures of males has three significant implications for prevention. First, continued study of these subcultures has the potential to illuminate processes that are similar in the cultural transmission of unhealthy norms, attitudes, and behaviors among females and males. Second, there are clearly groups of males, as well as females, who need selective and targeted prevention programs. To reiterate, eating problems and eating disorders are not "just a woman's health issue." The third implication concerns the value for universal and selective prevention of working with boys to develop a critical perspective on culture (Goldberg et al., 2000; Piran, 1999b, 2001). Piran (1999b; personal communication, February 8, 2001) found that getting healthy adolescent males involved in thinking critically about contextual influences on body image, and in taking constructive action to improve their subculture, was an important component of her prevention work with male *and* female students at an elite ballet school for adolescents (see chapter 8).

Body Dissatisfaction and the Drive for Bulk and Muscularity

The drive for bulk and muscularity is an intriguing psychological topic for establishing a critical perspective in males and for prevention of negative body image and eating problems in males (Goldberg et al., 1996, 2000). Studies have shown that many boys and men want to be more muscular without being fat (Furnham & Calnan, 1998; Neumark-Sztainer, Story, Falkner et al., 1999; Pope et al., 2000). On questionnaires these males report "body dissatisfaction," but this is a matter of feeling "too thin" or "too weak and puny." For example, in a study of weight and shape dissatisfaction in British males ages 16 to 18, Furnham and Calnan (1998) found that 31% wanted to lose weight and 38% wanted to gain weight. Those who wanted to gain weight had the highest drive to be bulkier, a finding corroborated by McCreary and Sasse (2000). Pope et al. (2000) presented evidence that this drive for bulk and muscularity reflects changes in Western, urbanized culture's ideal masculine shape that are parallel to the glorification of slenderness for women observed during the period 1960–1995 (see Silverstein & Perlick, 1995).

In the extreme this drive to be bigger, bulkier, and more muscular becomes part of a disorder called "muscle dysmorphia" (Pope et al., 2000). Muscle dysmorphia is analogous to AN. Psychological and social functioning are compromised by an obsessive concern about body shape (in this instance, being too small vs. being too fat), by an all-consuming need to become more larger and more muscular (vs. becoming thinner and taking up less space), by an iron determination to exercise and avoid fat (similar to AN), and by obsessive self-consciousness about appearance and body size (similar to AN). Pope et al. (2000) estimate that 10% of "hard core" male body builders who frequent health clubs and gyms have this form of body dysmorphic disorder (see *DSM-IV-TR*, 2000, pp. 507–510).

Several researchers (Andersen, Cohn, & Holbrook, 2000; Pope et al., 2000) have theorized that boys and men who internalize the muscular ideal from magazines, movies, and television (e.g., professional wrestling) are likely to be dissatisfied with their own appearance, muscularity, and power. A subset of these males, such as those who are insecure, perfectionist, and/or involved in power sports, will be highly motivated to lose fat and build muscle mass by working out excessively and by (ab)using illegal anabolic steroids and legal nutritional supplements (Pope et al., 2000; Wroblewska, 1997). Despite clear benefits in the short run, this process creates a high risk of binge eating, steroid abuse, obsessive social anxiety, and intense dysphoria when ideals are not realized (Andersen et al., 2000; McCreary & Sasse, 2000; Pope et al., 2000). Currently, there is only limited support for this broad theory. For example, we found that, controlling for body mass, boys ages 11 through 13 who internalized the muscular ideal were more likely to report weight control and muscle building techniques. However, the strength of these correlations was not as great as the relationship between internalization of the slender ideal and weight management behavior in girls of the same age (Smolak, Levine, & Thompson, 2001). Epidemiological research with over 2,200 adolescent boys (M age = 15) from Minnesota found approximately 5.5% reported having used anabolic steroids to gain muscle during the past year. Steroid use was correlated with dissatisfaction with shoulder size, with weight-related teasing by family members, and with use of unhealthy weight management behaviors in the past year (Irving, Wall, Neumark-Sztainer, & Story, 2002). Once again, evidence is limited, but it appears that male student athletes who are involved in sports emphasizing bulk and strength are more likely to use anabolic steroids (Bahrke, Yesalis, Kopstein, & Stephens, 2000; Goldberg et al., 2000).

Much more research is needed to support this sociocultural theory of the drive for muscularity in males and to understand the health implications of this motive. Nevertheless, its potential applicability to prevention and males is seen in a large-scale and well-designed study of the *Adolescents Training and Learning to Avoid Steroids* (ATLAS) program for male high school football players by Goldberg et al. (2000). This successful intervention and its sister program, ATHENA, for adolescent girls are described in detail in chapter 14.

As noted previously, we join Piran in arguing that this type of critical social perspective will be beneficial for males in subcultures at risk and for males and females in general (see chapter 8). We believe this type of critical perspective will give males a richer appreciation of cultural contexts that affect female body image and eating problems, and thus instill in males a stronger sense of their responsibility to create healthier contexts for females (Kelly, 2002a; Levine, 1994; Maine, 2000; Piran, 1999b).

FEAR OF FAT AND THE PREVENTION OF OBESITY

One cardinal feature of many forms of disordered eating, at least in Western societies, is an irrational, uncontrollable fear of fat and gaining weight. In part this fear reflects the harsh stigmatization of obesity and "fat" in modern, industrialized cultures. Consequently, a reasonable proximal goal for prevention of disordered eating is elimination or reduction of this fear in favor of more reasonable, flexible, and healthier attitudes about food, fat, weight, and shape (Berg, 2001; Irving & Neumark-Sztainer, 2002; Smolak et al., 1998b).

But how much, if any, "fear of fat," fear of weight gain, and weight dissatisfaction should be part of healthy attitudes about eating, weight, and shape (Heinberg, Thompson, & Matzon, 2001)? Numerous reviews by epidemiologists, physicians, and psychologists consistently show that pediatric obesity (i.e., in children and adolescents) and obesity in adults—and, in particular, central fat distribution (truncal obesity)—is associated with elevated blood pressure, hyperinsulinemia (and thus risk for diabetes), high levels of low-density lipoproteins (hyperlipidemia), and lowered physical fitness (Allison & Saunders, 2000; Dietz, 1998; Faith, Pietrobelli, Allison, & Heymsfield, 1997; Neumark-Sztainer, 1999; Pi-Sunyer, 1999; Power, Lake, & Cole, 1997; Tanofksy-Kraff, Hayden, Cavazos, & Wilfley, 2003). Given that obesity in people of all ages is a public health priority, shouldn't people in general and children in particular be more concerned about getting fat, not less concerned? Along the same lines, moderate to slight caloric restriction, resulting in either weight stabilization (even as children grow in height) or weight reduction, is a recommended part of many regimens for health risk reduction in overweight children, adolescents, and adults (Barlow & Dietz, 1998; National Heart Lung & Blood Institute [NHLB], 1998; Tanofsky-Kraff et al., 2003). But isn't calorie-restrictive dieting a risk factor for eating problems and eating disorders in children and adolescents?

These tensions and questions are part of a larger, challenging issue: Is prevention of eating problems necessarily at odds with prevention of obesity (Berg, 2001; Irving & Neumark-Sztainer, 2002; Neumark-Sztainer, 2003)? This is a critically important question because many people (e.g., parents, teachers, pediatricians, government officials) in a position to influence universal and selective prevention are much more concerned about the prevalence and health risks of obesity than they are about eating disorders (Austin, 1999; Faith et al., 1997). Many people are very alarmed by dramatic increases in the incidence of overweight and obesity among children and adults in the United States during the past 20 to 25 years (Troiano & Flegal, 1998; Neumark-Sztainer, 2003). Research indicates that the percentage of adults ages 20 to 74 with a BMI ≥ 30 (and thus are considered obese by many experts) has increased from 15% in 1976–1980 to between 27% and 33% in the mid to late 1990s (Irving & Neumark-Sztainer, 2002; National Center for Health Statistics, 2004). According to Neumark-Sztainer's (1999) review of the same data, in the late 1970s 7.6% of children and 5.7% of adolescents were obese (BMI 95th percentile). By the mid 1990s, 10% to 12% of children and adolescents ages 6 to 17 are obese, while nearly 20% are overweight (Irving & Neumark-Sztainer, 2002; Troiano, Flegal, Kuczmarski, Campbell, & Johnson, 1995).

Health Promotion

To date, and with some promising exceptions (see Gortmaker et al., 1999; reviewed in chapter 9), neither public health nor school-based programs to prevent obesity have been very effective (Gill, 1997; Robinson & Killen, 2001). Indeed, the secular trend toward increasing BMIs, extreme BMIs, and poor nutrition and increasing inactivity in youth across the socioeconomic spectrum underscores the failure of America's massive, well-funded, and sustained "war on obesity" (Berg, 2001; Cogan & Ernsberger, 1999; Dietz, 1998). One reason for this failure is that prevention programs have been unable to overcome the following myths that abound in the United States:

- Being thin is healthy, good, and beautiful; being fat is unhealthy, bad, and ugly.
- Dieting, accompanied by a dieting mentality emphasizing "safe" and "dangerous" foods, is a good way for people to manage their weight and to become slender or thinner.

- Fat people are unhealthy, ugly, and responsible for their condition because they lack self-control or have other psychological problems.
- At any size, your weight is a very important and very clear marker of your health status, and even small increments in weight are dangerous.

It is likely that these erroneous messages are the common ground underlying a set of interrelated problems for youth, especially young girls and women: chaotic eating and poor nutrition; eating disorders; obesity; and unhealthy weight management behaviors, including cigarette smoking and abuse of other stimulant drugs (Berg, 2001). As such, these ubiquitous messages are obstacles to the prevention of obesity *and* to the prevention of eating problems and eating disorders. The apparent conflict between prevention of eating disorders and prevention of obesity should therefore evaporate if specialists can devise a new paradigm for promotion of healthy eating, healthy exercise, and positive body image (Berg, 2001; Cogan & Ernsberger, 1999; Neumark-Sztainer, 1999; see also the Website www.BodyPositive.com). This paradigm emphasizes health promotion at every size (Berg, 2001; Burgard & Lyons, 1994; Robison, 2003), with health defined primarily in terms of multiple dimensions such as strength, stamina, resistance to illness, the energy to function well, emotional well-being, and positive social relationships. Weight-for-height, as determined by charts for children and adolescents, is a starting point for concern when BMI is too high *or* too low, and when other factors (e.g., ethnicity, location of fat deposition) are taken into account.

The health promotion at every size paradigm enables those concerned about obesity, eating disorders, and health in general to find common ground in these seven ways.

1. *In most instances the goals of prevention are measured in healthy attitudes and behaviors, not BMI or pounds on a scale*. Robison (2003), along with Deborah Burgard (see the Website www.BodyPositive.com), a leading proponent of the "Health at Every Size" approach to eating and weight issues, challenges the traditional height–weight charts by defining healthy weight "as the weight at which a person settles while moving toward a more fulfilling and meaningful lifestyle" (p. 4). Although this definition would be problematic for many people, including those with a developmental perspective, it does help remind us that as prevention specialists we want children, adolescents, and adults to develop:

- *a positive body image* that is supported by respect and appreciation for the diversity of human sizes and shapes;
- *an active lifestyle* that involves walking or biking instead of driving or using the elevator; relatively little time spent in a sedentary, snacking state in front of the television; and, where possible, regular moderate exercise that is done for fun (playfulness), fitness, and recreation;
- *good eating habits*, including increased consumption of complex carbohydrates such as fruits, vegetables, and grains, and decreased consumption (but not elimination) of red meat, saturated fats, salt, sugar, and soft drinks;
- *eating that satisfies hunger*; provides energy for health, growth, and well-being; and is regulated not by calorie-restrictive dieting and other externally imposed rules, but by hunger and satiety;
- *communal eating*, that is, ways to ensure that family and friends sit down and eat a meal in a friendly, nurturing atmosphere;
- *abstinence from cigarette smoking and use of other drugs* (e.g., appetite suppressants);
- *life skills to cope with stress and meet one's needs* in ways that do not include starving and/or anesthetizing feelings by eating large amounts or abusing drugs.

2. *Measures of weight (e.g., BMI) are relevant to health, but we must remember that weight has a complicated relationship to health, especially for females*. As noted previously in this chapter, there is a mountain of evidence that obesity is unhealthy for children, adolescents, and adults. Yet there are also data that encourage us to be careful about oversimplifying the relationship between body weight, body fat, and health. For example, Troiano et al. (1996) conducted a meta-analysis of prospective studies of the relationship between weight-for-height and all-cause mortality in White men and women with an average age of 50. Troiano et al. (1996) found that for men (17 studies, $N = 356,747$), increased mortality was associated with a BMI less than 23 or greater than 28. Across the 6 studies of women ($N = 248,501$), there was no meaningful relationship between BMI and mortality. One of the largest studies reviewed by Troiano et al. (1996) was part of a 10-year prospective study of BMI and life expectancy in 1.80 million Norwegians (see Waaler, 1984, as reviewed in Ernsberger, 1989). Waaler found an inverted-U relationship. Life expectancy of 25-year-old women was roughly the same (between 78–80 years) for women with BMI's between 20 and 34, and fell off in a more-or-less linear fashion below 21 and beyond 35. The curve for men looks similar, but truncated such that the plateau occurred between 21 and 28–29.

In general, we believe the data on obesity and on health promotion support the following reasonable principles:

- Health is improved substantially if one eats, exercises, and copes with life's challenges in ways that help one avoid becoming either too thin or too fat.
- Many, many people, including children and adolescents, have a BMI well within (and below) the so-called normal range, but still they are eating, exercising, and living in ways that are quite unhealthy.
- More research is needed (e.g., to determine the health risks of overweight and obesity in children, and to understand the relationship between body mass, ethnicity, and health), but reasonably useful statistical guidelines exist for the categories of "too thin" and "too fat" in children and adults (see chapter 2).

3. *Prejudice toward fat people is socially unacceptable and psychologically unhealthy for the culture.* In many industrialized, "modern" countries, being fat is a highly stigmatized condition (Puhl & Brownell, 2001; Rothblum, 1994; Yuker & Allison, 1994). Many people are convinced that because fat is bad and ugly, fat people in general and fat girls and women in particular are second-class citizens worthy of contempt, ridicule, or pity. In this widespread prejudice, obesity is seen as a natural, inevitable outcome of a process in which psychological weakness (e.g., gluttony) or psychological problems (e.g., depression fueled by low self-esteem) lead to binge eating, constant eating of high-calorie foods, and inactivity. This view persists even though considerable evidence demonstrates that overweight or obese individuals are either no different psychologically from nonoverweight people or slightly better adjusted (see, e.g., Allison & Saunders, 2000).

A wide variety of people, ranging from elementary school children to nutritionists to physicians to landlords and prospective employers, hold these prejudicial attitudes. Fat girls and women are often recipients of smirking stares, unkind comments, jokes about gluttony or ugliness, and other experiences of being demeaned and victimized (Burgard & Lyons, 1994; Neumark-Sztainer, Story, & Faibisch, 1997; Puhl & Brownell, 2001; Rothblum, 1994). Fat women are less likely to be hired than slender women, even if their job credentials, professional appearance, and personal hygiene are identical. It is extraordinary but painfully true that fat girls have a lower chance of being accepted to elite colleges, and when they are accepted to colleges in general, they are less likely to be financially supported by their own parents.

These beliefs, attitudes, and practices constitute unwarranted and unacceptable prejudice toward fat and fat people. No person, regardless of gender or age, should be subjected to teasing, taunting, or other forms of discrimination related to weight or shape. Elimination of this prejudice will also help to prevent obesity, as well as disordered eating. There is no evidence that prejudice helps fat people to lose weight and to develop a healthier lifestyle. Instead, prejudice contributes directly to body image problems, low self-esteem and depression, and avoidance of exercise, all of which increase the risk for unhealthy eating (including eating disorders) and further weight gain in heavy adolescents and adults (Burgard & Lyons, 1994). Widespread prejudice and ignorance about fat people and fat also causes many normal weight and even some underweight girls and women to feel fat, to be overly concerned with fat, and to avoid fat in ways that severely compromise the nutritional quality of their diet (Berg, 2001).

4. *The glorification of slenderness and calorie-restrictive dieting is a problem, not the solution*. As is the case for irrational beliefs about fat and fat people, the glorification of slenderness and dieting is not a healthy response to public health concerns about obesity (Berg, 2001; Ikeda, Mitchell, & Crawford, 2000). Both aspects of weightism—the prejudice that glorifies slenderness and vilifies fat and fat people—likely play a role in the tendency for overweight and obese youth to use unhealthy weight management strategies (Boutelle, Neumark-Sztainer, Story, & Resnick, 2002) and for many normal weight girls to feel "overweight" and "fat" (Field, Camargo, Taylor, Berkey, Frazier, et al., 1999). Many people, including children and adolescents, believe that the following are very good, not only for heavy people, but for people in general as part of management one's weight and avoiding illness: embracing a slender ideal, intentional dieting, and weight loss. We believe the data support a very different view as part of health promotion:

- Calorie-restrictive dieting is unhealthy and dangerous for children and adolescents who are not obese (Ikeda, 1998; Ikeda & Mitchell, 2001; Mallick, 1983).
- Obese adults may benefit from calorie-restrictive dieting, but they should use this form of weight management only (a) under professional supervision, and (b) after they have given informed consent following an explanation of the controversy about the value and risks of dieting (Brownell & Rodin, 1994; Devlin et al., 2000; versus Berg, 2001; Gaesser, 1996; Garner & Wooley, 1991).
- Obese children and adolescents may benefit from carefully monitored weight management programs that include calorie-restrictive dieting (Epstein, Valoski, Wing, & McCurley, 1994; Tanofsky-Kraff et al., 2003).

It is psychologically and physically unhealthy for children who are not obese to engage in calorie-restrictive dieting. In this respect, prevention of calorie-restrictive dieting may be common ground for prevention of obesity and disordered eating. A longitudinal study of nearly 700 ninth-grade girls showed that, regardless of initial weight and excluding those who were already obese, girls who engaged in strenuous, self-guided efforts to lose weight were more likely to gain weight over time and to become obese (Stice, Cameron, Hayward, Taylor, & Killen, 1999).

5. *Reducing "fear of fat" does not mean ignoring the needs of fat children.* This is true in three ways. First, reduction of myths and stigma pertaining to fat people will be of psychological benefit to children of all sizes (Ikeda & Naworski, 1992). Second, very large children should be evaluated for medical problems associated with obesity in children, including sleep apnea, Type II diabetes, and high blood pressure (Ikeda et al., 2000). Third, although there is evidence that carefully managed dieting can help some obese children to achieve sustainable weight loss and improved health (Epstein et al., 1994), great care should be taken in acknowledging that much remains to be learned about the most effective and ethical ways to help heavy children to become healthier. Programs that enable obese children to learn to manage their weight also need to emphasize factors that apply broadly to healthy development in youth. These include helping children to understand what they can and cannot change, to value themselves, to become more active and less sedentary, and to develop meaningful, constructive relationships and pastimes (Burgard & Lyons, 1994; Ikeda, 1998; Ikeda & Mitchell, 2001; Kater, 2004; Robinson & Killen, 2001; Story, 1999).

6. *Whatever one's size and shape, positive body image is an important part of health.* Many females and males living in Western, industrialized cultures have trouble establishing a positive body image. This is a serious public health issue because negative body image has a large number of negative implications for psychological, social, and physical well-being (Cash, 1997; Thompson et al., 1999). Therefore, *regardless of their size and gender*, it would be healthy for people to have multiple avenues for:

- differentiating body size from self-worth;
- learning to accept and value what one can and cannot change about one's physical characteristics, and appreciating the ways in which genetic constitution interacts with psychological and social factors to influence eating, size, and shape;
- appreciating the many good things our bodies do for us regardless of their size;
- developing one's own personal style as far as dress, sexuality, and self-expression go, and respecting and appreciating the uniqueness of others.

7. *A critical perspective toward culture will facilitate prevention of an array of problems related to nutrition, eating, and health.* American culture promotes a number of contradictory and unhealthy attitudes about food, weight, indulgence, and restraint (Battle & Brownell, 1996; Bordo, 1993; Levine & Smolak, 1996; see chapter 13). In addition, over the past 20 to 30 years the nutritional environment in the United States has become increasingly toxic. Specifically, there have been dramatic increases in both diet foods and calorie-dense foods, as well in portion sizes and time spent in front of the television or computer screen. People committed to health promotion should acknowledge their common need to help citizens of all ages and sizes, and especially children and adolescents, think critically about food, eating, weight, and beauty related messages conveyed through teasing, the mass media, sports, and other important aspects of culture. Cultural literacy and activism will help prevent obesity and disordered eating through a network of interlocking, positive changes in people and their

environments (Berg, 2001; Irving & Neumark-Sztainer, 2002; Kelly, 2002a; Neumark-Sztainer, 1996, 2003; Maine, 2000; Piran, 1999b, 2001; Thompson et al., 1999).

SUMMARY AND CONCLUSIONS

We have long advocated a feminist, ecological perspective as the basis for universal prevention of eating problems and eating disorders. This perspective has been criticized as irrelevant by those who champion a neurogenetic perspective, as sexist by those who feel that boys are ignored or blamed, and as dangerous by those who argue that fear of fat and the drive for thinness are necessary weapons in the war on obesity. Each of these concerns is revisited throughout the book, especially the contention that prevention should concentrate on identifying and intervening with those individuals who by virtue of genetics are at high risk for eating disorders (see chapter 14). However, this chapter sets the stage for consideration of specific sociocultural prevention models in chapters 4 through 8 by demonstrating that:

1. Many key features of the neurogenetic perspective lack consistent empirical support, and in general this paradigm cannot explain one of the most significant features of eating problems and eating disorders: the preponderance of female sufferers. Furthermore, much of the research on behavior genetics strongly supports, rather than negates, the importance of sociocultural factors.

2. Boys and men as a social category are not solely to blame for the large number of females with eating problems and eating disorders. However, within our patriarchal society, males have a responsibility to understand and to change those situations and actions that objectify females and contribute to negative body image and disordered eating as significant health problems for females. Conversely, prevention specialists have a responsibility to study and to help males because a minority are at risk for disordered eating and because a significant minority engage in binge eating and in unhealthy forms of weight and shape management. Moreover, there is increasing concern about the health implications of what seems to be a growing trend toward idealization of a hypermuscular, fat-free male body. Opportunities to develop a critical perspective on culture and to take action toward constructive change

are likely to be the factor that links females and males in improving each others' lives.

3. Extreme fear of fat and the idealization of thinness are not the answer to the crisis of obesity, just as minimizing the health risks of obesity will reduce the credibility of efforts to prevent eating disorders. We agree with those experts who argue that there are many theoretical, empirical, and practical reasons to integrate the prevention of eating problems and obesity (Berg, 2001; Irving & Neumark-Sztainer, 2002; Neumark-Sztainer, 2003). The paradigm of health promotion at every size is a very good place to begin the challenging task of bringing together prevention specialists from these two fields. This paradigm enables those concerned about obesity and eating disorders to build a common ground in working toward good nutrition, active lifestyles, freedom from sexist and weight-based prejudice, positive body image, ways to cope with stress that do not involved starving or binge eating, and reasonable means of changing weight when it becomes too high or too low.

II

GUIDES TO PREVENTION: MODELS AND RISK FACTORS

4

Developmental Psychopathology

Many clinically based theorists and researchers have described potential etiological factors in the development of eating problems and eating disorders. So, for example, Bruch (1973) discussed a potential desire to avoid sexual maturation and its attendant demands, whereas Johnson and Connors (1987) considered the possibility that early mother–infant interactions and subsequent development of an unhealthy attachment might contribute to, and perhaps even differentiate, AN and BN.

These arguments, and others, point to possible developmental factors in the onset and maintenance of eating disorders. Why, then, would we need a general model of developmental psychopathology (Cicchetti & Schneider-Rosen, 1986; Rosen, 1996)? What might a developmental psychopathology approach add to our understanding of eating disorders and the prevention of eating problems and disorders?

This chapter considers four components of a developmental psychopathology approach. First, clinically oriented theories, rooted in the medical model and case study methodology, have tended to emphasize the individual as pathological. The argument is that individuals with AN or BN have a disease or disorder that makes it difficult for them to function in society. This approach leads to a focus on individual factors, ranging from neurochemistry to temperament to trauma, as causative. Developmental psychopathology discusses such factors but, importantly, also incorporates a broad array of contextual factors, including schools, gender roles, and cultural norms, in explaining behavior. In considering these contextual factors, developmental psychopathology models often focus on transactions between the individual and her environments. These transactions not only involve reciprocal influence but also emphasize the ways in which behavioral outcomes are shaped by the expectations and interpretations of the involved parties.

Second, because it is self-consciously developmental in its orientation, developmental psychopathology attempts to trace trajectories or pathways of development. In line with developmental theory generally, the principle of equifinality maintains that there can be multiple pathways to one outcome. A highway analogy is appropriate here. To get to Columbus, Ohio, from our college, you can take at least four different highways. They will all get you to Columbus. But some are faster than others, some are prettier, and some are more dangerous during particular seasons or times of day. And they all land you in slightly different parts of Columbus, although you can get to any part of Columbus from any of them. Continuing a highway analogy, one could start out on one route to Columbus but, by choosing (more or less intentionally and knowledgably) different turns, one might end up in Cleveland, Indianapolis, or Morgantown, West Virginia. So it is, too, with development. What starts off as one path may veer into several trajectories that might lead to very different outcomes.

Third, developmental psychopathology models look for molar as well as molecular change. The idea here is that there is an underlying organization, a molar level, to behavior. This molar level will be periodically reorganized during development. This leads us to focus on the possibility of qualitative as well as quantitative shifts in development, for example, in the cognitive–affective meaning of "fat" or "control." Thus, this model alerts us to pay close attention to developmental transitions and the special risks they might engender (Smolak & Levine, 1996).

Finally, developmental psychopathology raises several methodological issues. These include issues of research design, measurement, and ethics. These issues are relevant not only to basic research concerning the etiology of eating problems but also to the development and evaluation of prevention programs.

CONTEXTS OF DEVELOPMENT

Developmental psychology has a long history of examining the contexts of development as well as the contribution of individual characteristics to the process of development. Pioneering work by Bronfenbrenner

(1979) and Lerner (1990) set the stage for these complex, multilayered models. However, even prior to their work, developmental psychologists had moved away from an either/or, nature versus nurture approach and toward an interactionist and even transactional approach to behavior and development (see, e.g., Overton, 1985; Piaget, 1967; Sameroff & Chandler, 1975).

Bronfenbrenner's Model

According to Bronfenbrenner (1979), a child is embedded in several layers of contexts. The layer analogy is meant to represent the proximity of the context to the child. Contexts in closest proximity are most likely to have almost daily impact on the child's life. They are also likely to mediate the effects of the more distal contexts. Consequently, these more proximal levels, such as family influences, have typically received the most attention from researchers. This means that several factors that may be important in the etiology of eating disorders and eating problems—including the effects of societal assumptions about gender and ethnicity—have received relatively little research attention.

More specifically, Bronfenbrenner argues that five "layers" of development constitute the "ecology" of child development. The first layer is the child herself. Here Bronfenbrenner acknowledges the role of genetic and physiological individual differences on the development of the child. Factors relevant in the etiology of eating disorders might include a genetic or neurochemical predisposition to negative affect. As discussed in chapter 3, although other factors (e.g., temperament) have been offered as potentially innate contributors to eating disorders, research linking genetics and neurochemistry to the onset of eating disorders is in its infancy and is generally inconclusive. Thus, emphasis has been, and continues to be, on sociocultural factors such as family, peers, and media as potential causes of eating disorders. This approach makes Bronfenbrenner's model particularly appropriate as a framework.

The next layer is the microsystem. This is the context that has immediate effects on the child and includes the parents and siblings as well as day care and school experiences. The activities and interactions that occur in this context are likely to have a direct influence on a child's behavior. However, the child's behavior also directly influences the nature of the microsystem. This transaction has become evident in clinical studies of eating disorder clients in which it is difficult to ascertain how much of family dysfunction is attributable to living with someone with a severe eating disorder and how much predated the onset of the disorder. Less dramatically, if a child has a tendency to display more than average amounts of negative affect (Bates, 1987), her family interactions may be marked by discord, pressure to behave differently, perceived lack of parental support, and ultimately, perhaps, mutual withdrawal.

The third level is the mesosystem. This represents the interactions of the various components of the microsystem, thereby explicitly demonstrating the interplay among the environmental influences on the child. For example, what goes on at school influences what happens at home and vice versa. Furthermore, school and home can send congruent or conflicting messages to a child about abilities, values, and roles. There are several interesting examples of this in the field of eating disorders. First, the likelihood that a girl internalizes the societally defined standard that "thin is beautiful" is increased if she is exposed to that ideal in multiple contexts such as peers, family, and media (Levine, Smolak, & Hayden, 1994; Smolak & Levine, 2001b). Second, the family's reactions to problems that occur at school are likely to moderate the effects of the school issues. For example, a majority of girls report being sexually harassed at school (American Association of University Women Educational Foundation, 2001). If parents advise girls to just "ignore" the harassment or suggest that such harassment is a normative part of growing up, the girl may internalize the objectification inherent in the harassment. This, in turn, may lead to shame, negative self-esteem, and body hatred, all of which might contribute to the development of eating disorders (Fredrickson & Roberts, 1997).

The fourth level is the exosystem. These are contexts that affect children and adolescents more indirectly. Children are not part of these contexts every day although they may sometimes be part of them. Relatives not living in the child's home, pediatricians, and parents' workplace are all examples of exosystems. Health care is an interesting example of this type of context. With decreasing availability of programs to treat eating disorders, both in their subthreshold and full-blown forms, the need for prevention becomes even more pressing (see chapter 1).

Finally, there is the macrosystem. This contextual level includes the values and beliefs of a society as expressed both formally in laws and informally in unspoken social expectations. Elements of this level are often referred to as "cultural." If a child is growing up in two cultures, then both cultures, as well as the relationship between them, affect the child's development. It is very challenging to operationalize these contexts. This is probably one reason why the effects of gender and ethnic discrimination have received so little attention in the eating disorders literature (Smolak & Murnen, 2001; Smolak & Striegel-Moore, 2001). Yet, qualitative research (e.g., Thompson, 1994; Piran, 2001) and some quantitative research (Piran, 2002) suggest that experiences of racial and ethnic discrimination may contribute to negative affect, negative body image, and eating problems.

Bronfenbrenner's model is not the only theory postulating multilayered ecological contexts of development. It is, however, an effective means of specifying such layers and of considering their possible implications for prevention (see chapter 15).

Implications of an Ecological Approach for Prevention

This model has at least four important implications for prevention: (a) changes in the health care system of the United States necessitate increased prevention efforts; (b) contexts of development are interrelated and prevention must address those connections; (c) the more distal levels of context must be considered in prevention efforts; and (d) the dynamic, reciprocal nature of development, including the schema people use to organize and interpret behavior, must be acknowledged in prevention programs.

Health Care Systems. As discussed in chapter 1, one rationale for prevention is that the health care systems of most nations do not have the resources to provide treatment to anywhere near all of the people who need it. In the United States no more than 50% of people with clinical symptoms of mental illness currently receive treatment (U.S. Office of the Surgeon General, 1999), and there is no reason to believe that the percentage of eating disorders sufferers receiving treatment is any higher. Indeed, given the culturally syntonic nature of many eating disordered attitudes and behaviors (Gordon, 2000), and given the secrecy that often surrounds eating disorders, particularly BN, it would not be surprising if the percentage is much lower.

Health care providers are becoming more reluctant to pay for inpatient, long-term care for eating disorders clients (Garvin & Striegel-Moore, 2001). In the United States there are currently less than 50 inpatient programs for eating disorders, and some states have none.

Furthermore, many health insurance and HMO programs severely limit the number of days of treatment for which reimbursement is available.

In addition to heightening the need for prevention, the nature of the health care in the United States, Canada, the United Kingdom, and many other countries has also influenced our understanding of eating disorders in at least two important ways. First, the prominent role of physicians and drug companies in determining the diagnosis and treatment of eating disorders has undoubtedly contributed to the growing emphasis on finding neuroscientific causes and pharmacological treatments (e.g., Kaye & Strober, 1999; Mitchell, 2001). Until mental health broadly defined becomes equal to physical health in terms of status and funding, this trend will likely continue. Second, studies with clinical samples have led many to the erroneous belief that eating disorders are rare, and perhaps virtually nonexistent, among certain ethnic groups and socioeconomic statuses (Striegel-Moore & Smolak, 2002). Although it is indeed possible that the prevalence of specific forms of eating disorders varies by ethnicity and social class (Crago et al., 1996), it is equally plausible that use of the health care system varies by ethnicity and social class. Both ability to pay and willingness to trust the health care system—perhaps particularly the mental health care system—may account for the apparent lower use of treatment options by ethnic minority and poor populations (Garvin & Striegel-Moore, 2001).

Connected Contexts. Bronfenbrenner's model emphasizes the interconnections among the various contexts of development. Indeed, the mesosystem is defined in a way that highlights these connections. Yet, eating disorders researchers have only occasionally considered the influence of one context on the other, much less the effect of the interaction of two or more contexts on an individual's development. This oversight is striking because what happens in one context clearly does influence what goes on in another. This is evident, for example, in the effects of divorce, which negatively impacts a parent's ability to provide support at home, monitor peer relationships, and be an active partner in the child's education. This, in turn, affects the child's behavior in all three of these realms.

In a related vein, Garmezy (1983) suggested a triad of influences on the likelihood that a child will develop pathological behaviors. Garmezy argued that the child's own characteristics, the family, and the availability of nonfamilial support can contribute to a child's resilience in the face of risk factors. These factors may have additive effects. A child lacking familial and peer support is probably at greater risk than a child lacking only one of these. However, the factors may also affect each other such that one can offset or attenuate the other. Thus, a coach's message that a girl needs to lose weight might overwhelm her mother's message that the girl's weight is all right, particularly if the girl is very invested in succeeding in the sport. This may be one reason why some sports show higher levels of body image and eating problems (Smolak, Murnen, & Ruble, 2000), although, presumably, parent support for "doing what it takes" to succeed would increase the likelihood of the child developing a problem.

Programs aimed at preventing eating disorders must take into account the interactions among contexts in two ways. First, insofar as it is possible, eating disorders programs must aim at multiple contexts (Neumark-Sztainer, 1996; Piran, 1998). Programs that focus only on the individual underestimate the influence of the variety of sources of social messages about thinness, attractiveness, dieting, and eating disorders. Similarly, programs aiming at only one context (e.g., parents) may be missing equally influential contexts (e.g., peers) that continue to put the girl at risk. This is especially problematic if the program fails to reach some parents or if the parents become unable to enforce or convey the messages they learned in the program. Not surprisingly, then, cigarette and other drug prevention programs that target multiple social contexts have typically enjoyed more success than those simply aimed at the individual or at one context (Hawkins, Catalano, & Arthur, 2002; Tobler et al., 2000).

Second, prevention programs should aim to provide members of one context with the tools to work with and possibly influence members of another context. Thus, teachers might be given information on how to discuss teasing about body shape with parents or how to help students reduce "fat talk" among themselves and in their families. Parents might be provided with information to help them change school policies about teasing. Girls and parents can be taught how to lobby teachers and mass media to present more positive images of women and of people of a variety of sizes. This type of guidance will be particularly crucial in programs that do not have the resources to include all contextual levels. A good example of a prevention program that uses social resources effectively in this way is the work of O'Dea and Abraham (2000), which is discussed in detail in chapter 7.

Distal Influences. It has long been accepted that there are substantial gender differences in the prevalence of AN and BN, as well as of the individual symptoms (e.g., body image disturbance, fear of fat, dieting) that comprise these disorders (see chapter 8). Although the gender differences in BED are probably less pronounced, girls and women still appear to suffer from this disorder more commonly than do men and boys (see Smolak & Murnen, 2001, 2004, for a review). There also appear to be some differences in the occurrence of eating problems across different American ethnic groups (see Douchinis et al., 2001, and Smolak & Striegel-Moore, 2001, for reviews). For example, AN appears to be more rare among African Americans than White Americans, although binge eating appears with comparable frequency in the two groups and obesity is more common among Blacks.

These gender and ethnicity findings, particularly when considered along with cross-cultural data, suggest that broad cultural factors may play an important role in the development of eating problems. One such factor, cultural differences in ideal body type, has received considerable research attention (Douchinis et al., 2001; Smolak & Striegel-Moore, 2001). It is now widely accepted that African American culture accepts a less stringently thin ideal body type for women than does the European American culture. This ethnic difference is evident even in childhood such that, for example, a larger percentage of Black than White girls will report a desire to be heavier, whereas more White girls report an interest in losing weight, particularly once BMI is controlled (Douchinis et al., 2001; Smolak & Levine, 2001b)

Research on other ethnic group differences and how they might be related to the development of eating disorders is more limited. Gender and ethnicity should be thought of as summary terms that capture a variety of possible influences (Striegel-Moore & Smolak, 2001). Differences in gender roles, expression of emotion, sexual harassment and assault, the meaning of food and eating, emphasis on appearance, and health care access may all contribute to differences in rates of eating disorders. Perhaps even more important is the need for more attention to the potential role of discrimination and minority status in the development of eating problems (Piran, 2002; Smolak & Murnen, 2001; Smolak & Striegel-Moore, 2001). Factors such as acculturation have received some attention, although the data are confusing and conflicting because of inconsistent methodology and poorly delineated theories. For example, sometimes acculturation is defined as acceptance of the "majority" culture; in other studies, it is defined as ethnic identity. Theories relating acculturation to eating disorders have not carefully considered the meaning of acculturation in various ethnic groups. Some cultures share the White American investment in thinness; others do not. Adopting White American culture would have different meanings for girls raised in the former versus those raised in the latter. More research is also needed as to how discrimination in particular contexts might contribute to negative affect and a limited sense of control or effectiveness. These, in turn, might contribute to binge eating or other eating disorders.

There are, then, severe limitations in the research that might guide prevention efforts. Nonetheless, the extant data as well as conceptual advances in the field suggest several aspects of broad cultural factors that should be considered in prevention programs (Nichter, Vukovic, & Parker, 1999; Smolak, 1999). First, it is clear that not all topics are of equal interest to all ethnic groups. Black educators and parents, for example, may be much more concerned about obesity than about the internalization of the thin ideal. Thus, the points of intersection between obesity prevention and eating disorders prevention may be of particular interest to them (see chapter 3). Second, program organizers and facilitators need to be open to and prepared for discussions of cultural factors. People designing and implementing programs should make an effort to be familiar with their audience (see chapter 10). Third, program organizers and facilitators should be open to and prepared for discussions of racism. Feminist research has clearly demonstrated the importance of considering girls' experience with sexist and racist behavior in developing effective prevention (see chapter 8).

Developmental Reciprocity. In the developmental process, the child and the environment influence each other. Each is constantly changed by this interaction (transaction). This means that development is a truly dynamic process, one that is not adequately captured by static interaction processes. More specifically, it means that the risk of developing eating problems is not static. Under certain circumstances, a child who was relatively high risk may become lower risk or vice versa. For example, if the child changes schools, the expectations for thinness, including its importance, to which she is exposed, might change. This, in turn, may affect her body satisfaction. Research also shows that young women in certain contexts (e.g., sororities) are more likely to learn that binge eating and purging are acceptable behaviors and hence are more likely to engage in them (Crandall, 1988). Thus, changes in behavioral expectations are part of the reciprocal process.

For example, we generally consider a secure attachment of infant to mother to be a protective factor against the development of psychopathology, including eating disorders (Altman et al., 1997; Johnson & Connors, 1987). There is now evidence that attachment status has substantial continuity from infancy into adulthood (Hamilton, 2000; Waters, Merrick, Treboux, Crowell, & Albersheim, 2000). However, research also clearly indicates that, even in relatively low-risk samples, attachment status can change from secure to insecure in the face of a variety of familial stressors, including divorce (Hamilton, 2000; Lewis, Fiering, & Rosenthal, 2000). Under these circumstances, the risk of developing psychopathology may be raised. Less is known about the circumstances under which insecure attachments change to secure attachments, although a reduction in significant stressors is probably helpful. This gap in knowledge reflects the general tendency of psychologists to focus more on risk than on protective factors.

The reciprocal, dynamic nature of development presents many challenges to prevention researchers. Not only do we need to be sensitive to the developmental level of the audience (Smolak, 1999; see chapter 10), but we also need to consider the probability that the precise nature of children's risk changes over time. This has several implications for prevention programs. First, and in line with an ecological perspective, prevention programs need to aim to reduce the occurrence of factors that might increase the risk of a child developing eating disorders. Providing children with coping mechanisms that they can use in the face of stressors may be part of this. Several prevention programs that include life skills as an element have been successful in changing knowledge, attitudes, and behavior related to eating problems (see chapter 9). But this emphasis on the individual child is not enough. Prevention programs should try to actually reduce some of these risk factors, including sexual abuse, weight- and shape-related teasing, and presentation of thinness as a body ideal.

Second, programs need to be more than a one-time intervention. The nature of risk changes with development or because of nonnormative factors (such as a change in the most popular "look" for young girls). This means that a one-time program cannot address or even anticipate all possibilities. Furthermore, children's ability to understand and act on risk factors that might be discussed in a program changes. Thus, repeated discussions, across grades, about body image, negative affect, teasing, and other factors, coupled with the continuing presence of a resource person (see chapter 11) allow for the possibility that relevant changes will be noticed and addressed. Third, programs need to find ways to make parents, educators, and physicians more aware of factors that might increase or decrease a child's risk of developing an eating disorder. More research is needed before we can do this effectively, but there are models for this work in the field of preventing substance use and abuse (see chapter 10).

DEVELOPMENTAL TRAJECTORIES

There is no single pathway to healthy development, nor is there a single pathway to psychopathology. For example, probably at least half of all victims of child sexual abuse do not develop a major psychiatric disorder (Finkelhor & Browne, 1986). Among those who do, some will develop an anxiety disorder, some an affective disorder, some posttraumatic stress disorder (PTSD), and some eating disorders (Kendall-Tackett, Williams, & Finkelhor, 1993). Mediating factors such as familial support, nature of the sexual abuse, and personal beliefs about the abuse (e.g., regarding blame) may contribute to these differences (e.g., Smolak & Murnen, 2002; Wooley, 1994). Thus, even a negative experience as powerful as child sexual abuse does not guarantee a particular outcome.

The concept of developmental trajectories has been at least partially reflected in the multidimensional models of eating disorders, which acknowledge that a wide range of factors can contribute to the development of eating disorders (e.g., Garfinkel & Garner, 1982; Johnson & Connors, 1987; Striegel-Moore & Smolak, 2000). Furthermore, some authors have tried to stipulate different combinations of factors that might result in different outcomes (e.g., Smolak & Levine, 1996; see Table 4.1). On the other hand, some theorists, in accordance with the principle of equifinality, have shown how different pathways can lead to comparable outcomes. For example, Stice, Nemeroff, and Shaw (1996) demonstrated that binge eating can be rooted in either calorie-restrictive dieting or negative affect.

It might seem that theories emphasizing multidimensional approaches or different trajectories would confuse prevention efforts. These models should not be seen as validating a "throw everything

TABLE 4.1
Paths to Eating Problems During the Early Adolescent Transition

Predispositions	Precipitator or Triggers	Developmental Tasks	Mediators	Outcomes
Individual Personality Thinness schema Perfectionism Need for social approval Body dissatisfaction Dieting Self-esteem ↑ Interacts with ↓ *Systems* Family enmeshment Family hostility Peer pressure Teasing	*Individual* Awareness of ending childhood: puberty, school changes, parent relationship changes *Stressful or Unanticipated Life Events* Sexual abuse or harassment *Social Systems* ↑ Peer interaction ↓ Parental support and	Adjusting to adult physical (reproductive, body size, strength) features Begin heterosocial relations Begin realistic career exploration ("tracking" toward high school) Assess relationship with family vs. peers Gender role intensification	Simultaneity of task demands (particularly for least adaptive outcomes)	*Most Adaptive* In the absence of individual predispositions, tasks may be positively interpreted→body satisfaction, positive self-esteem, mature interpersonal relationships, achievements motive *Moderate* With presence of thinness schema and nonsimultaneous tasks, simple dieting, without notable pathology. With thinness schema, simultaneous events→disturbed eating with

		dieting and reduced self-esteem, due to body dissatisfaction
Family attitudes and behaviors concerning weight & shape	influence ↓ Teacher support ↑ Pressure from coaches, teachers ↑ Exposure to media messages	*Least adaptive* Presence of thinness schema and three simultaneous, especially early, tasks→subthreshold eating disorders Presence of several personality predispositions and three simultaneous task→eating disorders

Note. Adapted from "Adolescent Transitions and Eating Problems" (p. 214) by L. Smolak and M. P. Levine, in L. Smolak, M. P. Levine, & R. H. Striegel-Moore (Eds.), *The Developmental Psychopathology of Eating Disorders: Implications for Research, Prevention, and Treatment*, 1996. Copyright © 1996 by Lawrence Erlbaum Associates. Reprinted with permission.

against the wall and see what sticks" type of approach. Any prevention program needs a clearly stated underlying model and carefully defined goals (see chapter 1). Just as a multicontext approach is probably the most effective, prevention programs that cover several different risk and protective factors may have a positive effect on a wider range of girls and boys. Of course, time and financial resources also influence the scope of the prevention program. Program developers also need to consider the relative costs and benefits of emphasizing particular risk or protective factors (Kraemer et al., 1997). For example, might describing purging behaviors have an iatrogenic effect in some situations while serving as a deterrent in others (Mann et al., 1997)? Could emphasizing body acceptance contribute to obesity in some contexts (Heinberg et al., 2001)? Or could the institution of an action-oriented media literacy group for high school girls have limited benefits or even negative consequences when the costs of locating and training the right facilitator and of arranging for regular meetings in a private space are prohibitively high (see chapter 8)?

Some prevention programs try to select "at risk" participants for selective or targeted prevention (see chapter 14). Some programs also provide educators and parents with lists of characteristics (warning signs) to use to identify at-risk girls. These efforts have considerable empirical backing and validity because there are, of course, several risk factors for eating disorders that have received considerable empirical support (Stice, 2002; see chapter 5). Nevertheless, because there are a variety of pathways to eating disorders, it is probably impossible, in a short list, to cover all possible cases. It is, therefore, important to emphasize to the audience that, although the list includes "likely" risk factors, there are girls who do *not* fit the profile but who may develop eating problems. A common example is the statement that White girls are considerably more likely than Black girls to have poor body image, to engage in calorie-restrictive dieting, and to develop AN. However, Black girls can and do develop AN. It is possible that some eating problems among Black girls have been overlooked because of the failure to acknowledge multiple pathways and, instead, to focus on more common pathways.

In addition, parents and educators should be informed of factors that might shift a girl's risk status. Changing schools, moving up to the elite levels of a sport emphasizing appearance, or joining a new and more appearance-conscious peer group might make a girl more susceptible to social messages regarding thinness and hence to internalization of the thin ideal and to development of eating problems. Similarly, developing a peer group that is *less* invested in thinness, or a hobby that is unrelated to appearance, or a supportive relationship with an adult woman might lessen a girl's chances of developing eating problems.

MOLAR CHANGES IN DEVELOPMENT

Even elementary school girls show more weight and shape dissatisfaction than do boys. They are also more likely to report more concerns about being or becoming fat and to engage in weight loss attempts (see Smolak & Levine, 2001b; Smolak, Levine, & Schermer, 1998b, for reviews). Yet, it is exceedingly rare for prepubertal girls to develop AN or BN. Rates of both, and particularly AN, begin to increase in early adolescence but do not peak until late adolescence or early adulthood (ages 20–24). It is quite rare for either AN or BN to onset after early adulthood (Hoek & van Hoeken, 2003; Lucas, Crowson, O'Fallon, & Melton, 1999; Woodside & Garfinkel, 1992). These trends suggest that there are structural changes in biochemistry or personality or coping skills that facilitate the development of eating disorders at some points but not at others.

Structural changes and reorganizations may be precipitated by a traumatic experience. However, developmental psychopathology models tend to focus more on *normative* restructuring that occurs during the developmental transitions. Both early and late adolescence include transitions. Table 4.2 outlines the major components of a transition. By definition, transitions begin with a developmental precipitator such as puberty or moving away from home. This precipitator, or, more accurately, group of precipitators, renders existing coping mechanisms and supports less effective. Thus, for example, moving from elementary to middle school means a loss of familiar teachers and comfortable school routines and a change in peer group. This, in turn, means that these cannot easily serve to help the child adjust to new academic demands. The child must find another way of dealing with the new academic and social demands.

This search will involve the examination of existing coping mechanisms to discover which may be retained as a basis for new ways of adapting to developmental demands. Retention of such elements of previous coping styles accounts for the continuity that is evident across the early adolescent (and other) transitions (e.g., Caspi & Moffitt, 1991;

TABLE 4.2
The Components of Developmental Transitions

Predispositions	Precipitators	Deconstructing	Reconstructing	Outcomes
Individual Features • Cognitive • Personality • Coping Styles **Family** **Social Support Network** **Social Contexts** • Media • Violence • Harassment • Sexism • Racism NB: Many of these may continue after the transition is completed	**Normative changes** • Physical • Cognitive • Self-structure • Coping ability • Family relationships • Friendships • School or work changes • Social responsibility **Nonnormative change** (examples) • Parental death or divorce • Chronic or life threatening illness • Rape NB: If changes are cumulative (occur in a 1 year period), their effects may be greater	The appearance of the precipitators renders the existing cognitive, personality, social, and coping mechanisms inadequate. Hence, they are gradually examined and broken down. Changes that are normative may become nonnormative if they are unusually early or late developmentally. Under such circumstances or when the changes are cumulative, the deconstruction process may be rapid and overwhelming, leaving the person with few effective coping mechanisms.	With aid from others (peers, parents, other adults), new cognitive, self, and social structures emerge. Some of this process is also accomplished through introspection and through trial and error (the "moratorium" process of identity development). Cumulative, stressful change, too little support during the transition, or poor pre-existing structures (individual or contextual) may undermine the reconstruction process. NB: Several types of structures are being reconstructed	Development is a life-long process and there are several transitions. Success in one transition tends to predict success in another. However, each transition is unique, and it is possible that a particular one will be unusually challenging for an individual. The *context* of a particular transition is crucial to its outcome.

Hayward et al., 1997). In addition, new ways of coping will be investigated and tried. Some of these, such as alcohol, other drugs, and sex, may carry negative consequences. Other developments, such as learning more problem-oriented, instrumental approaches to challenges, may be protective. Thus, it is a combination of old and new elements that will result in the reorganized personality structure. This new structure will be more or less adequate to address developmental challenges. When it is no longer sufficient, a new transition will begin. Such developmental transitions will continue throughout adulthood (Levinson, 1986).

Within an ecological context, it is worth noting that these transitions do not occur in a vacuum and do not simply reflect the individual's developmental history. The early adolescence transition provides an interesting example of this. The meaning of differential pubertal timing for boys and girls appears to reflect cultural factors. In the United States, early maturation is associated with psychopathological outcomes for girls but not for boys (Graber, Peterson, & Brooks-Gunn, 1996). Indeed, early maturation is often found to be protective for boys. However, research in Norway suggests that this trend is not universal. In Norway, any off-time maturation is associated with pathology. Unlike American boys, early maturing Norwegian boys scored higher on measures of depression than did on-time maturers. These differences in findings may reflect societal differences in the nature and idealization of the masculine role and the tolerance for deviant development (Wichstrøm, 1999).

Change can occur in any number of developmental realms, including the physical, personality, or cognitive aspects. For example, physical shifts have been implicated in the relationship of early adolescence to eating disorders. Perhaps the hormonal shifts of puberty make girls more susceptible to negative affect or mood instability and hence to eating disorders. Some authors have proposed that pubertal hormones might account for the appearance of a gender difference in depression in middle adolescence. Depression and eating disorders are comorbid and might be linked by hormonal influences. Yet, there is no prospective evidence linking hormones to eating disorders, and the sparse evidence linking pubertal hormones to depression (e.g., Brooks-Gunn & Warren, 1989) suggests a small and possibly temporary effect. Thus, it does not appear to be primarily a hormonal reorganization that accounts for the adolescent period as a peak age of onset for AN and BN.

However, another aspect of pubertal development may be related to increased risk for eating disorders. This factor is the effect of secondary sex characteristics, and probably breast development in particular, on social and personal self-definition. Girls report that they are more likely to be teased about breast development than any other aspect of puberty (Brooks-Gunn, Newman, Holderness, & Warren, 1994). This teasing may be a form of sexual harassment. Inasmuch as sexual harassment is associated with the development of eating problems (e.g., Larkin, Rice, & Russell, 1999; Murnen & Smolak, 2000; see chapter 8), this social interpretation of and reaction to girls' pubertal development may precipitate eating problems.

Similarly, the addition of over 20 pounds of body fat during puberty (Graber, Brooks-Gunn, & Warren, 1999) may increase body dissatisfaction and lead to initiation or intensification of weight loss efforts. Indeed, it was the BMI increase that accounted for what appeared to be an early maturation effect in one longitudinal study (Graber et al., 1994). These effects are not due to BMI per se but rather to the societal vilification of fat, particularly on the female body, that is transmitted to girls via media, parental, and peer messages (Smolak & Levine, 2001b; see chapter 3).

Perhaps what is most crucial about the adolescent transitions, at least in relation to the development of eating problems, is the intensification of gender role demands. During childhood, a certain amount of gender role flexibility is tolerated, particularly for and among girls. Adolescents are actually less tolerant of cross-gender behavior than are children. This is probably particularly true within the heterosocial realm. Girls who want to get dates must look attractive; in many instances this means, among other things, being thin or at least not appearing to be fat. And, while physical attractiveness is increasing in importance, other opportunities for success are decreasing for girls (relative to boys). For example, despite large increases in the number of high school girls participating in high school sports, the numbers are still much smaller than for boys. And in the vast majority of careers, full-time adult women workers make substantially less money than full-time men workers (Smolak & Murnen, 2001). As adult gender roles become clearer and more mandatory, girls are pushed more to rely on attractiveness, and hence thinness, to succeed.

The focus on developmental transitions has at least two important implications for prevention efforts. First, it means that universal prevention might aim to prepare girls for the adolescent transitions. Preparation for the early adolescent transition, particularly in terms of coping with sexual harassment and gender role intensification, might reduce rates of not only eating problems but also depression (and social anxiety). Eating problems, body image disturbances, and depression are intimately linked during early and midadolescence (e.g., Stice & Bearman, 2001; Wichstrøm, 1999) and preventing one may impact all of them. If one can prevent or delay the onset of dieting, the risk for obesity might also be reduced (Stice et al., 1999). Thus, helping girls adjust to the transition may have multiple positive outcomes.

Second, delineation of the challenges facing girls helps attune us to what elements of the ecology of late childhood and adolescence might be ripe for intervention. Again, reducing sexual harassment and sexual objectification in general, or at least indifference to these practices, increasing opportunities for success, and deemphasizing appearance might all help reduce body dissatisfaction and eating problems among adolescent girls (see chapter 8).

METHODOLOGICAL IMPLICATIONS

The developmental psychopathology approach carries with it several methodological implications, not only in terms of risk and protective factor research, but also in prevention program design and evaluation (Smolak, 1996, 1999). We have already noted some of these, for example, the need to consider multiple rather than simply common pathways to eating disorders. There are three broad themes that bear reiteration here, however, with special regard for their methodological implications.

First, we need to consider new sources of risk and protection. Traditionally, prevention programs have reflected risk factor research and have thereby focused on the individual. It has been particularly common for the programs to focus on body dissatisfaction, weight loss techniques, and individual "resistance" to sociocultural messages glorifying them (see, e.g., Killen et al., 1993). There are exceptions to this, most notably in the work of Niva Piran (see chapter 8), which has emphasized the importance of contextual change. Both risk factor research and prevention work need to examine this contextual approach more thoroughly, particularly looking at the role of context-specific cultural values and expectations (see Levine & Piran, 2004). Such work will help clarify the meaning of some of the ethnic and gender differences so evident, yet so poorly understood, in the literature (Smolak & Murnen, 2001; Smolak & Striegel-Moore, 2001; Striegel-Moore & Smolak, 2002).

Second, eating disorders are developmental phenomena, that is, they change across time. Thus, one-time (cross-sectional) evaluations of risk–outcome relationships are not generally appropriate (Kraemer et al., 1997; Smolak, 1996; Stice, 2002). Similarly, interventions may well need to include multiple presentations with at least "booster" sessions after the initial exposure (see Botvin, 2000). Finally, in order to truly evaluate the *preventive* effects of a prevention program, evaluation must involve multiple assessments spread across the putative risk period for development of the problem (Smolak & Levine, 2001a; see also chapters 1 & 11).

Finally, part of what changes across time is the *meaning* of eating disorders symptomology as well as risk and protective factors (Smolak & Levine, 2001b). Therefore, measures must reflect not only the vocabulary of the targeted age group but also the molar structures. Research concerning the Dutch Eating Behaviors Questionnaire (DEBQ; Van Strien, Frijters, Bergers, & Defares, 1986) provides an interesting example. The DEBQ contains three subscales: restrained eating, emotional eating, and externally-induced eating. This instrument has been widely used in research with adult samples. Several researchers have modified the language of the scale and administered it to children under age 12 (see, e.g., Carper, Fisher, & Birch, 2000; Hill & Robinson, 1991). Such modifications appeared to be successful, at least in terms of the internal consistency of the scales. Yet, following interviews with six children, Braet and Van Strien (1997) reported so much concern with children's understanding of the concepts in the scale that they opted to devise and use a parental report version of the DEBQ. More research is needed to fully appreciate the meaning of constructs like "dietary restraint" or "emotional overeating" among young children. A developmental psychopathology model would predict important differences among adults, adolescents, and children.

SUMMARY AND CONCLUSIONS

The idea that eating problems and disorders *develop* is not new, but the implications of a developmental perspective have not always been fully articulated, particularly with regard to prevention. These implications are summarized in Table 4.3. A developmental psychopathology model helps move us away from a medical model of pathology that focuses exclusively on the risk factors that reside within the individual, be they genetic vulnerability or poor coping skills or negative temperament.

Developmental psychopathology, of course, recognizes the possible role of such individual characteristics. However, it also emphasizes the *contexts* of development. These contexts range from the immediate microsystem that subsumes influences that the child encounters daily (including parents, siblings, and day-care workers) to the macrosystem level that focuses on broad cultural values including sexism, weightism, and racism. These contextual levels are reciprocal and interactive. Indeed, within Bronfenbrenner's (1979) Ecological Model, there is a level, the mesosystem, that represents the interactions among influences.

All of these levels have some influence on the development of eating problems. This is the focus in chapter 5, which addresses the established risk factors that may serve as guides for the content of prevention

TABLE 4.3
Implications of a Developmental Psychopathology Model
for Primary Prevention of Eating Disorders

- There are multiple, interlocking, reciprocal contexts of development. These contexts range from the immediate familial environment to broad cultural influences.
- All of these contexts need to be considered in designing primary prevention programs. Programs that address multiple contexts will be more successful. This includes attention to the broad cultural influences that are summarized as "gender" and "ethnicity."
- Inasmuch as developmental contexts are constantly changing, programs that acknowledge changes by having "booster" sessions or follow-up programs are likely to be more successful.
- There are multiple pathways to a single outcome. A pathway is never fixed and an outcome is never inevitable. This is one reason prevention is possible.
- Prevention programs that try to intervene along several different trajectories are likely to reach a wider range of children.
- Because we are intervening along a trajectory, program evaluation needs to assess immediate changes in risk and protective factors as well as long-term rates of eating problems and disorders.
- Developmental changes occur at both molecular and molar levels. The molar level means that there are likely to be developmental changes in the ways children, adolescents, and adults understand eating-related constructs (e.g., binge eating, healthy exercise, moderation in eating). This, again, means that program constructs will need to be repeated at different phases of development.
- Molar changes also imply that developmental transitions (i.e., the periods during which old structures are disassembled and new ones constructed) are times of special risk and vulnerability.

programs. The most successful prevention programs are likely to be those that address several different levels that are specific to the target audience (Piran, 1998; Smolak, 1999). Furthermore, programs that focus only on the individual are likely to leave toxic environments relatively untouched and thereby to limit their own long-term success (see chapters 9 & 10).

Developmental psychopathology also points to the multiple developmental trajectories that might lead to eating problems and disorders. There is not just one way to develop an eating disorder. Therefore, prevention programs need to try to address multiple pathways. Furthermore, as pathways are changeable and, in fact, always changing, one-time interventions, even if several months in duration, are not likely to have permanent effects. Instead, program messages will need to be reiterated at later times.

Changes in the comprehension of key eating-related constructs also necessitate multiple exposures to program messages. Young children's understanding of binge eating or of "eating in moderation" is going to differ from that of adults in important ways. This means that a message delivered by educators or parents to children at age 6 cannot have the same complexity or even the same meaning as one "received" at 12, which, in turn, is likely to be heard differently at ages 16 or 20.

Developmental psychopathology models, then, require that prevention programs consider the ecology of development, the nature of developmental change, and the possibility of multiple trajectories. Although this approach may increase the complexity of the prevention task, it also points the way toward increasing the long-term effectiveness of prevention efforts.

5

Risk Factors as Guides to Prevention Program Design

If you were going to design a program to prevent the development of eating disorders, where would you start? Let us assume that, like many experts (see chapter 9), you have already decided that you want to develop a classroom-based curriculum. How would you determine the focus of the lessons? Or, if you decided on a media literacy program (see chapter 13), what is the basis for that decision? Why media literacy rather than, say, self-esteem enhancement or academic support or employment opportunities, as have been the focus of programs aimed at preventing other adolescent problems (e.g., Allen, Philliber, Herrling, & Kuperminc, 1997)?

The most common answer to these and related questions is "risk factor research" (see, e.g., Killen, 1996; Stewart, 1998). Perhaps because most program designers work from a scientist-practitioner model, we expect to begin the process of prevention by using scientific methods to identify potential causes of eating disorders. A prevention program would then seek to reduce or eliminate those "causes" so as to reduce the incidence of the disorder (Mrazek & Haggerty, 1994).

Those "potential causes" constitute risk factors, although not all risk factors are causes, at least in the "necessary" and "sufficient" sense of the word. A *risk factor* is any variable whose presence increases the likelihood that the disorder in question will develop (Kraemer et al., 1997). Some risk factors are fixed, that is, they cannot be modified. Gender is an example of this. Others are modifiable, as gender role might be. In all cases, the risk factor predates the onset of the disorder, that is, the risk factor is "preeminent."

This chapter considers those risk factors that are most promising in terms of empirical support and of modifiability. Because this is such an important matter for prevention and for the field of eating disorders in general, we first analyze a number of important issues in deciding what is and what is not a viable risk factor on which to focus prevention efforts. In addition, this chapter discusses the implications for prevention of research on protective factors or sources of resilience.

PROBLEMS WITH EXPERIMENTAL AND PROSPECTIVE DATA

The criteria of modifiability and preeminence imply that one of two types of data is required to establish a variable as a risk factor (for a rich discussion of this complex matter, see Jacobi, Hayward, de Zwaan, Kraemer, & Agras, 2004). One must present either prospective, longitudinal data, establishing that the putative risk factor predates and predicts the disorder, or experimental data indicating that manipulation of the potential risk factor affects the likelihood of developing the disorder. Both of these approaches can be difficult to use in the study of psychopathology in general and eating disorders in particular.

There is no doubt that experimental data are the "gold standard" of the scientific method. Experimental approaches are as close as we can come to guaranteeing internal validity, that is, establishing a causal relationship between the independent and dependent variables. On the other hand, ecological validity can be an issue. Furthermore, ethical considerations preclude the manipulation of some variables. Similarly, prospective, longitudinal data are the "gold standard" of developmental research. From a scientific perspective, however, longitudinal data are typically correlational in nature, making it difficult to isolate a particular cause–effect relationship. In addition, longitudinal data may reflect the development of one particular cohort, a special problem when sociohistorical factors may be playing a role in development. Finally, ethical issues are also a problem here. At what point in the natural history of a disorder is the researcher ethically obligated to intervene?

These tend to be general issues in the use of experimental and longitudinal designs. In the case of eating disorders research, we face four additional challenges: (a) the clinically significant outcome variables have a low prevalence; (b) the relationships among individual symptoms, subclinical syndromes, and eating disorders are unclear; (c) sexual abuse and sexual harassment may be important contributors; and (d) sociocultural influences probably vary from setting to setting.

Prevalence of Eating Disorders

As shown in chapter 2, AN, BN, and BED are rare disorders. Furthermore, although some women suffer from AN with bulimic features, and some women develop BN after suffering from AN, and some women develop either BN or AN after a period of having EDNOS, we cannot assume that the individual eating disorders are the *same* disorder in any meaningful way; that is, we cannot reasonably assume that they have identical risk factors or causes. Ideally, then, we would design research projects so that we could identify, or at least have the opportunity to identify, the risk factors for AN versus those for BN versus those for BED or other types of EDNOS.

Assume, then, that you are interested in designing a longitudinal study examining the risk factors for BN, which you assume occurs at a rate of 3% (a fairly high estimate; see Hoek & van Hoeken, 2003) among White and Hispanic girls. The evidence indicates that the full syndrome of BN usually begins in late adolescence or early adulthood, between, say, 18 and 24. In studies as short as 3 years in duration, attrition rates sometimes exceed 30% (Smolak, 1996). Furthermore, attrition is typically not random; rather, girls with more psychological, familial, and behavioral problems are more likely to drop out of studies. Thus, to end up with 30 cases of BN, a number likely to ensure respectable power for most statistical analyses, one needs to have 1,000 participants at the end of the study. Although this number may be somewhat reduced by particular analytic techniques, such as random regression, it may also be increased by unknown features of the sample. If the aim is to finish the study with 1,000 girls, then an expected attrition rate of 30% mandates an initial sample of 1,429 participants. This is, of course, often not feasible in terms of money or staff.

Continuum of Eating Disorders

Given the relatively low prevalence of eating disorders, researchers have two options. One is to select high-risk samples. This may preclude the detection of some of the earliest risk factors for eating disorders.

The second is to use possible symptoms or precursors of eating disorders as the outcome or criterion variables. Weight concerns, body dissatisfaction, internalization of the thin ideal, and sociocultural pressures to be thin are examples of established risk factors for eating disorders (see Stice, 2002, and Jacobi et al., 2004, for reviews). Many longitudinal studies have used variables such as these as criterion variables (e.g., Cattarin & Thompson, 1994; Davison, Markey, & Birch, 2003; Smolak, Levine, & Gralen, 1993). Researchers have also used scores on measures, such as the EAT or EDI, that are capable of discriminating eating disorders clients from other groups (e.g., Attie & Brooks-Gunn, 1989). Still others have used symptoms, such as purging or binge eating, as outcome variables in longitudinal research (e.g., Stice & Agras, 1998).

Although body dissatisfaction, dieting, purging, and binge eating are clearly related to eating disorders, they are just as clearly not synonymous. As discussed in chapter 2, some elements of eating disorders may occur on a continuum, but there are also important differences between body-dissatisfied or dieting women who develop eating disorders and those who do not. Thus, understanding risk factors for body dissatisfaction, dieting, or even binge eating does not ensure that we have identified those for eating disorders. On the other hand, it is worth emphasizing that dieting, binge eating, and purging are dangerous behaviors in and of themselves. Even when they do not culminate in eating disorders, they may create serious health problems, especially in developing children. They may, therefore, be worth targeting in prevention programs because of their inherent risks and only secondarily as a possible way of preventing eating disorders.

Sexual Abuse and Sexual Harassment

Researchers and theorists have long proposed that sexual abuse is related to eating problems and disorders. Indeed, empirical data indicate that there is some relationship, although the specifics of the relationship remain elusive (Connors, 2001; Smolak & Murnen, 2002). Establishing whether or not sexual abuse is a true risk factor for eating disorders or problems presents some special difficulties.

First, there is the question of accessibility of memories of abuse to the victim. There is a long and ongoing debate concerning "repressed" memories (Brown & Burman, 1997; Loftus, 1997). The issue here is whether it is possible for memories of child sexual abuse to be so suppressed that the victim is unable to recall the events, although the events may still influence her behavior. Furthermore, there are questions about whether such repressed memories can eventually be recalled, how such recovery of memories might occur, and how the memories might be verified.

In line with the question of recovery of memories of abuse, it is not clear with whom victims might share their memories. Wooley (1994) noted that women therapists are more likely to report that clients have raised the issue of child sexual abuse. It is possible that victims are often unwilling to discuss their experiences with men, an effect that might be exacerbated in a scientific versus a clinical setting.

Research concerning child sexual abuse has been hampered by inconsistent definitions and inadequate measures (Smolak & Murnen, 2002). Measures that ask whether someone has been abused assume that the respondent identifies the incident as abusive. This is typically problematic, especially in cases of abuse that do not involve penetration. On the other hand, listing all possible types of sexual abuse runs the risk of leaving out something or leading the respondent to interpret the events in new, and unexamined, ways.

Finally, it is probably impossible to do prospective research involving child sexual abuse and perhaps sexual abuse more generally. Parents who know (or suspect) their child is being abused are unlikely to consent to the child's participation, and children who are being abused and have been threatened with punishment for telling are unlikely to report the abuse. Should a young child report ongoing abuse, the researcher is morally (though perhaps not legally) obligated to intervene, hence influencing the "natural" relationship between abuse and the development of eating disorders.

Similarly, children are unlikely to conceptualize sexual harassment as harassment. Indeed, young girls are socialized to accept the harassment as teasing and to ignore the perpetrator (Brumberg, 1997; Stein, 1999). Measures of sexual harassment developed with adults are probably not particularly useful with children (Murnen & Smolak, 2000). Thus, it will be difficult to prospectively investigate the relationship between sexual harassment and eating problems, although correlational research suggests a concurrent relationship (e.g., Harned, 2000).

Site Influences

Research consistently links sociocultural factors, including media, peer teasing, and peer or parent modeling, to the development of body dissatisfaction and eating problems (Thompson et al., 1999). It is fairly common to find that levels of these factors vary from one research site to another. Indeed, this is part of the basis of cross-cultural, ethnic group, or gender differences. It is also likely that the meaning of these variables differs from one group to another or one setting to another (Piran, 2001). So, for example, peer comments about weight and shape may hold a different meaning in a setting where such teasing is common than in a setting where such teasing is quite rare. Or peer comments may have a different effect if they occur in relative isolation compared to occurring along with messages about fat and thin from peer modeling, parental comments and modeling, sibling teasing, and mass media.

In a recent prospective study involving two data collection sites, one in Arizona and one in California, a significant site by ethnicity effect emerged (The McKnight Investigators, 2003). At the Arizona, but not the California, site Hispanic girls were at greater risk of developing eating disorders than girls from other ethnic groups. One could consider such an effect to be noise or even error in the data. However, one might also argue that the meaning of being Hispanic varied between California and Arizona. For example, both country of origin and immigration status differed for the two sites. When arguing a sociocultural perspective, then, we must at least investigate the various levels (macrosystem, exosystem, mesosystem) of social influence and their specific meanings in individual contexts, rather than assuming that an important variable based on theory and previous research is unaffected by the context in which it occurs (Piran, 2001; see chapters 4 and 8).

RISK FACTORS FOR THE DEVELOPMENT OF EATING PROBLEMS

Despite these and other difficulties in conducting risk-factor research, several risk factors have been identified. The risk factors for females are shown in Table 5.1. As might be expected, there is more consensus about some risk factors than others. Furthermore, the nature of the data supporting the different factors varies; we have tried to capture this variation in Table 5.1 also. The table reflects data from four types of studies.

TABLE 5.1
Risk Factors for the Development of Body Dissatisfaction, Eating Problems, and Eating Disorders

Variable	Experimental Support	Prospective Support	Correlational Support	Clinical Report
Body dissatisfaction	XX	XX	XX	XX
Weight concerns	XX	XX	XX	XX
Internalization of thin ideal	XX	XX	XX	XX
Dieting		XX	XX	XX
Media influences	XX	XX	XX	XX
Peer teasing		XX	XX	XX
Peer modeling			XX	
Paternal comments			XX	
Maternal comments			XX	
Paternal modeling			XX	
Maternal modeling			XX	
Child sexual abuse			XX	XX
Sexual harassment			XX	XX
Serotonin, dopamine, norepinephrine levels			XX	
Negative affectivity	XX	XX	XX	XX

The first are classical experimental designs in which the researcher actively controlled and manipulated levels of the independent variable, including a control group (e.g., Irving, 1990). Experimental research does include some prevention/intervention work in which, for example, attempts were made to reduce internalization of the thin ideal and hence reduce bulimic symptoms (e.g., Stice, Chase, Stormer, & Appel, 2001). The second type is prospective designs in which one variable or set of variables "predicts" levels of another variable measured at a later time (e.g., The McKnight Investigators, 2003). The third category consists of cross-sectional, correlational studies, which include a variety of types of data, some qualitative and some quantitative. The common thread is that the data in these studies were collected concurrently and without any of the variables (except, in some instances, psychiatric status) being controlled by the researcher. Finally, the clinical reports are commonly case studies or small group studies that reflect impressions and experiences of participants and clinicians, rather than, for example, standardized measures. It is worth noting that, although clinical reports are often disparaged for "lack" of methodological rigor, these are the studies most likely to involve true cases of eating disorders. When extant data are exclusively concurrent correlations and clinical reports, only factors that have been identified in several studies are included. Note that if a variable has been identified as a potential risk factor in correlational or clinical reports but has consistently failed to emerge as a significant variable in prospective or experimental research, it is not included here (see Stice, 2001b, 2002). Self-esteem, perfectionism, and early menarche are examples of such variables. Interestingly, BMI is also such a factor. It is frequently assumed that higher BMI is associated with the development of eating disorders, but several longitudinal studies have not found this link (see Stice, 2001b, 2002, for reviews).

Table 5.1 does not, however, clearly delineate what the dependent variable is in each case. As noted earlier, it is rarely the case that clinically diagnosed eating disorders are the outcome variable in experimental or prospective research. More details concerning supporting studies can be found in Connors (2001), Groesz et al. (2002), Jacobi et al. (2004), Shisslak and Crago (2001), Smolak and Levine (2001b), Smolak et al. (2000), Smolak and Murnen (2001, 2002), Stice (2001b, 2002), Thompson and Stice (2001), and Thompson et al. (1999).

Finally, it is important to reiterate that the vast majority of eating disorders risk-factor research involves samples that are female and White. Whether these or different risk factors will emerge for boys and for members of ethnic minority groups is very much an open question (e.g., Smolak, Levine, & Thompson, 2001; Smolak & Striegel-Moore, 2001; see also Ricciardelli & McCabe, 2004, p. 182). Table 5.1 reflects these biases in the data.

Many of these risk factors are interrelated and some are most certainly proxies for others (Jacobi et al., 2004; Kraemer et al., 1997). Furthermore, it is possible that some, such as engagement with mass media, only have an effect in the presence of others, such as weight concerns. Finally, despite the existence of many multidimensional models of eating disorders, the sequence or chain of effects—for example, what leads to body dissatisfaction and then to dieting and then to symptoms such as purging and then to clinical eating disorders (if this is indeed a viable sequence)—remains poorly defined.

Weight Concerns and Body Dissatisfaction

Of all of the variables used in prospective studies, variables that tap into body dissatisfaction and concerns about being or becoming too fat are probably the most consistent predictors of eating disorders and their components (e.g., Killen et al., 1994, 1996; Leon et al., 1995; The McKnight Investigators, 2003). This relationship has been uncovered repeatedly when participants are at least middle school age (approximately 11 or older) at the time of the initiation of the study.

These variables also, however, may reflect components of eating disorders themselves. Body dissatisfaction and weight concerns are too widespread to argue that they are simply proxies for eating disorders, but it is possible that some of the girls are in the early phases of an eating disorder (see chapter 2). If so, the variable has a different meaning than if the body dissatisfaction occurs substantially before any symptoms appear. In the future, researchers need to carefully control for this possibility. It is also the case that body dissatisfaction and weight concerns are clearly in place by the beginning of middle school. Thus, much more research is needed to address the causes of body dissatisfaction. This will be crucial in developing universal elementary school programs (Smolak, 1999; Smolak & Levine, 2001b).

Sociocultural Factors

Both peer teasing and media influences are related to body dissatisfaction and eating problems. These are factors that are amenable to change in terms of either levels of their occurrence or girls' ability to cope with their influences. This is also true of sexual harassment. The empirical support for these and other sociocultural factors strongly points to the likelihood that prevention can and will work in the area of eating disorders (see chapter 1).

Biological Influences

In chapter 3 we considered the challenges of understanding biological factors involved in the development of eating problems and disorders. There are currently no prospective data linking hormonal or neurotransmitter levels to the onset of eating disorders, nor are there any longitudinal outcome studies of girls who are presumably at high risk because they have a mother or sister with an eating disorder.

One could potentially consider studies of therapeutic drugs to be experimental studies of biological factors. If one could say definitely how a particular drug works (i.e., if one could identify the precise site of the drug's action) and if we knew the precise neurological or neurochemical underpinnings of a behavior or behavioral syndrome, we could link the two. But, although researchers have marshaled considerable evidence for the "role of serotonin" in disordered eating, the knowledge necessary to link drugs, mechanisms of action, and eating disorders is not currently available (see chapter 3). Furthermore, the data concerning the general effectiveness and specific actions of therapeutic drugs are very mixed (see Mitchell, 2001, for a review). Indeed, drugs do not appear to be particularly effective in the treatment of AN, although relapse rates may be reduced. Similarly, although the selective serotonin reuptake inhibitors (SSRIs, such as fluoxetine) help decrease binge eating and vomiting in BN clients, they do not typically result in the disappearance of these symptoms (Mitchell, 2001).

Another general category of biological influence, genetic influences, is equally confusing. As discussed in chapter 3, the data are too mixed to permit a conclusion (see, e.g., Fairburn et al., 1999). Moreover, even if one takes a less skeptical position, the behavior genetic work seems to offer a clearer statement about the role of the environmental factors in the cause of both full-blown eating disorders and components such as the drive for thinness (Bulik, 2001, 2004) than it does about what exactly might be inherited to create an increased risk for eating disorders.

PROTECTIVE FACTORS IN THE DEVELOPMENT OF EATING DISORDERS

It is possible that some factors actually *reduce* the likelihood of developing eating disorders, even in the face of substantial risk factors. This issue of what makes children resilient has long been of great interest to researchers in developmental psychopathology (Garmezy, 1983). If such protective factors were identified, prevention programs might aim to introduce or strengthen them.

In general, it appears that girls are better able to negotiate the stresses and demands of adolescence if they have high self-esteem, multiple sources of achievement, a mentor, and an opportunity to express their voices (e.g., Brown & Gilligan, 1992). Volunteer work and other activities that foster positive bonds between youth, adults, and their communities have also been useful in promoting adolescent mental and behavioral health (see, e.g., Catalano, Berglund, Ryan, Lonczak, & Hawkins, 2002). The common thread here is the girls are equipped or supported in ways that allow them to focus on something other than thin bodies as a means to social and even career success. As part of these efforts, girls are also encouraged to critique and influence the sources of the messages that lead to thin ideal internalization (see chapters 8 and 13).

Although some authors have tried to link these messages of social support, empowerment, and multiple opportunities for success to the prevention of eating disorders (e.g., Crago, Shisslak, & Ruble, 2001), there is actually little evidence for their effectiveness or centrality in prevention efforts. Indeed, the data from a number of studies are mixed as to whether low self-esteem or negative self-concept is a risk factor for eating disorders (compare Stice, 2001b, 2002, to Jacobi et al., 2004). On the other hand, Piran's successful intervention program did involve providing girls with a forum to express their voices and with empowering experiences in changing their own subculture (Piran, 1999a, 2001; also see chapter 8).

One factor that has received some support as protecting against development of eating problems is athletic participation (Geller, Zaitsoff, & Srikameswaran, 2002; Smolak et al., 2000). In particular, participation in non-elite high school sports may have a protective influence. This is consistent with the argument that providing alternative success experiences, particularly involving one's body, may help to prevent eating problems (Geller et al., 2002). On the other hand, studies of athletic participation underscore the complexity of risk-factor research. Meta-analytic research also shows that some sports that emphasize a thin ideal create greater risk for the development of eating disorders (Smolak et al., 2000). Thus, some forms of athletic participation may constitute risk factors, whereas others are protective factors in the etiology of eating disorders.

Murnen, Smolak, Mills, and Good (2003) found that elementary school girls' active rejection of the media image of thin, sexualized women is associated with a more positive body image. Interestingly, it was the group of girls who were unsure whether they liked or disliked the image who had the poorest body image. The girls who actively endorsed the image fell in between these two groups in terms of body image. This relationship, as well as the causes of active rejection of the media image, deserves further scrutiny.

Feminist theory also suggests that empowering girls to express their opinions and feelings, that is, to have "voice," may protect against the development of eating disorders (see chapter 8). Research on this issue is very limited, so we have not included it in Table 5.1. Nonetheless, the limited work available (e.g., Piran, 1999a, 2001; Smolak & Munsterteiger, 2002; Steiner-Adair, 1986) indicates that this is a potential protective factor worthy of more research (see chapters 8, 9, and 13).

CONCLUSIONS AND FUTURE DIRECTIONS

We want first to reiterate the position outlined in chapter 1: It does not seem to us that prevention efforts need to wait for complete identification of the sequence, interactions, and relative contributions of all major risk factors in the development of eating disorders. Prevention efforts in other fields, such as breast cancer and heart disease, certainly are not guided by empirically confirmed etiological models that explain anywhere close to 100% of the variation in the health outcomes. Eating disorders prevention should not be constrained by such an unrealistic demand either (see chapter 7).

Having said this, it is reasonable to look to the empirical literature for clues as to what factors might be emphasized in a prevention program (see Jacobi et al., 2004; Stice, 2002). Certainly the research concerning risk and protective factors provides designers of prevention programs with possible candidates for prevention and intervention. Furthermore, prevention or reduction of some of the potential risk factors, including body dissatisfaction and weight concerns (including dieting), are worthwhile in and of themselves as they are associated with a variety of problems, most notably depression (Stice & Bearman, 2001; Stice, Hayward, Cameron, Killen, & Taylor, 2000; Wichstrøm, 1999).

Three directions in risk and protective factor research seem particularly important to prevention efforts. First, there needs to be more attention to protective factors that are amenable to change within a prevention program. This may allow many prevention programs to adopt a more positive tone, avoiding the public relations pitfalls of seeming to "blame" boys, parents, schools, and so on. Second, risk and protective factor research should focus on younger children, in order to better understand the roots of the body dissatisfaction and weight concerns that, by middle school, are powerful predictors of eating disorders and their components. Finally, more research is needed to examine ethnic group differences as well as gender differences in the etiology of eating problems and disorders. Researchers particularly should attend to the role of ethnic discrimination in such research (Smolak & Striegel-Moore, 2001).

In thinking about etiological and prevention research, it is very important to remember that these are complementary, not adversarial. Prevention research can make critically important contributions to the risk and protective factor literature. Well-designed prevention work can, as discussed in chapter 11, serve as an experimental evaluation of the causal role of particular factors (Jacobi et al., 2004; Kraemer et al., 1997; Stice, 2001b, 2002).

The relationship between risk/protective factor research and the design of actual prevention programs is a complicated one because the programs are guided by particular paradigms that accord more or less attention to certain types of factors. Two interrelated paradigms have the clearest, most direct relationship to the factors listed in Table 5.1: the Cognitive Social Learning (or Social Cognitive Theory) paradigm and the Cognitive-Behavioral paradigm. These are the focus of chapter 6.

6

Social Cognitive Approaches

There is overwhelming evidence that sociocultural factors create and maintain the beliefs, emotions, and behaviors that make up the continuum of eating problems and eating disorders (see chapter 5). In other words, risk factors such as the female gender role, negative body image, the idealization of slenderness, unwarranted and uncontrollable fear of fat, and rigid dieting are learned to a significant degree. As discussed in chapter 4, what an individual learns is affected by a variety of ecological influences that operate at different levels of organization (e.g., family, neighborhood, school, culture). The processes by which people learn involve direct rewards and punishments, observation of what actual people do and feel, and interpretation of information gleaned from what other people say, as well as from mass media, books, and so forth. Therefore, some researchers in the field of eating problems have drawn on either cognitive social learning theory (now called *social cognitive theory* or SCT; Bandura, 1986) or cognitive-behavioral theory (CBT) to develop prevention programs for children and adolescents. In fact, most of the research on universal, selective, and targeted prevention of eating problems and eating disorders have been guided by one or both of these models (Levine & Piran, 2001, 2004; Piran, 1995). There is a long tradition of research in which SCT has been applied with moderate success to prevention of cardiovascular disease, substance abuse, and teenage pregnancy (Baranowski, Perry, & Parcel, 2002; Botvin, 2000). The substance abuse research is considered in detail in chapter 10. Use of CBT methods for prevention is a logical outgrowth of the effectiveness of cognitive-behavioral therapy in the treatment of depression and various psychological problems, including negative body image and disordered eating (Cash, 1996; Fairburn, 1997; Wilson, Fairburn, & Agras, 1997). This chapter introduces the essential components of the SCT and CBT models for prevention.

SOCIAL COGNITIVE THEORY

Basic Concepts

SCT sees normal (adaptive, healthy) and abnormal (maladaptive, unhealthy) "behavior" in terms of reciprocal transactions between three types of factors: (a) cognitive and emotional processes within the person; (b) behavioral patterns and potential competencies; and (c) the environment or context (Bandura, 1986, 1997; Baranowski et al., 2002). A wide variety of important processes take place within the person. These range from physiological tendencies (e.g., stress reactivity), to styles for interpreting personal successes and failures, to the capacity for self-reflection on the way one thinks about the environment. Environment encompasses factors outside the person that affect the person's behavior. Behaviors refer to competencies and skills, including those involved in learning new things and learning to improve.

Each set of factors encompasses content and processes. For example, with respect to the phenomenon of dieting, personal variables include the content of specific beliefs a person has about "dieting," as well as the psychological processes that this person employs in constructing and testing those beliefs. From the perspective of the person, learning is an active process of constructing organized sets of beliefs, expectations, feelings, and behaviors. There are genetic predispositions and other biological constraints on learning, but SCT focuses on the ways in which the personal construction of knowledge, expectations, emotions, and behaviors are shaped and modulated by the physical, social, and cultural environment. But the influences connecting the person and environment (and behavior) are reciprocal, because personal knowledge, styles of information processing, expectations, and imagination all operate to select certain aspects of the environment as being relevant. Moreover, the person's habitual activation of or selection of specific behaviors eventually creates changes in the physical and social environment. The concept of reciprocal determinism is consistent with developmental psychopathology's emphasis on integrated transactions between the person and the environment, and especially the environments created by other people (Smolak & Levine, 1994a; see chapter 4).

We illustrate some key features of SCT by applying it to the development and maintenance of calorie-restrictive dieting. In combination with weight concerns, calorie-restrictive dieting is a risk factor for disordered eating (Jacobi et al., 2004) and an important health concern in its own right (Neumark-Sztainer, 1995). According to SCT, the behaviors involved in calorie-restrictive dieting to lose weight are guided by various forms of knowledge, some of which contribute to learned values and expectations (Bandura, 1986; Killen, 1996). Consider, for the purposes of illustration, a fictitious White, middle-class adolescent named Jennifer. She is 13 years old. Based on what she has been told, on what she has observed, and on what she has inferred, Jennifer is convinced of the following: (She "just *knows*" that) "Dieting plus exercising is the best way to lose weight"; "Girls who want to diet successfully can do it if they really bear down and work hard at it"; and "Milk is fattening so you should drink diet soda instead whenever possible." With respect to *values*, Jennifer holds that: "Being thin means you are in control, and control is important to me"; "Fat is ugly—like older, flabby women are ugly—so I'd rather smoke cigarettes and not live as long than get fat"; and "Approval from my mother and from boys for being thin really matter a lot to me."

SCT proposes that experience and knowledge result in three important types of *learned expectations* (Bandura, 1986). *Stimulus–stimulus* expectations correspond to the well-known concept of classical conditioning. The inherently neutral "fat" has taken on enormous emotional significance for Jennifer and her friends because their culture cultivates a contingent association between this word and the experience or threat of unattractiveness, rejection, failure, and inferiority (Rothblum, 1994). *Behavior–outcome* expectations refer to beliefs about the consequences of behavior in specific environments. Jennifer has learned to expect that dieting behavior will result immediately in social approval for "self-control" and later in weight loss that in turn evokes more social approval. Finally, *person–behavior* expectations, also known as *efficacy* expectations, reflect the expressly cognitive nature of SCT. Jennifer values social approval, she knows that her brother and certain boys at school will unmercifully tease any girl who appears to have gained weight, and she expects that dieting behavior will produce social approval from a variety of people who matter to her. However, according to SCT, Jennifer will not begin dieting in any serious way unless she believes herself to be capable of the component behaviors, including the ability to deal with obstacles, ambiguities, and frustrations that arise in the process of dieting (Bandura, 1997).

In summary, if Jennifer values social approval and expects that the social context will punish weight gain and reward weight loss, and if Jennifer believes herself to be capable of effective dieting, then the probability of dieting is high (Killen, 1996). In thinking about the impact of the social environment on knowledge and expectations, SCT focuses on three types of learning that are relevant to prevention.

THREE TYPES OF SOCIAL LEARNING

Direct Experience

SCT is, in part, a behavioral approach, so it acknowledges the importance of learning through direct experience, with reinforcements and punishments emanating from the environment (Bandura, 1986). For example, outcome expectations and efficacy expectations are established or reinforced when Jennifer's diet and subsequent weight loss do indeed result in compliments from parents and friends. Jennifer may also learn that her own thoughts and verbal statements, such as "I feel so fat today," are reinforced because they help forge closer connections with peers who are also seeking to make sense of pubertal weight gains in a culture that worships slenderness (Nichter, 2000).

Observational Learning

Human beings have perceptual and other cognitive mechanisms that enable them to learn a tremendous amount through observation. Values, motives, specific standards for behavior, the three types of expectations, and components of behavior can all be acquired through observation of real people in their immediate environment, and through exposure to symbolic others in movies, magazines, and books (Bandura, 1986). From observing her peers, parents, and mass media, Jennifer easily extracts a wide variety of cultural messages that serve as the basis for values, incentives, expectations, and subsequent information processing (Gordon, 2000; Levine & Smolak, 1996, 1998). For example:

- If you are female, what you look like is more important than your personality, your skills, and your passions.
- Women are naturally self-conscious and anxious about many different parts of their bodies, and especially their weight.
- A slender appearance is a crucial part of being sexy, physically fit, successful, and good.
- Any woman can be slender and successfully manage her weight and shape if she just works hard at it and purchases the right products.
- Fat is a sign of failure, loss of control, and an unhealthy lifestyle.

Symbolic Communications

Learning involves not only changes in behavior and skills, but also the development of knowledge that guides expectations, values, choices, and the intentional application of behaviors for changing the environment and the self (Bandura, 1986). The ability to construct symbols and then to use them in producing and receiving communications is a very important aspect of our cognitive capacities. Thus, SCT incorporates the fact that people learn a lot from information imparted through language. The informative, persuasive, and guiding elements of language are key features of the social processes called parenting, teaching, coaching, and mentoring (Bandura, 1986). Some linguistic communications are indirect or less direct, almost constituting a form of symbolic modeling with abstract models (e.g., "other people"). For example, Jennifer easily makes abstract but emotionally potent inferences about "fear of fat" from a lecture in her middle school health class about obesity as a "potentially fatal disease."

Other linguistic communications are direct attempts by people to educate and socialize the person. In these instances, ideas and judgments are voiced directly to the person in hopes of persuading them to think and behave in certain ways. Several forms of this type of persuasive communication are relevant to body image and disordered eating. Some statements function as punishments and reinforcements for certain behaviors. One Sunday morning, before church, Jennifer's mother said to her, "Oh, sweetie, take that dress off—it makes you look heavy. Try the one I bought you last month. It is so much more flattering to you." But more often the communication is a direct attempt to offer information, to give advice, and to persuade. The wrestling coach told Jennifer's friend, "Chuck, you're at 143 pounds now. You've got a real shot at the conference championship if you wrestle at 135 instead of 150. Here's a few ways you can lose those pounds by the day after tomorrow. Listen up, you want to be a 'winner' and I know you can do this . . ."

At age 13 Jennifer herself has heard, for example, all of the following:

- (From mother, in response to Jennifer's concerns): "I know you're worried about how your body is changing, honey. Every girl gains weight during puberty, but you're like me, so you'll just need to stop eating dessert for a while and start exercising a lot more. Otherwise you'll have a problem with fat like your aunt."
- (From father, as Jennifer is eating a few cookies after school): "Those cookies are good, I know. But you need to learn to take only one or two, or just skip them, because boys don't want see a girl who eats too much."
- (From a harried mother, late at night as Jennifer helps with the weekly shopping): "What are you thinking, picking out that bread for us?! It's incredibly fattening. A girl in our family has to avoid those kinds of foods entirely, or we just get these thighs. You know what I mean. . . ."

Research Background

Many studies indicate that social cognitive factors are correlated with eating problems (see chapter 5). The vast majority of these studies concentrate on the sources and content of influential messages and the extent of their concurrent and predictive relationship with the criterion variables. For example, in several 1-year longitudinal studies of late adolescent girls and young women, Stice (1998a, 2001a) examined the impact of perceived pressure to be thin—emanating from family, friends, dating partners, and the media—and internalization of the slender beauty ideal. Perceived pressure predicted the onset of binge eating and purging, while both variables predicted significant increases in body dissatisfaction, dieting, and negative affect. As is typical of such research, Stice's work leaves unanswered the question of which social learning processes are creating the influential pressures.

Mass media are important sources of both observational learning and persuasive, symbolic communications in regard to cultural values, gender roles, eating, and weight management (Levine & Harrison, 2004; Levine & Smolak, 1996, 1998). Women who are congenitally blind have a more positive body image and healthier eating patterns than women who lost their sight later in life and women who were sighted (Baker, Sivyer, & Towell, 1998). Cross-sectional surveys (e.g., Levine et al., 1994) and experimental presentations of images of the slender ideal (Groesz et al., 2002) indicate that (a) many adolescent girls compare themselves to the slender, glamorous women found ubiquitously in magazines, TV, and movies; (b) this comparison makes them feel worse about their own weight and shape; (c) this comparison motivates them to try to lose weight, sometimes in very unhealthy ways; and (d) the probability of this social comparison process and its negative effects is greater in adolescent girls and young adult women who have internalized the societal ideal and who are already feeling negative and anxious about their weight and shape. Surprisingly, given the great deal of attention that mass media have received, how exactly they exert their various influences is as yet poorly understood (Levine & Harrison, 2004; Levine & Smolak, 1996, 1998).

Application of SCT to parent and peer influences has been more fruitful. A number of studies (e.g., Byely, Archibald, Graber, & Brooks-Gunn, 2000; Pike, 1995) contradict the intuitively appealing proposition that parental modeling is an important influence on body image and dieting, although such modeling does contribute to development of more extreme body dissatisfaction and eating problems in postpubertal girls (Benedikt, Wertheim, & Love, 1998; Stice, 2002; Thompson et al., 1999). When it comes to normative weight and shape concerns, as well as eating problems, direct parental messages about body shape, weight, and dieting are more important than modeling (Benedikt et al., 1998; Strong & Huon, 1998; Smolak, Levine, & Schermer, 1999). In contrast, several studies indicate that, among adolescent girls at least, peers do serve as models of weight concerns and dieting (Wertheim, Paxton, Schultz, & Muir, 1997; see Paxton, 1999, for a review). We found that, in early adolescence, a girl's perception of her friends' investment in dieting, as measured by how often friends talk about weight loss and how many friends are on a diet, had a small but significant relationship to her motivation to become thinner and her level of eating disturbance (Levine et al., 1994; see also The McKnight Investigators, 2003). Unlike the situation for parents, direct exhortation to diet and direct comments about weight are rare among female friends (Paxton, 1999).

There is no doubt that one important form of social learning involves direct comments, including teasing, about weight and shape (Thompson et al., 1999). Sometimes these comments constitute response-contingent punitive feedback, as when Jennifer's father makes a loud joke at the dinner table after she takes what he considers too much spaghetti. In other instances, teasing or critical comments are unrelated to any particular behavior or characteristic. They are designed to bother or intimidate or objectify the target (see chapter 8), or to draw attention to the cleverness of the source.

The negative impact of teasing and critical commentary on body image, and subsequently on dieting and disordered eating, is well established (Thompson et al., 1999). It is likely that a substantial portion of the correlation for females between increasing body mass and increasing body dissatisfaction is explained by the fact that in many modern societies getting fatter evokes insensitive teasing and criticism. However, although heavier girls are more likely to be teased, teasing is a strong predictor of body dissatisfaction independent of BMI. There is also a cumulative effect in that teasing, like mass media images of the slender beauty ideal, has a more negative impact on people who are already anxious and self-conscious about their bodies. Another aspect of teasing that makes it an important target for prevention is the finding that a wide array of people are a source of this negative social influence, including parents, siblings, peers, and coaches (Thompson et al., 1999).

In summary, there is a good deal of evidence for the role of social cognitive learning in the development and maintenance of negative body image, and eating problems. Nevertheless, lack of empirical data makes it challenging for prevention specialists to determine which social cognitive processes are operating, individually or in combination, at which stages of development.

COGNITIVE-BEHAVIORAL THEORY

Basic Concepts

Transactions between the person and the environment are a key feature of SCT's principle of reciprocal determinism. This theory has "cognitive" in the title because one extremely important aspect of what the person brings to situations is a style of perceiving and interpreting the information provided by the "environment." Cognition and information processing encompass psychological processes such as perceiving, remembering, thinking, problem solving, and hypothesis testing. Certain ways of processing information become habitual styles that influence the way we automatically and unconsciously interpret and react to situations. This constitutes a transaction, not an interaction, because cognitive styles help determine the very nature of the "situation" itself (see chapter 4).

Cognitive psychology has had a major impact on the understanding and treatment of psychological disorders, including eating problems and eating disorders (Cash, 2002; Fairburn, 1997). One striking aspect of eating disorders is the tenacity with which sufferers cling to extreme, often dichotomous convictions about the value of thinness, the horror of fat, and the importance of weight and shape for self-concept and self-esteem (Fairburn, 1997). These beliefs are also salient aspects of the cultural contexts that contribute to the continuum of eating problems and to the high prevalence of negative body image, calorie-restrictive dieting, binge eating, and so forth (Gordon, 2000; Smolak & Levine, 1994a). As cognitive-behavioral techniques have been fairly successful in the treatment of panic disorder, depression, and bulimia nervosa, cognitive-behavioral theory (CBT) has influenced the development of prevention programs. There are many different cognitive-behavioral approaches to negative body image and disordered eating. Our introduction to CBT incorporates the work of Thompson et al. (1999, chapter 11), Cash (1996, 1997, 2002), Fairburn (1997; Fairburn, Shafran, & Cooper, 1998), and Vitousek (Garner, Vitousek, & Pike, 1997; Vitousek & Hollon, 1990).

Schema. We "know" a lot of things: what a horse is (as distinct from a cow), how to write a check, and that we are not fast runners. What does it mean when a person says out loud or to themselves "I *know* I am fat and ugly" or "I *know* my hips and thighs are too big and I hate them"? In cognitive psychology, what we "know" or "believe" or "feel" refers to a schema. A schema is a mental structure that helps people to organize their interactions with the world in a stable, consistent, and meaningful fashion.

CBT emphasizes the problems inherent in and created by negative body image. In female adolescents, negative body is clearly a risk factor for disordered eating and depression (see chapter 5). The correlations between body image and either actual size/shape or others' judgments of one's attractiveness are low. This suggests that body image is determined by the interplay between cognitive-emotional factors and the social experiences highlighted in, for example, teasing and mass media standards of beauty. According to the cognitive perspective, body image is a schema that includes one's assumptions, beliefs, thoughts, and feelings about one's appearance (Cash, 1996, 1997, 2002; Thompson et al., 1999).

People do not necessarily apply this schema to every situation, but it may be activated by a wide variety of situations: meeting another person for the first time; looking in the mirror; hearing one's mother talk about food; shopping for a new pair of jeans; going to the beach with friends; viewing a love scene in a movie. Activation of this body image schema generates thoughts, interpretations, and conclusions that people typically describe as internal dialogues (Cash, 1996, 1997). The way we talk to ourselves influences how we feel and what actions we take and avoid. According to Fairburn (1997), in females at risk for disordered eating, negative body image reflects a disparity between one's self-perception and an overinvestment in the importance of low(er) weight and a thin(ner) shape. Rigid thinking about this discrepancy leads to harsh internal dialogue ("This is awful. I am getting fat and totally losing control"), which motivates intense and rigid dieting. This increases the probability of binge eating in response to stress. In the presence of extreme weight and shape concerns, and of loss of control over feelings, binge eating may lead to purging, and the stage is set for cycles of negative affect, dieting, binge eating, and purging (Fairburn, 1997). Over time, with reinforcement by repetition and by strong feelings, the internal dialogues and concomitant distress become automatic. This gives them a sense of being undeniable truths instead of working assumptions or testable hypotheses.

Thus, a schema brings together, in a structured form, various aspects of thinking and feeling (Beck, Rush, Shaw, & Emery, 1979). The schema also organizes various components of body image such as weight, shape, appearance, health, and strength. As an illustration, consider parts of the schema that underlies Jennifer's negative body image. Assume that this schema has been activated by a specific environmental stimulus, in this case a phone call from her friend Maggie, inviting Jennifer to go swimming with friends. Almost automatically, Jennifer has several painful memories about how fat she feels her swimsuit makes her look, including a family picnic at which her younger brother yelled, "Hey, look at Jennifer's 'blubber butt' swimsuit!" Jennifer also imagines the other boys and girls staring at her body. She can almost hear their (her own?) negative evaluations out loud, and she thinks to herself, "This would be fun if it wasn't for my stupid, flabby body. Why was I too lazy to lose that weight over the winter?"

Jennifer's schematic memories, images, and self-statements are connected to negative feelings such as embarrassment, anxiety, and irritability over how unfair the world is and how inadequate she is at managing her weight. Jennifer's memories, thoughts, and dysphoria are also directly connected to exaggerated and painful generalizations such as "No boy would ever want to be near a girl with my huge stomach and thighs" and "I'll never be able to control my eating and lose the weight necessary to look beautiful." Underlying such generalizations are fundamental assumptions or basic expectations: "It's critically important to be in control all the time, and if you are too fat, everyone will know you are out of control"; "I'm just not thin and pretty, and the only thing that matters if you are a girl is whether you are pretty"; and "Life will never be any good if I can't lose this awful weight."

Maggie has called with a friendly invitation to have fun, but Jennifer's schema transforms this stimulus into an "opportunity" to focus obsessively on what she considers her gross physical flaws. Based on Jennifer's mental set, Maggie's invitation becomes a cue for self-consciousness and anxiety. Sensing Jennifer's discomfort, Maggie tries to be helpful by saying, "Jen, you don't have to go in swimming if you don't want to, but come anyway so we can all talk." Jennifer hears this as, "Maggie knows how gross I look in a suit, and she's trying to give me a way not to take my wrap off." Thus, schema activation results in Jennifer's attending to features of the conversation that support her schema (Vitousek & Hollon, 1990).

Most likely, anyone who repeatedly talked to herself the way Jennifer does would develop and deepen a negative body image. Jennifer may the reject the invitation with an excuse that leaves Maggie perplexed and frustrated. Or Jennifer may accept, but end up awkwardly and anxiously enduring the experience because all she concentrates on is her own shape and weight in comparison to the other girls. Her tension and isolation make others uncomfortable, and thus Jennifer's negative body image schema is reinforced by her reactions ("That felt awful" and "People avoided me because I'm fat and dumpy"), as well as, potentially, by the responses of the other adolescents, who do leave her alone or who occasionally stare, wondering what is wrong and why she is not having fun.

This example also illustrates the connections between a personal body image schema and other cognitive structures pertaining to weight, success, and self-concept (Fairburn, 1997; Thompson et al., 1999; Vitousek & Hollon, 1990; Williamson, Stewart, White, & York-Crowe, 2002). What Jennifer thinks and feels about her body is linked to her larger self-schema, including her overall sense of self-worth, her beliefs about what characteristics she should ideally possess, her (in)adequacy in other domains (e.g., as a student, a daughter, an athlete), and what her parents and other significant people expect of her. In this regard Jennifer's body image may be much more important to her than her ability at science, her sense of herself as a caring or religious person, and other potential components of self. Her body image schema is also deeply intertwined with specific constructs such as "birthday cake" (tempting but bad), "anxiety" (painful and isolating, but food helps), and "sports" (fun but I'm too slow because I'm not thin enough). Finally, her body image schema influences how she makes sense of interpersonal relationships. If the connections between these structures and processes are elaborate, then stress and failure in realms seemingly unrelated to body image could result in heightened negative feelings about the body, which in turn sets the stage for further processing of information in terms of the negative body schema.

In summary, Jennifer's "negative body image" represents one aspect of a set of cognitive processes that influence her beliefs, feelings, and behavior. She has a bias that makes it easy for her to perceive the world—and to think rapidly and selectively—in ways that reinforce and extend her negative feelings about parts of her body. Schematic processing of this sort provides the short-term benefits of simplicity, stability, and certainty. However, as is evident in Jennifer's life, a cognitive style of this sort creates a lot of distress and makes her resistant to corrective experiences (Vitousek & Hollon, 1990).

Paralogical Errors. Some aspects of Jennifer's beliefs have a basis in physical and social facts: She is indeed a slow runner; all too many boys look only at a girl's breasts and buttocks; thinner girls are indeed more popular than fatter girls. Nevertheless, her body image schema and its connections with other cognitive structures generate distorted, dysfunctional forms of thinking called *paralogical errors* (Beck et al., 1979; Cash, 1997; Garner et al., 1997). Examples include all-or-none statements ("I'm in control or I'm a total pig"), perfectionism ("I must *always* be in control and I must *never* expose myself to embarrassment"), unfair comparisons ("I am so disgusting compared to the model in that ad"), minimization ("OK, I've heard from friends that several boys want to go out with me, but I'm sure everyone really thinks I look gross"), and magnification ("My pants felt tight today. I just know I'm going to gain all kinds of weight, and my life will be awful"). Self-consciousness, anxiety, and despair are logical outcomes of this type of thinking. So are useless preoccupations, such as worrying about how everyone else looks, obsessively checking one's appearance in the mirror, or constantly asking others if they think you look too fat. Thinking in this manner also motivates Jennifer to avoid dancing or swimming because of perceived fatness, to think seriously about beginning to smoke cigarettes in order to manage her appetite, and to begin to skip breakfast to reduce her overall caloric intake. The emotional and behavioral outcomes of this process combine to reinforce and perhaps extend Jennifer's negative body image schema.

Hypothesis Testing and Behavioral Change. Cognitive-behavioral therapists—and, by extension, those who apply CBT to prevention—believe that people can be helped to change their body image schema, as well as related schema for dieting, exercising, food, eating, and so on. Advocates of CBT, whether they are therapists or prevention specialists, argue that these changes will improve body image and increase the probability of healthier eating and exercising. Consequently, we consider this approach in some detail.

Using an *ABC* model, advocates of CBT help people learn to monitor and analyze the connections between *A*ctivating events (situations that trigger operation of the body image schema), *B*eliefs, and emotional and behavioral *C*onsequences (Cash, 1997, 2002; Stewart, 1998). "Beliefs" is a general term referring to perceptions, thoughts, interpretations, and internal dialogues. Self-monitoring of the *ABC*s demonstrates that, although the consequences seem to arise automatically from the activating events, beliefs play a major causal role. These beliefs can be tested for their logic, their empirical validity, and their functionality. With guidance, an individual can learn to detect dysfunctional beliefs, dispute them, and develop new beliefs and behaviors that are healthier.

A variety of techniques are used to challenge dysfunctional beliefs. We can think of this "cognitive restructuring" as adding *D*isputation to form the heuristic *ABCD* (Cash, 1997, 2002). Like self-monitoring and cognitive analysis, disputation is a skill to be learned and practiced as a form of talking back to one's dysfunctional inner dialogues. Psychoeducation challenges absolutist assumptions such as "physically attractive people have it all"; "one's outward physical appearance is a sign of the inner person"; and "rigid dieting is the only way to improve my body shape, because it's the only way to lose weight" (Cash, 1997, pp. 91–92; Fairburn, 1997). Reasoning through dialogue enables people to examine the emotional value or functional utility of, for example, constantly worrying about appearance, or dressing to hide perceived flaws, no matter how uncomfortable the clothing. If a person assumes that appearance is the key quality affecting one's life, this could be put to the test by gathering evidence about the body size and shape of people (e.g., relatives, teachers, coaches, historical figures) who have made a real difference in one's life. The tendency to minimize positive aspects of one's body, and thus positive feelings about one's body, can be reduced by exercises like constructing and then saying aloud a number of affirmations. All of these cognitive techniques are buttressed by a variety of other practical techniques. These include ways to interrupt negative internal dialogues, ways to relax and think more clearly as one addresses one's body image, advice about setting up contingencies to reward progress toward one's body image goals, and strategies for approaching and coping with situations that previously evoked avoidance (Cash, 1997, 2002).

Research Background

In comparison to SCT, the empirical foundation of cognitive-behavioral theory is limited by a relatively small number of studies and by the formidable methodological challenges involved (see, e.g., Cooper & Fairburn, 1993; Huon, 1995). One commonly used procedure for studying psychopathology and information processing is the Stroop task (Huon, 1995). If a person has multiple and emotional connections to "weight" and "shape," then it should be harder to say aloud the color "red" when the word "fat" is printed in red than when the word "rat" or "far" is printed in red. A predisposition to pay attention to the word "fat" should activate a set of connections that interfere with rapid, selective processing of the color "red." In general, there is some support for this proposition, although the phenomenon is found more consistently if weight and shape concerns are defined broadly to encompass a high drive for thinness, and if the key stimuli are food-related (e.g., cake or butter) rather than body-related (e.g., hips or weight; Huon, 1995).

Altabe and Thompson (1996) found that, compared to participants who thought about body-related information in general, undergraduate females instructed to think about characteristics relevant to their *own* body image and self–ideal discrepancies were more likely to remember this information later. This encoding effect for self-related information occurred even though they were not expecting the subsequent memory task. Another study of incidental memory showed that undergraduate female athletes who were preoccupied with weight and shape tend to remember ambiguous self-referential sentences about body size (e.g., "see your hips in the mirror") as having specific *negative* information about themselves (e.g., "see your large hips in the mirror"). This negativity bias was not found for sentences pertaining to performance or health (Jackman, Williamson, Netemeyer, & Anderson, 1995). Cooper (1997) demonstrated that eating disorder patients were more likely than nonclinical women to interpret negative events, but not positive events, in terms of their preoccupation with weight and shape. As predicted by schema theory for self-concepts, this attributional style applied only to negative events affecting the self; it was not used in explaining events affecting other people. Although the data are limited and not entirely consistent (see, e.g., Tantleff-Dunn & Thompson, 1998), these studies support the cognitive theory that negative body image is a mental representation that acts like a schema in focusing attention and guiding the organization and recall of information (see Thompson et al., 1999; Williamson et al., 2002).

As noted earlier, body image is a multidimensional cognitive structure. Self-discrepancy theory explores the psychological ramifications of different domains and perspectives of the self (Higgins, 1987). This theory yields several key predictions. The greater the difference between one's perceptions of one's "actual" body (actual–own self) and one's mental representation of the ideal body defined by personal wishes (ideal–own self), the greater the probability of negative body image and bulimic behavior (Strauman, Vookles, Berenstein, Chaiken, & Higgins, 1991). People are motivated to achieve consistency between their various self-representations, so the actual–ideal/own discrepancy will also be correlated with disappointment and dejection. These negative emotions intensify negative body image. Thus, over time, large actual–ideal/own discrepancies create vulnerability to the sort of emotional problems and self-defeating behaviors seen in BN. Self-discrepancy theory also predicts that anorexic tendencies will be more closely connected to a difference between the actual–own self and one's conceptions of one's duties and responsibilities as defined by others (the ought–other self).

Strauman et al. (1991) found support for these predictions in their examination of body image, disordered eating, and self-representations in female college students. Moreover, the predicted relationships emerged apart from the strong connection of negative body image and eating problems to an endorsement of the slender beauty ideal (see Thompson & Stice, 2001). Szymanski and Cash (1995) developed a measure of self-representations as applied to specific physical attributes such as facial features, strength, and weight. These researchers also found that the actual–ideal/own discrepancy was the best predictor of general and situational body dissatisfaction, as well as maladaptive appearance-related beliefs. However, contrary to the self-discrepancy theory, the actual–ought discrepancy, not actual–ideal, was the better predictor of bulimic symptoms. Marsh (1999) conducted a 7-month longitudinal survey of nearly 800 Australian boys and girls ages 11 to 16. Twelve silhouette figures, arranged across a continuum from slender to rotund, were used to determine actual self-representation and a combination ideal–ought self-representation. Using structural equation modeling, Marsh found substantial support for the predictive value of the discrepancy between the perceived actual self and these two self-representations. The more slender the ideal–ought self and the heavier the perceived actual self at Time 1, the greater the likelihood of an increase over time in concern about being and feeling fat.

Self-discrepancy theory is intuitively appealing on many levels, but it has a long and controversial history (Marsh, 1999). Prevention researchers need to acknowledge that many questions remain about which discrepancies are most important for explaining different facets of disordered eating, and whether negative body image and eating problems are best predicted by discrepancies in the physical realm or in broad psychological characteristics (Forston & Stanton, 1992; Marsh, 1999; Strauman & Glenberg, 1994). Nevertheless, self-discrepancy theory has enough empirical support to merit the attention of prevention specialists who are very concerned about the negative effects of unrealistic cultural standards of beauty, gender role, control, and so forth. Self-discrepancy theory is potentially very useful for understanding many different components of disordered eating, including the processes by which internalization of the slender beauty ideal from various sources (e.g., peers, mass media) results in harsh self-evaluations and chronic negative emotions (Thompson et al., 1999).

TWO PROGRAMS

In other areas of health promotion, application of social cognitive principles such as reciprocal determinism has resulted in comprehensive, multidimensional prevention programs (Baranowski et al., 2002; Perry, 1999). In the field of eating problems and eating disorders prevention, applications of SCT and CBT have been narrower (see, e.g., Killen, 1996; Neumark-Sztainer, Butler, & Palti, 1995). In general, SCT-based interventions have consisted of 6 to 12 weeks of 30- to 60-minute lessons implemented in school classrooms by psychologists or teachers. Table 6.1 presents the prototypical content of those lessons. Students are provided with the knowledge, values, expectations, skills, incentives, and support seen as necessary to help them resist psychosocial influences that increase risk for the spectrum of eating problems (see chapter 5), and to adopt healthier patterns of eating and exercise (Levine & Piran, 2001, 2004; Levine & Smolak, 2001). The lessons weave all

TABLE 6.1
Prototypical Content of Lessons in the Disease-Specific Pathways Approach to Prevention

1. Specific exercises for understanding and improving body image.
2. Instruction in analyzing and changing unhealthy "beliefs" about one's own weight and shape.
3. Instruction in nutrition and exercising as they pertain to healthy weight control.
4. Information about the clash between developmental factors (e.g., pubertal weight gain) and cultural contexts that idealize thinness and vilify fat and fat people.
5. Information about the dangers of calorie-restrictive dieting.
6. Instruction in individual strategies for analyzing and resisting specific cultural factors such as mass media and peer inducements to diet.
7. Information about the nature, dangers, and identification of eating disorders (e.g., bulimia nervosa).
8. Encouragement of individuals to take action in changing environments that foster eating problems and eating disorders.[a]

Note. Most "disease-specific pathways" approaches are based primarily on Social Cognitive Theory or Cognitive-Behavioral Theory. This table is adapted from Levine and Piran (2001).

[a]This element applies the principle of reciprocal determinism, which includes the proposition that individuals can plan for behavioral changes that will modify their environment in ways that will, in turn, have a positive effect on individual behavior (Bandura, 1986).

three types of social learning processes into classroom activities and homework assignments.

Chapter 9 reviews research on the effectiveness of universal prevention programs for negative body image and eating problems. There are over 75 studies, so it is impossible to provide much detail about each one. Consequently, in the next sections we describe in detail two programs that were somewhat successful and that illustrate, respectively, application of the SCT and CBT approaches to prevention and to research (see also Killen, 1996).

The Weigh to Eat! Program

The Weigh to Eat! curriculum (Neumark-Sztainer, 1992; Neumark-Sztainer et al., 1995; see also Appendix B) is based on SCT. This program attempts to prevent unhealthy dieting and binge eating by providing students ages 14 through 16 with the knowledge and skills to (a) resist unhealthy peer and media influences; (b) improve their own body image, eating and exercise patterns, and self-esteem; and (c) establish new peer-group values and norms to reinforce individual changes. Improvement of eating expressly includes healthy ways to manage weight. In addition, teachers receive two training sessions so they can support the program during class time and during informal conversations with students.

Lessons. Jewish-Israeli high school girls and boys (mean age = 15.3) participated in the program or in a no-program comparison condition, although only data for the girls were reported by Neumark-Sztainer et al. (1995). The program consists of 10 lessons delivered in weekly, hour-long sessions during regularly scheduled classroom time. Program content and the associated social learning mechanisms are presented in Table 6.2 (modeled after Piran, 2001, p. 224).

Key Change Processes. According to SCT, four conditions are necessary for developing healthy behavior. First, the individual must be motivated. Second, the person must have the requisite knowledge and skills. Third, the person must have a strategy for change and the means to guide herself or himself through the necessary steps of setting goals, monitoring progress, and making goal-oriented adjustments. And, finally, the person must believe in her or his capacity for change, that is, the person must have the necessary efficacy expectations (Bandura,

TABLE 6.2
Social Cognitive Theory and *The Weigh to Eat!*
(Neumark-Sztainer et al., 1995) Prevention Program

Factor	Content Themes	Mechanisms for Learning
Personal	Biopsychosocial changes of adolescence Gender differences Nutritional needs and challenges Healthy weights and healthy diets Healthy weight management Body image	Education and direct symbolic communications • Teacher presentations • Student discussions • Student problem-solving and guided discovery Observational learning • Symbolic modeling in readings and discussion
Behavioral and Environmental	Eating disorders Critical thinking about mass media Developing a healthy diet and healthy exercise/activity patterns Resisting social pressures for negative body image and unhealthy eating Developing new personal and group norms and values	Direct experience and behavioral management • self-monitoring of eating and exercising Education and direct symbolic communications (same as above) Observational learning (same as for Personal factors) Direct experience and behavioral management • self-monitoring • goal-setting • role-playing • behavioral projects as homework

Note. The Weigh to Eat! program (Neumark-Sztainer, 1992) is the basis for the prevention program described in Neumark-Sztainer et al. (1995).

1986, 1997; Baranowski et al., 2002; Kohler et al., 1999). In accordance with the principle of reciprocal determinism, all of these conditions must be supported by environmental conditions, including influential people.

The Weigh to Eat! program tries to change knowledge, attitudes, and behavior through a combination of symbolic communications, behavioral programming, and guided discovery (see Table 6.2). The teacher and students work together from a teacher's curriculum guide (Neumark-Sztainer, 1992) and a complementary student workbook. The program relies heavily on symbolic communications, primarily through brief presentations by the teacher and the many handouts contained in the workbook. Every lesson involves class and/or small-group discussions, including group problem solving, for example, how to change environments so as to cue healthier eating. With respect to the cognitive aspects of healthy development, students not only receive a lot of information, they gather and interpret it via homework assignments. One such assignment requires students to interview other people about weight and shape satisfaction, and then to examine one's own impression of those people to determine if people in general are too hard on themselves when it comes to body image.

Findings. Students were assessed prior to program implementation, 6 months following program completion, and again 18 months later. The 6-month follow-up assessment indicated that, compared to the control group, the program had a positive effect on nutritional knowledge, regular meal patterns, and exercising. A true prevention effect also appeared. Girls who were not using unhealthy weight management methods or were not binge eating at baseline were less likely to begin these unhealthy behaviors during the 6 months following the program if they had participated in the program. The prevention effect for binge eating was maintained at the 2-year follow-up, whereas the other positive effects on knowledge and behavior were no longer significant. For girls who were already engaged in binge eating and/or unhealthy weight management, the program had no significant effect on these behaviors, although there was some evidence of a positive effect at 6 months and 12 months for overweight girls.

The Warneford Hospital Curriculum

British psychiatrist C. G. Fairburn is the leading proponent of cognitive-behavioral therapy as the evidence-based treatment of choice for BN and BED (Fairburn, 1997; Wilson et al., 1997). Anne Stewart and her colleagues at Warneford Hospital, Oxford (UK), worked with Fairburn to develop a program designed to prevent negative body image and disordered eating in adolescent girls ages 13–14 (Stewart, 1998; Stewart, Carter, Drinkwater, Hainsworth, & Fairburn, 2001). The Warneford program tries to reduce risk factors that (a) are supported by research; (b) are amenable to change through cognitive-behavioral techniques; (c) could reasonably be affected in a school setting; and (d) are part of the developmental psychology of girls 13–14, an age group at risk for development of abnormal eating habits and behaviors.

The specific goals of the Warneford program reflect the cognitive-behavioral model provided in Stewart (1998, p. 108). A major goal is to reduce dietary restraint and concerns about weight and shape. These phenomena are seen as especially likely when girls develop feelings of low self-esteem and helplessness in response to factors that make it difficult for them to meet the developmental challenges of early adolescence.

Lessons. A large sample ($n = 459$) of British girls ages 13–14 attending one of three different schools participated in the Warneford program. Another large group ($n = 386$) from three similar schools in the same geographic region served as a no-program comparison condition. Assignment of schools to condition was not random, but all schools were girls only, and there was no initial difference between experimental and comparison groups in BMI.

The Warneford program contains six lessons delivered in weekly sessions (45 minutes maximum) during regular classroom hours. The lessons were administered by a psychology graduate student who had no particular expertise in eating disorders. She was assisted by eating disorder professionals on the research team, and they all worked from an unpublished manual devised for regular classroom teachers by Stewart and Carter (1995; described in Stewart, 1998). Program content and associated cognitive-behavioral mechanisms for learning are presented in Table 6.3. To supplement the program all teachers in the intervention schools received an hour of education concerning developmental and sociocultural pressures faced by adolescent girls, and how teachers can facilitate identification and referral of eating disorders.

Key Change Processes. Many of the topics and change processes in this program are similar to the social cognitive approaches of Neumark-Sztainer et al. (1995; see Table 6.2) and Killen (1996). The Warneford program is more cognitive because the girls were taught how to identify and challenge beliefs and automatic thoughts about shape and weight. There were also specific behavioral exercises designed to reduce dietary restraint.

Findings. The Warneford program appears to be modestly successful in the short run, as indicated by assessment 1 week after the last lesson. However, a 6-month follow-up provided only a small amount of evidence pointing to sustained improvements. The program produced significant, lasting increases in knowledge about program content. More important, there were small improvements in scores on the Eating Atti-

TABLE 6.3
Cognitive-Behavioral Theory and The Warneford Hospital (Stewart, 1998) Prevention Program

Theoretical Feature	Content Themes	Mechanisms for Learning
Changing schema	Challenging popular beliefs and attitudes about dieting Individual differences in weight and shape, influenced in part by heredity Positive body image Thinking critically about influences of family, peers, and teasing	Presentation of cognitive-behavioral principles Exercises, including guided discovery, to identify and challenge beliefs and automatic thoughts about weight and shape Homework assignments to identify positive attributes of the self Symbolic modeling
Promoting healthy eating and exercising; avoiding dieting	Body weight regulation and the effects of dieting Nondieting approaches to healthy eating The wide range of healthy weights Nature and consequences of eating disorders Identifying and helping people with eating disorders	Presentation of information Instruction and practice in the ABC model of changing unhealthy eating and dieting Self-monitoring Behavioral exercises as homework, including assigning new behaviors to test effects Active encouragement to make changes in eating and exercising Planning for future changes and challenges (a la relapse prevention)

(Continued)

TABLE 6.3
(Continued)

Theoretical Feature	Content Themes	Mechanisms for Learning
Developing skills	Understanding and coping with sociocultural (including media) pressures for thinness Understanding and coping with developmental stresses of early adolescence	Exercises, including group discussion and guided discovery Presentation of information Symbolic modeling Instruction in goal-setting Role-playing and guided practice for learning stress management skills
Increasing healthy sources of reinforcement and self-esteem	Ways to promote competence and enjoyment outside of appearance and perfectionism in appearance and achievement	Presentation of information Group discussion and guided discovery Self-monitoring and clarification of one's own positive attributes

Note. The Warneford Hospital program is described in Stewart (1998) and in Stewart et al. (2001). Mechanisms for learning correspond to the theoretical feature; they do not apply one-to-one to the adjacent content theme.

tudes Test that were maintained at 6-month follow-up. The program also had a small but sustained effect on reducing dietary restraint, but, in contrast to the work of Neumark-Sztainer et al. (1995), this effect was particularly significant for those considered "dieters" at baseline. The Warneford program did have a small but significant positive effect on global eating disorder scores, and on specific shape concerns and eating concerns at posttest, but these desired changes were not maintained at follow-up. Furthermore, in contrast to expectations, the program had no effects on weight concern, self-concept, and eating disorder behaviors.

SUMMARY: KEY FEATURES OF SLT AND CBT PROGRAMS

One goal of describing the SCT and CBT perspectives in detail is to enable a fuller description and comparison of the outcome studies reviewed in chapter 9. Therefore, we conclude by considering the prototypical features used to describe and classify those outcome studies.

Disease-Specific Targets for Intervention

Social cognitive approaches attempt to intervene in causal pathways that are seen as specific to the development of eating problems and eating disorders. In general, programs based on the SCT and CBT models are looking to disrupt the processes that run from sociocultural influences through negative body image to weight concerns, dieting, and binge eating. Typically, negative body image is defined narrowly as body dissatisfaction encompassing the idealization of slenderness, the belief that one is too fat, a fear of fat, and the drive to become thinner. Program elements try to decrease these disease-specific risk factors while increasing healthy attitudes and behavior related specifically to body image, eating, and exercising. As noted previously, Table 6.1 presents eight prototypical elements of SCT/CBT programs. In our later description and comparison of outcome studies (chapter 9), we rate how many of these are present in each study.

It is possible to categorize prevention programs in terms of superordinate models, but most programs have features of several different prevention models (see chapters 4, 7, and 8). For example, although it is debatable whether low self-esteem is a causal risk factor for eating disorders (Stice, 2001b; see chapter 5), it is widely believed to be (Shisslak, Crago, Renger, & Clark-Wagner, 1998). People who develop eating disorders invariably have low self-esteem, and low self-esteem is a general risk factor for psychopathology (see, e.g., Fairburn et al., 1998). Therefore, a number of SCT/CBT programs (e.g., Neumark-Sztainer et al., 1995) try to improve global self-esteem. Similarly, some programs (e.g., Neumark-Sztainer et al., 1995; Stewart et al., 2001) teach skills for coping with stress, including the normative challenges of adolescence. From a disease-specific perspective, adolescent girls with eating disorders are thought to turn to dieting and weight and shape concerns in order to simplify challenges to their sense of control and structure (Fairburn, 1997; Stewart, 1998; Vitousek & Hollon, 1990). However, program elements concentrating on self-esteem and general coping skills are considered features of the Non-Specific Vulnerability-Stressor (NSVS) model (Levine & Piran, 2001), which is discussed in the next chapter.

Structure of the Program

The scientist-practitioner model of clinical psychology and psychiatry has been a major influence on the development of SCT and CBT (Bandura, 1986, 1997; Fairburn, 1997). One manifestation of this clinical model explicit in both perspectives is the principle of collaborative empiricism (Beck et al., 1979). This means that an expert (e.g., a doctoral-level clinical psychologist) applies theory and research to "work with" (i.e., variously direct, teach, coach, and guide) an individual or group of people so as to help people understand themselves better and make desired changes.

In the realm of prevention, this clinical perspective results in programs that are directed to children and adolescents from the "top down" by mental health professionals, expert health educators, or adult classroom teachers. Although activities allow for individualized information and for unpredictable group discussions, the content and structure of the lessons is determined in advance according to the general outcomes of research and theory on risk and resilience, and according to general theories of health promotion (Piran, 1995, 1998). Program structure is formalized in a manual containing lesson plans, handouts, and homework assignments (e.g., Levine & Hill, 1991; Neumark-Sztainer, 1992; see also Appendix B). As seen in the work of Neumark-Sztainer et al. (1995) and Stewart et al. (2001), program activities are varied and potentially very engaging for the student participants. Nevertheless, the program and adult(s) directing it are clearly the locus of knowledge, authority, and change.

Moreover, even though program participants often function as a class or work in small groups, individual behavior is the focus of change (Piran, 1995, 1998; see also Levine & Piran, 2001, 2004). This is consistent with a medical model, with many forms of psychotherapy, and with most forms of Western education. This means that, typically, there is an emphasis on *individual* changes in skills, expectations, and values, as well as *individual* resistance to unhealthy sociocultural influences. Presentation of information about "sociocultural factors" necessarily addresses social values (e.g., idealization of slenderness) and social practices (e.g., weight- and shape-related teasing). However, with only a few exceptions (see, e.g., Smolak, Levine, & Schermer, 1998a, 1998b), the top-down, disease-specific approaches tend not to work directly to establish or reinforce healthier *group* norms and values, *group* dynamics, and *group* actions.

Levels of Intervention

The top-down, disease-specific programs evaluated by Neumark-Sztainer et al. (1995) and Stewart et al. (2001) suggest that universal prevention in an educational setting can produce some beneficial, short-term effects. This is quite consistent with other research (Levine & Piran, 2001, 2004; Levine & Smolak, 2001; see chapter 9). An immediate candidate for program improvement is the fact that in most SCT and CBT programs (see also, e.g., Killen, 1996; Santonastaso et al., 1999) student "cognition" and "behavior" are basically the sole focus of intervention. One wonders why most of the SCT and CBT prevention programs have not really applied the ecological perspective contained in the fundamental SCT principle of reciprocal determinism (Bandura, 1986, 1997; Baranowski et al., 2002). If behavior, cognitions, and attitudes are a function of environment, and the environment is also a function of behavior, then prevention and health promotion will be facilitated if experts and students learn how to improve those sociocultural factors that constitute a key part of disease-specific processes: peer interactions, teachers and parents as role models, mass media, the school environment in regard to weight and shape messages, and so on (Austin, 2000; Levine & Smolak, 2001, 2002; Neumark-Sztainer, 1996; Piran, 1998; Smolak, 1999; see chapter 4). The limited focus of SCT programs to date is especially bewildering because multidimensional interventions have for many years been standard practice in the application of SCT to prevention of cardiovascular disease and substance use/abuse (see Perry, 1999; Weissberg, Barton, & Shriver, 1997; see also chapter 10).

7

The Non-Specific Vulnerability-Stressor Model

As discussed in chapter 6, social cognitive and cognitive-behavioral models of prevention presume that in order to prevent eating disorders, one must identify specific risk and protective factors for those disorders and then intervene to block or disrupt the destructive pathways. This has led proponents to use cognitive social learning mechanisms (direct instruction, live and symbolic modeling, guided practice) to reduce weight concerns, body dissatisfaction, calorie-restrictive dieting, and negative emotions (see chapters 5 and 9). This approach is compelling because of its logical appeal and because it has been applied with some success in preventive medicine and in the prevention of cigarette smoking and alcohol abuse (see chapter 10). In addition, the disease-specific perspective has helped to illuminate some specific risk factors for eating disorders and problems (Stice, 2001b, 2002; see chapter 5), and it has produced a few promising prevention programs (see chapters 6 and 9). However, it has also delayed progress in prevention because a number of influential experts in the field of eating disorders believe that "We're just not ready to do good prevention work because we don't know the *specific* developmental pathways to disordered eating."

An important group of community psychologists and prevention specialists disagree with this "disorder-targeted" (or "disease-specific") perspective (Albee & Gullotta, 1997; The Consortium on the School-based Promotion of Social Competence [The Consortium], 1994; Cowen, 2000; Weissberg & Greenberg, 1998). They argue for a much broader approach to preventing disorder and to promoting individual and community health. In our previous work we called this perspective the *Non-Specific Vulnerability-Stressor* model (NSVS; Levine & Piran, 2001, 2004; Levine & Smolak, 2001). This chapter outlines this broad model, provides an example from eating disorders prevention, and considers the implications of the model for evaluating current prevention efforts and developing more effective programs.

THE GENERAL MODEL

Generic Risk Factors

The NSVS model is founded on three types of data. First, a large body of research demonstrates that similar, generic sources of stress and vulnerability are part of the pathways for multiple forms of psychopathology, such as eating disorders, depression, substance abuse, and anxiety disorders. Mental disorders, behavioral problems, and ill health in general flourish where people have too much stress, too little respect for themselves and for others, too few meaningful relationships and too little perceived social support, and too few personal, social, and physical resources for meeting their needs. Studies in developmental psychopathology (Masten & Coatsworth, 1995), health promotion (Blum, 1998), stress and mental illness (Dohrenwend, 1998), community psychology (Albee & Gullotta, 1997; Cowen, 2000; Elias, 1995), and prevention science (Coie et al., 1993) all support this proposition. Thus, prevention will be facilitated when stress, prejudice, social exploitation, alienation, and powerlessness are reduced while coping skills, self-esteem, meaningful interactions, and opportunities for competence and meaningful work are increased (Albee, 1983; Bloom, 1996).

In this regard it is also well known that mental health problems (e.g., eating disorders and mood disorders) and risky behaviors (e.g., substance abuse) tend to co-occur. For example, Kandel and Davies (1982; reviewed in Compas & Hammen, 1994) found that in girls ages 14 to 18, depressed mood was related to more delinquency, absence from school, lower grades, and use of cigarettes, alcohol, and other drugs. In the realm of eating problems, frequent dieting behavior, vomiting, and use of laxatives by adolescent girls are associated concurrently with a variety of health risk behaviors such as initiation of smoking, drinking, and other drug use (see, e.g., French, Story, Downes, Resnick, & Blum,

1995; Neumark-Sztainer, Story, & French, 1996). Similarly, in a recent longitudinal study of young adolescent girls, Stice and Shaw (2003) found that eating pathology and elevated levels of negative emotions made independent contributions to the prediction of smoking initiation 1 year later. Moreover, research has shown that there is considerable symptom overlap across categories of disorder. Agitation, irritability, poor concentration, and negative thoughts about the self are likely to occur in a variety of syndromes and disorders, including depression, anxiety, and eating problems (Compas & Hammen, 1994; Fairburn, 1997). DiClemente, Ponton, and Hansen (1996) add that many high-risk behaviors—and here we could include calorie-restrictive dieting—co-occur and follow a similar developmental trajectory of increasing prevalence and increasing intensity during adolescence. This is particularly true in the United States, where most adolescents are given many broad choices, often with little supervision and support. Consequently, according to the NSVS model, prevention programs will be more efficient if they are designed to affect broad, generic risk factors instead of disease-specific pathways (Greenberg, Domitrovich, & Bumbarger, 2001).

Durlak (1997) provides substantial evidence for an emphasis on generic risk factors. He reviewed nearly 1,200 outcome evaluations of prevention and health promotion in eight areas, encompassing behavioral problems, drug use, and physical health. Stress, low SES, parental psychopathology, and comorbid (multiple) problems were consistent correlates (predictors) across all eight areas. Other correlates in at least six of the eight areas were impoverished neighborhoods, poor quality schools, marital discord, punitive childrearing, and peer modeling of negative, unhealthy behaviors. Durlak's (1997) review supports an ecological perspective by highlighting the generalized negative effect of community, school, peer, family, and individual factors (see chapter 4). Risk exists at multiple levels, and the same risk factors are connected with multiple negative outcomes.

Resilience and Positive Development

The second set of findings at the heart of the NSVS model complements the focus on generic risk with an emphasis on the importance of generic correlates of positive development and nonspecific sources of resilience. In Durlak's (1997) large-scale review, five broad categories of variables emerged as consistent protective factors across all eight major behavioral and health outcomes: (a) healthy social norms within the community (e.g., about cigarette smoking and drinking alcohol); (b) effective social policies (e.g., enforcement of laws governing nonsale of alcohol and tobacco to minors); (c) good parent–child relationships; (d) personal and social competence; and (5) direct social support for children or for significant adults in children's lives. Also consistent with an ecological perspective was the finding that the remaining variables associated with positive outcomes in the behavioral realms (e.g., drug use) were high quality schools, positive peer models, and individual self-efficacy.

Resilience occurs when positive, and not negative, developmental outcomes are seen in children and adolescents who would be expected to fare poorly because they are faced with multiple adverse circumstances and other risk factors. So, technically, resilience refers to positive outcomes and to the processes underlying positive development, particularly the dynamic transactions between people and their environments. Kumpfer's (1999) literature review lists sources of resilience for high-risk youth that are quite consistent with the generic protective factors identified by Durlak (1997). Therefore, assuming that they are not covariates of some as yet unidentified master source of resilience, it is very likely that these variables are important for prevention and health promotion in general. Kumpfer (1999) and Durlak (1997) agree that resilient children and adolescents have positive values and skills in several interlocking realms, including spirituality broadly defined (e.g., purpose and hope in life), cognition (e.g., academic and problem-solving skills), social skills, emotional stability (e.g., self-management and empathy), and physicality (e.g., health and physical talents). These sources of resilience are fostered by secure attachments within the family or with at least one person within the extended family or community. Such attachments nurture prosocial skills and interests, in part by providing positive role models and high expectations for competence. In a related vein, resilience is encouraged when family members or community structures provide children and adolescents with opportunities for meaningful social involvement and meaningful, constructive activities (Kumpfer, 1999).

Community, Resilience, and Health

This emphasis on the ecology of health connects the study of risk and resilience to the third area supporting the NSVS model. This area is variously known as Youth Development Programs (Roth, Brooks-Gunn,

Murray, & Foster, 1998), Developmental Assets (Benson, Leffert, Scales, & Blyth, 1998), and Applied Developmental Science (Lerner, Fisher, & Weinberg, 2000). These approaches share a fundamental concern about the social disorganization implied by statistics indicating that approximately 20% to 25% of children and youth have significant psychological and behavioral problems, while an equal percentage are engaging in various risky behaviors (Dryfoos, 1997). Consequently, each of these approaches asks: What generic community, family, and personal factors support the positive development of youth?

The nature and nurture of positive development is complex and potentially very controversial. Nevertheless, these approaches concur with the conclusion of the Carnegie Council on Adolescent Development (1989; cited in Roth et al., 1998) that positive development incorporates an interest in and the skills for positive social relationships, lifelong learning, meaningful work, a strong sense of identity, good health, and responsibility for one's self and others. Lerner et al. (2000) organize these outcomes as broad attributes that they call the "Five Cs": Competence, Connection, Character, Confidence, and Caring (Compassion).

Roth et al. (1998) note that "youth development programs are best characterized by their approach to youth as resources to be developed rather than as problems to be managed, and their efforts to help youth become healthy, happy, and productive by increasing youths exposure to external assets, opportunities and supports" (p. 427). In general, young people need safe places, challenging experiences, people who care about them on a daily basis, and the opportunity to serve and be part of meaningful groups of people.

These ideas are the cornerstones of the theory of personal and contextual "developmental assets" proposed by Peter Benson and colleagues at the Search Institute in Minneapolis (e.g., Benson et al., 1998; French et al., 2001). Contextual assets include various types of external support from family and community, which increase youths' experience of empowerment, caring, connection, and constructive use of time. Personal assets subsume a commitment to learning, social competencies, and a positive identity. According to the Search Institute's wideranging literature reviews and its own empirical research, developmental assets are correlated with higher levels of physical health and lower engagement in many unhealthy behaviors, such as violence, gambling, substance abuse, early sexual activity, and depression (Benson et al., 1998; Leffert et al., 1998). In 1996–1997 researchers at the Search Institute surveyed over 95,000 girls and boys attending Grades 6 through 12 in over 213 cities across the United States (French et al., 2001). For girls and boys, the *absence* of binge eating, purging, and weight loss behaviors was associated with a strong experience of contextual assets (family support, positive family communication, feeling valued by the community, positive peer and adult role models, and constructive use of time at home) and personal assets (engagement in school, valuing restraint over indulgence, skills for avoiding trouble and risky behaviors, sense of purpose, self-esteem, and optimism). Within the limits imposed by correlation-based, cross-sectional research, these findings are consistent with the developmental assets model.

PROXIMAL GOALS FOR PREVENTION

According to the NSVS model, numerous forms of disorder and ill health will thrive at the individual and social level wherever limitations (vulnerability, risk, stressors) predominate over strengths (protective factors, support, developmental assets). Thus, proponents of this model intervene at multiple ecological levels in order to reduce stressors in children's lives, to teach "life skills" for coping effectively with stress and for attaining positive personal and social goals, and to increase sources of positive socialization and other forms of social support for youth (Albee & Gullotta, 1997; Elias, 1987).

Generic Life Skills

At the individual level, youth can be taught a variety of strategies for healthy functioning in many areas of life. Botvin (2000) developed a drug prevention program for middle school students that uses cognitive social learning techniques (see chapter 6) to work with problem-specific influences and to teach generic life skills such as decision making, problem solving, and stress management, as well as some general social skills such as assertion. Based on findings from his long-standing, extensive research program, this combination of social influence training and competence enhancement produces 40% to 80% reductions for the rate of tobacco use in seventh graders. Changes have also been durable. This influential research program is discussed in detail in chapter 10.

Social Competence

One particularly important domain of life skills that is not very thoroughly addressed in Botvin's program is "social competence." Major facets of social competence are, for example, (a) a positive sense of self-worth; (b) confidence in one's ability to interact with people and take on new challenges; (c) respecting the diversity and value of others; (d) empathy and perspective taking; and (e) understanding social cues and interpersonal complexities (The Consortium, 1994; Elias, 1995). These social attitudes and abilities are facilitated by the following skills for managing the self in social interactions: goal-setting; consideration of multiple strategies; planning a sequence of goal-directed activities; and self-monitoring the effectiveness of one's social actions (Caplan & Weissberg, 1989).

The Consortium (1994) reviewed evidence from several meta-analyses suggesting that school-based social competence programs can have a moderately positive effect on adjustment. More recently, Weissberg and Greenberg (1998) reviewed several long-term, longitudinal studies indicating that boys and girls participating in social-competence promotion programs were less likely than control participants to engage in substance use and in antisocial behavior against people and property. But Weissberg and Greenberg (1998) also caution that training in positive, adaptive social behavior does not necessarily reduce the incidence of specific problems such as high-risk sexual behavior or substance use (see also Caplan & Weissberg, 1989). For example, Elias et al. (1986) worked intensively with fifth-grade teachers to help boys and girls learn social problem-solving skills. Twenty lessons focused on attending to one's own and others' feelings in a situation; thinking about your goals and generating alternative solutions and consequences; and developing both the expectancy that obstacles can be overcome and the understanding that some solutions sometimes do not resolve the problem. In the first half of the school year these forms of social competence were developed through role playing, discussion, and practice. In the second half of the year the teachers and children were helped to apply the lessons, as well as to keep records to review what worked and what did not. Four months after the year-long program, students who had received both instruction and application training coped significantly better (than comparison participants who received no intervention or just the first half) with the stressful entry into middle school, particularly in terms of coping with peers and avoiding problems with materials and school personnel. Interestingly, there was little effect of the social competence program on substance use and abuse.

The reviews by Weissberg and Greenberg (1998) and by Botvin (2000) strongly suggest that prevention of eating problems and eating disorders will be facilitated by a combination of the generic and the disease-specific approaches (see also Smolak et al., 1998a). This issue is developed further in chapter 10.

Multiple Levels of Intervention

Proponents of the NSVS model agree with developmental psychologists (see chapter 4) that an ecological perspective is necessary for understanding and improving behavior. In fact, Albee unabashedly contends that prevention, like other forms of health promotion, is fundamentally about multidimensional, systemic, social change (see, e.g., Albee & Gullotta, 1997; see also Levine & Piran, 2001, 2004; Piran, 1999b, 2001). The Search Institute offers a model for engaging—and integrating—various levels of a community in order to empower its citizens, including its youth, to promote social and individual developmental assets (Benson et al., 1998).

Social competence programs have typically applied this principle across various levels of the school setting. For example, the Social Competence Promotion Program for Young Adolescents (SCPP-YA; Weissberg et al., 1997) consisted of 27 sessions of instruction in social problem solving, a 9-session substance-abuse module, and a 9-session module on AIDS and pregnancy prevention. The program sought to make social competence the norm within the school, so classroom lessons were systematically reinforced by training teachers to model problem solving in their daily behavior and as they implemented the curriculum. The researchers also worked with parents and with school staff in order to improve the policies and practices of the school and the broader community. Relative to controls, adolescents participating in the SCPP-YA had improved problem-solving skills, better relationships with peers, fewer conduct problems, and were less inclined to use alcohol and other drugs. The positive findings of this program, which combines problem-specific and generic life-skill targets, are consistent with the positive effects of multilevel prevention programs originating from the social cognition (Perry, 1999; see chapter 10) and feminist-empowerment-relational models (Piran, 2001; see chapter 8).

A PROTOTYPICAL PROGRAM

To date, only a few programs for the prevention of eating problems and eating disorders have incorporated some combination of life skills, social competence, and multidimensional intervention. One encouraging example is *Everybody's Different*, a program developed by Australian researcher Jennifer O'Dea (1995, cited and evaluated in O'Dea & Abraham, 2000; O'Dea, personal communications, February 6, 2000, and January 30, 2002; see also O'Dea, 2002c).

Everybody's Different

O'Dea and Abraham (2000) argue that disease-specific, information-based approaches designed to build resistance to negative sociocultural factors are not only ineffective, they are potentially dangerous because they glamorize unhealthy lifestyles and inadvertently offer unhealthy weight-management techniques (see also O'Dea, 2000, 2002a). Consequently, the goal of *Everybody's Different* is "to improve body image by building general self-esteem" (O'Dea & Abraham, 2000, p. 45).

Although O'Dea does not conceptualize her work in terms of the NSVS model, it is closely connected to this perspective by its focus on health promotion through self-esteem development and by its use of life skills (e.g., learning to communicate effectively, to appreciate and respect uniqueness, and to deal constructively with stress) to improve both self-image and respect for other people. In this regard, the program was integrated into the ongoing health curriculum as a unit concerning personal development. Prevention of eating disorders and body image were not mentioned as goals of the program to either teachers or students, and every effort was made to dissociate program evaluation (e.g., via the EDI) from program participation. Hence, the confounding effects of demand characteristics and student bias were reduced.

Lessons. Australian girls and boys (ages ranged from 11.1 to 14.5 years; $N = 470$) were randomly assigned to the program or a no-program condition, based on school classes. *Everybody's Different* contains nine 1-hour lessons that are implemented by the regular classroom teacher. The content of the program and mechanisms for change are presented in Table 7.1 (see O'Dea & Abraham, 2000, Table 1, p. 45, and O'Dea, 2002c, Table 1, p. 92). *Everybody's Different* is only one component of *Body Basics*, a large, multidimensional nutrition education program that has been implemented in two thirds of Australian high schools (O'Dea, 2002a).

Key Change Processes. As noted earlier, *Everybody's Different* intentionally provides no direct instruction about weight, healthy eating and exercising, calorie-restrictive dieting, and disordered eating. Instead, this program creates opportunities for youth to create and reinforce a (more) positive self-image. This is accomplished through development of tolerance and appreciation for individual differences (i.e., uniqueness), through an emphasis on multiple aspects of self-image (vs. overvaluation of a thin or muscular appearance), and through peer support. Group activities, discussions, games, and homework assignments promote an understanding and appreciation of the fact that everybody is different and nobody is perfect. Thus, the focus is on knowledge, values, and skills that foster a general, multifaceted sense of self-worth, which in turn should anchor healthy body esteem.

O'Dea and Abraham (2000) maintain that positive changes in self-esteem and in the values and skills necessary to resist unhealthy social and peer pressures will be facilitated by group-oriented and student-centered learning in a cooperative, nonthreatening setting. The classroom teacher initiates each lesson, but examples, connections, and personal relevance are discovered and elaborated by the students themselves. Students cooperate in a variety of activities, including games and drama. One life skill promoted in these interpersonal exchanges consists of ways to seek and receive positive feedback from significant others. In addition, activities for feeling connected to and safe within one's body are practiced at school and at home.

Findings. Students completed a number of validated and standardized self-report assessments before and after the 3-month program, as well as 12 months later. At posttest and relative to the control group, EDI body satisfaction significantly increased for boys and girls who had participated in the program. In addition, during the intervention the increase in the number of girls who were currently trying to lose weight was less for program participants (2%) than for controls (8%). During the 12-month follow-up, girls in the comparison group who were of normal weight lost a significant amount of weight, whereas girls participating in the program did not. For girls in the program, pre-to-posttest

TABLE 7.1
Non-Specific Vulnerability-Stressor Model and the Everybody's *Different* Prevention Program

Factor	Content Themes	Mechanisms for Learning
Life Skills and Social Competence	Dealing with stress as one important means of feeling good in your body	Relaxation tape and training; guided imagery; guided group brainstorming and discussion
	How other people affect our self-image. Learning interpersonal skills to seek and accept positive feedback from others	Hand outline activity Creating and presenting a self-advertisement
	Dealing with relationships	Video and role playing
	Communication skills, for expressing emotions and for solving problems	Games, activities (e.g., role playing), and group discussion
Self-Esteem	Identifying and valuing one's unique features	"I am OK" self-esteem building activity
	Understanding self-image and threats to it	Creating and presenting a self-advertisement
	Broadening self-image to a wider array of physical and personal attributes	[Teaching style that promotes self-esteem]
	Challenging perfectionism and "all-or-none" thinking Promoting respect and appreciation for diversity Prejudice and teasing are unacceptable	Activities (in class and as homework), games, and discussion
	Understanding gender stereotypes to frame the value of being an individual	Posters and student-led discussion (e.g., of mass media)
Ecological Intervention	Positive feedback and other support from friends and family	Assignments done at home, involving friends and family (parents, siblings, and grandparents); modeling by peers in the classroom
		Specific inclusion of males and females in the activities and discussions
	Teacher training for promoting student self-respect and tolerance via teaching style and teacher's comportment in the classroom	2 hours of one-on-one training with each teacher, followed by post-lesson individual discussion of each lesson with each teacher

Note. Sources are O'Dea and Abraham (2000), O'Dea (2002c), as well as O'Dea, personal communications, February 6, 2000, and January 23, 2002.

increases in body satisfaction were also evident in improved self-ratings for physical appearance and improved perceptions of how mother and fathers would rate their physical appearance. The positive changes in how girls believed their fathers would rate their physical appearance were still strong at the 12-month follow-up. Moreover, the program was successful in the short and long term in decreasing concerns about physical appearance, athletic competence, and social acceptance. An important finding of O'Dea and Abraham's (2000) study was that the benefits occurred in all weight groups, including overweight students.

These positive effects support a NSVS approach to prevention for both girls and boys, but more research is clearly needed. There were no significant changes in EDI subscale scores other than body dissatisfaction, although girls in the program who were categorized as "high risk" on the basis of low self-esteem and high anxiety scores did reduce their drive for thinness from pre- to posttest. This benefit and the relative improvements in body satisfaction for all program participants dissipated at 12-month follow-up. In addition, there was a significant pre-to-follow-up increase of 9% in the number of girls in the intervention group trying to lose weight, whereas the comparable figure for the control group was 6% (a nonsignificant increase). In previous reviews (Levine & Piran, 2001; Levine & Smolak, 2001) we characterized this negative finding as "troubling," given O'Dea's emphasis on the potential of disease-specific SCT approaches for unintentional harm. However, O'Dea (personal communication, January 30, 2002) disagrees with this interpretation. She notes that there was no significant between-group difference in dieting, and that the increase in dieting was observed only after the program terminated and girls in the program (but not the comparison girls) continued to gain weight, as one would expect in early and middle adolescence. Thus, O'Dea interprets the rebound effect as supporting the need for continuing intervention based on her model (see chapter 9).

SUMMARY: PROTOTYPICAL FEATURES OF NSVS PROGRAMS

Emphasis on Non-Specific Targets for Intervention

As noted in chapter 6, the "disease-specific" SCT and CBT approaches do, in fact, incorporate elements of the NSVS model (see, e.g., Stewart, 1998). The converse is true to some extent, as there are to date no prevention programs that completely exclude disease-specific elements such as personal and social factors influencing positive body image or the idealization of thinness. *Everybody's Different* is the purest application of the NSVS model. It clearly tries to reduce risk factors, and increase sources of resilience, that are not specific to eating problems and eating disorders, while purposefully ignoring disease-specific factors such as dieting behavior and fear of fat (see Table 7.1). Nonspecific targets for this program and for other interventions with significant elements of the NSVS model include, for example: life skills such as social competence and coping with stress; multiple ways of increasing self-esteem; and promotion of physical fitness and physical competence (O'Dea & Abraham, 2000; Phelps et al., 1999; Seaver, McVey, Fullerton, & Stratton, 1997, evaluated in McVey, Davis, Tweed, & Shaw, 2004).

Table 7.2 presents four prototypical elements of the NSVS approach. Of the four, the first two (self-esteem building and life-skills development) do not overlap with key elements of the social cognitive approaches (chapter 6) and the feminist-empowerment-relational model (chapter 8). In our later description and comparison of outcome studies (chapter 9), we rate whether none, one, or two of these distinguishing elements are present in each study.

Structure of the Program

Like social cognitive theory's emphasis on reciprocal determinism (Bandura, 1986; Perry, 1999), the NSVS model explains disorder and health in terms of the interplay between individual, social, and environmental factors. In fact, the NSVS model adopts the type of participatory-

TABLE 7.2
Prototypical Elements Comprising a Non-Specific Vulnerability-Stressor Approach to Prevention

1. Specific personal and interpersonal exercises for understanding and improving self-esteem, internal locus of control, and/or individual identity. This includes dimensions of self-concept that are explicitly unrelated to appearance or "image."
2. Instruction, at the individual and peer group levels, in ways to increase life skills such as stress management, assertion, and decision making.
3. Substantial student (and system) input into the understanding of the issues and the creation of positive changes.
4. Creation of more supportive environments—with healthier norms and fewer stressors—by changing the attitudes and behaviors of peers, parents, teachers, and/or significant adults in the lives of students. This subsumes goals such as the elimination of weight-related teasing and other forms of objectification.

Note. This table is adapted from Levine and Piran (2001).

ecological perspective that is a pillar of community psychology in North and South America (Dalton, Elias, & Wandersman, 2001) and of the Health Promoting Schools movement in Europe (World Health Organization, 1999) and Australia (O'Dea & Maloney, 2000; see also chapter 15). In practical terms, this means much more than an acknowledgement of the role of contexts in shaping attitudes and behaviors. Program developers and evaluators operating from a participatory-ecological perspective plan carefully to work with "stakeholders" at various ecological levels (e.g., teachers, students, parents) in order to identify the key contextual issues and the most promising, multidimensional avenues for lasting change. This collaboration becomes a consultation rooted in trust, respect, and relationships, all of which are framed by an understanding of the professional consultant's place within the ecology he or she is seeking to influence. Thus, according to the NSVS model, the prevention specialist must avoid the role of "outside expert" delivering a prefabricated program based on general, decontextualized principles. Instead of being a "scientist-practitioner," the specialist functions as a "participant-conceptualizer," helping to improve environments and to empower people, not only with classroom "lessons," but also through the very processes of collaborative ecological assessment and collaborative establishment of prevention programming in interlocking systems (Dalton et al., 2001). This approach is discussed and illustrated in more detail in chapters 8, 10, 12, and 15.

In practice, Piran's (1999a, 1999b, 2001) feminist-empowerment-relational approach to prevention of negative body image and disordered eating has been much truer to the participatory-ecological principles of community psychology (see chapter 8). *Everybody's Different* (O'Dea & Abraham, 2000) is obviously a "prefabricated" program based on positivist psychosocial theory and "applied" from the "top down" by an expert. Nevertheless, O'Dea carefully constructed this program so as to avoid imparting extended "lessons" and predetermined, didactic knowledge. Instead, she used many open-ended, discovery-based activities in order to make students—and their peers, parents, and teachers—the locus of change in the construction of healthy knowledge, attitudes, and skills (see Table 7.1).

Levels of Intervention

The explicit ecological perspective of the NSVS model emphasizes the importance of providing healthy contexts for youth and for significant adults in their lives (see chapter 4). Consequently, O'Dea and colleagues worked closely with educators to create positive changes in different levels of social influence (O'Dea & Abraham, 2000; O'Dea & Maloney, 2000; O'Dea, personal communication, January 30, 2002). The classroom "lessons" and "homework" were designed to improve peer and parental factors influencing self-esteem and body image. In addition, classroom exercises for students were facilitated by regular classroom teachers, who received several hours of individual training prior to program implementation, as well as individual feedback after each lesson. However, in O'Dea's research and in the few other controlled evaluations of programs with significant elements of the NSVS model (see chapter 9), the values and behaviors of individual student participants remain the focus of change efforts and of assessment. Those who advocate an NSVS perspective (e.g., Shisslak et al., 1998) face the same challenge seen in the shortcomings of the SCT and CBT approaches to prevention of eating problems and eating disorders: reconciling a strong theoretical emphasis on the transactions between individuals and their ecologies with the need to make and assess changes in those social contexts.

Our developmental model, which combines the disease-specific and NSVS models, focuses on the need for multidimensional, integrated efforts to help young girls negotiate the normative and often simultaneous stressors they face in making the transition from late childhood to early adolescence (Smolak, 1999; Smolak & Levine, 1996, 2001b; Smolak et al., 1998b). We argue that, based on a nonspecific community mental health perspective, this type of intervention should help prevent the high levels of anxiety, depression, and substance use that often accompany and sustain the spectrum of serious eating problems. At the moment, universal prevention programs are a long distance from this basic goal. This critically important issue is discussed in detail in chapter 12.

A comparison of the SCT and NSVS models indicates that both perspectives tend to yield programs that operate from the top down to influence the knowledge, attitudes, and behaviors of participating individuals (Levine & Piran, 2001, 2004; Piran, 1995). Furthermore, neither type of program has devoted a great deal of attention to one of the most salient aspects of disordered eating, namely the startling gender difference. In the next chapter we consider an alternative perspective that emphasizes gender, locates knowledge and the processes of change primarily within the participants, and insists on changing some of the systems that shape the lived experience of girls and young women.

8

The Feminist-Empowerment-Relational Model: A Critical Social Perspective

There was a television commercial, airing in 2001, showing a man standing in the middle of a ladies' clothing store, awkwardly holding a purse for his wife while she goes to try on clothes. The voiceover says, "At least you can eat like a man." This hot dog commercial illustrates that men and women live in different "cultures." In the universe defined by this commercial—indeed, in most realms of the symbolic universe of television—women are concerned with clothes and carry purses, while men eat hot dogs and would rather not even touch a purse. The not-so-implicit message is that it is demeaning for a "real" man to do a female thing like hold a purse. In 30 seconds the advertiser has reminded us of the differences between men and women in terms of behavior, including eating, as well as status.

Recognition of such differences is the starting point for much of feminist psychology. Although liberal and postmodern feminist theories are represented in psychology (e.g., Tavris, 1992), cultural feminism has been the dominant approach. Psychologists have routinely argued that women have a "different voice" than men, a voice rooted in a developmental process that is more relationship-oriented than independence-oriented (Chodorow, 1978; Gilligan, 1982; Miller, 1976). Unlike men, who are socialized to be assertive and even aggressive, thereby establishing and fiercely defending their independent functioning, women are raised to be sensitive to the needs of others and to value relationships over self. In a patriarchal society, women's experiences and values have lower status (de Beauvoir, 1952). Women's interests and needs are often belittled and treated as secondary to those of men. Cultural feminists (e.g., Wolf, 1991) often suggest that greater respect for women's perspectives, especially for women's emphasis on relationships, will at least partially remedy the negative effects of the lower status of women and their experiences.

Cultural feminism, unlike, for example, liberal feminism, is willing to acknowledge gender differences in behaviors. Indeed, some feminist theorists celebrate gender differences and advocate creation of rituals and systems that support women's experiences and values (Belensky, Clinchy, Goldberger, & Tarule, 1986; Piran, 1999b; Wolf, 1991). Given the differences in a wide range of behaviors, it is not surprising to cultural feminists that men and women display different behavioral problems, including differences in eating problems and disorders. In the same vein, the pronounced gender differences in eating problems and disorders have made feminist perspectives important in understanding their etiology, treatment, and prevention.

GENDER AND EATING DISORDERS

Few disorders defined by *DSM-IV-TR* (2000) show gender differences as large as those found for AN and BN. With a ratio of 9–10 women for every man diagnosed, the gender differences for AN and BN are substantially larger than for depression, panic disorder with agoraphobia, autism, drug abuse, and antisocial personality disorder, all of which are considered gendered disorders (*DSM-IV-TR*, 2000). Individual symptoms of AN and BN, such as body dissatisfaction even when weight is within the normal range, are more common among girls and women than among boys and men, although the differences are not as pronounced as those for AN and BN (see chapter 2). Behaviors that are related to AN and BN as concomitants, symptoms, or risk factors, including intense weight concerns, dieting, and purging behavior, are also more common among girls and women than among boys and men (Smolak & Levine, 2001b). In fact, the differences between women and men are greater in terms of taking action to alter body shape and weight than in body dissatisfaction (Muth & Cash, 1997). In general, girls and women are more intensely and personally invested in body shape and in appearance than are males.

If body dissatisfaction is defined in terms of satisfaction with weight and shape (as opposed to hair or facial features), gender differences emerge in elementary school (see Smolak & Levine, 2001b, for a review). Gender differences in dieting and exercising to lose weight also emerge in elementary school, and these differences are often fairly large, even at this young age. For example, in a sample of 9- to 11-year-old White American children, 33% of the girls and 17% of the boys worried "very often" about being too fat (Gustafson-Larson & Terry, 1992). In a study of 8- to 10-year-olds, 55% of the girls and 35% of the boys were dissatisfied with their size (Wood, Becker, & Thompson, 1996). Although data are quite limited, similar childhood gender differences emerge in various countries (e.g., Australia, Great Britain) as well as in American ethnic groups (e.g., African Americans; Dounchis et al., 2001; Smolak & Levine, 2001b). Despite lower rates of body dissatisfaction among Black than White girls in the United States, Black girls have poorer body esteem than do Black boys. Gender effects apparently cross ethnic and cultural lines (Smolak & Levine, 2001b). As discussed in chapter 3, studies concerning males, body image, eating problems, and muscularity underscore the gendered nature of body image and eating disorders. It is not that boys and men do not have weight, shape, and eating concerns and problems. Rather, their body image and eating problems tend to be different from the problems girls have (e.g., Parkinson, Tovée, & Cohen-Tovée, 1998; Schur, Sanders, & Steiner, 2000; but see Thompson, Corwin, & Sargent, 1997).

Explaining Gender Differences in Eating Problems

The consistency and magnitude of gender differences in body image and eating problems mandate that any etiological theory address gender. Ironically, however, gender differences are often assumed rather than explained. Many biological models, for example, do not explain why women's brains might predispose them, but rarely men, to AN and BN (see chapter 3). Similarly, because many studies of sociocultural factors include only females in their samples, it is often unclear which putative risk factors occur at a higher rate or frequency among girls, or why and how the risk factors might be processed differently by girls.

That said, the single most common approach to explaining the special vulnerability of girls and women to eating problems and disorders is to suggest that girls are exposed to some experiences that boys are not. Media images of women, for example, are an important influence on girls' body image (Groesz et al., 2002; Levine & Smolak, 1996; Thompson et al., 1999). Peer discussions of body shape and weight are more common, and more influential on body image, among girls than boys (Nichter, 2000; Paxton, 1999; Vincent & McCabe, 2000). Sexual abuse and sexual harassment, both of which victimize girls more often than boys, also appear to be important factors in the gender differences in body image (Connors, 2001; Harned, 2000; Larkin et al., 1999; Murnen & Smolak, 2000).

Gender differences in individual risk and protective factors do not tell the whole story. For example, Vincent and McCabe (2000) found that adolescent boys actually reported more negative comments from peers about their bodies than did girls. Yet, girls had significantly higher body dissatisfaction and a higher drive for thinness. Smolak, Levine, and Thompson (2001) reported that boys ages 12 through 14 were aware of and internalized an "ideal," muscular male body image. However, this process was less related to body dissatisfaction, weight loss, and attempts to build muscles than girls' awareness and internalization of a thin feminine ideal body shape was to girls' body dissatisfaction and weight loss efforts. Murnen and Smolak (2000) found that frequency of sexual harassment experiences was related to body esteem in elementary school girls but not boys.

Such findings suggest that the interpretation and meaning of body-related messages differ for boys and girls. Apparently, the different experience of growing up female compared to growing up male somehow sensitizes girls to body-related messages. Objectification theory, articulated by Fredrickson and Roberts (1997), provides a framework for understanding how this process might occur. Together with feminist therapy principles (e.g., Piran, 2001; Wooley, 1994), objectification theory also provides ideas for developing prevention programs.

OBJECTIFICATION THEORY

Objectification theory (Fredrickson & Roberts, 1997; McKinley, 2002) is built on the assumption that society conceptualizes and treats men's and women's bodies differently. Women's bodies are seen and thought of as passive objects for the viewing pleasure of others, particularly men, whereas men's bodies are seen as active, for accomplishing things such as sports or heavy labor. The fact that women's bodies are to be looked at means that they must be available as well as pleasant and even pleasurable to the eye. Girls and women learn these lessons early and are reminded of them throughout their lives. They look to other people, particularly men, for approval of their appearance. Gradually, girls and women internalize the evaluative gaze of others, which leads adolescent girls and women to self-consciously monitor their own bodies from an outside perspective so as to better maintain an attractive appearance. This is known as *self-objectification* or *objectified body consciousness*.

This section examines three components of objectification theory. First is the proposition that women's bodies are sexually objectified in modern societies. This objectification is pervasive enough to be taught to and to affect even relatively young girls. Second, we examine evidence that self-objectification does occur. Finally, we consider self-objectification theory's explanation of the development of negative body image and eating problems. Fredrickson and Roberts (1997) view eating disorders as one of the major problems growing directly out of objectification.

Sexual Objectification

The idea that bodies carry culturally laden meaning is neither new nor unique to psychology (Bordo, 1993; Foucault, 1979). The bodies of prisoners and slaves, for example, have been conceptualized and treated differently from those of the ruling elite. The horrific example of the Tuskegee syphilis studies, in which Black men were intentionally left untreated for this fatal disease, underscores the cultural meaning of the body of a poor person from an ethnic minority group. Social status has consistently been a factor in determining the meaning and treatment of bodies.

And so it is, too, with men and women. Women hold lower status than men do. Women make less money, are less likely to hold high political office, and are less likely to be CEOs than men are. Women are also much more likely to be victims of men's violence than men are to be victimized by women. Part of the greater financial and political power of men is that women are typically defined in relation to men. This is analogous to the definition of ethnic minority members in terms of the White majority's values, behaviors, and beliefs (McLoyd, 1999).

Women's bodies are culturally defined as being intended for men's enjoyment. There is a pervasive, consistent, and strong message that girls and women who meet the cultural definition of beautiful are highly paid; in fact, they are often among the highest female earners in the United

States. Women in advertisements are posed in ways that enhance their sexuality while emphasizing their accessibility and reducing their individuality (Bordo, 1993; Kilbourne, 1994). So, for example, women's breasts or legs might be shown without a face. Indeed, women's bodies are pictured without heads more frequently than are men's bodies. Women might be posed lying on beds with their legs spread or sucking on some vaguely (or not so vaguely) phallic object. Even the women—and young girls—who are supposed to appeal to preteen girls are often pictured in provocative clothes and poses, baring midriffs or exposing breasts.

The importance of women's role as objects to be looked at by men is evident in the products marketed to and for women. What is the male equivalent of *Victoria's Secret*? What is the male equivalent of the Wonder Bra? Americans, predominantly women, spend over $8 billion on make-up and beauty products every year (The World's Priorities, 2001). Americans, again particularly women, also buy diet and exercise products, to the tune of at least $30 billion, to try to achieve the desirable thin body (Papazian, 1991). Even more dramatically, breast enhancement and liposuction are now the most common plastic surgery procedures. The clients are overwhelmingly female (Sawrer, 2001).

Plastic surgery may be the only way for many women to achieve the dominant culturally sanctioned image of women as thin with large breasts. The unrealistically thin image that continues to dominate print media, television, and movies is an image (an object) designed for viewing. It is not an image associated with good health, sports participation, intelligence, educational attainment, or motherhood. Indeed, the women presented by mass media are often posed so as to appear passive, vulnerable, and available rather than active, busy, and self-contained (Bordo, 1993; Kilbourne, 1994).

Other behaviors, most notably sexual harassment and sexual violence, reflect the culturally approved availability of women's bodies. Even elementary school boys feel entitled to comment on girls' bodies in ways that girls are apparently not comfortable commenting on boys' bodies (Murnen & Smolak, 2000; Stein, 1999). Certainly boys are teased about their bodies. However, the perpetrators tend to be other boys, as they jockey for hierarchical status among themselves (Stein, 1999). But, generally speaking, boys have status over girls, at least in terms of their ability to remark on and touch girls' bodies without the girls' permission.

This effect is even more dramatic in terms of sexual violence. Child sexual abuse, relationship violence, date rape, and stranger rape are all most commonly perpetrated on girls and women by boys and men (Connors, 2001). When boys are the victims, the perpetrator is still more likely to be a man than a woman. Sexual terrorism theory (Sheffield, 1995) suggests that the effects of rape go beyond the effects on the individual woman who is victimized. The threat of rape serves to keep women in their lower status position, depending on men for protection from other men.

Sexual evaluation and commercial exploitation of women's bodies (as occurs routinely in the media, including the multibillion-dollar pornography industry), sexual harassment, and sexual violence are all part of a continuum of the sexualization of women's bodies (Fredrickson & Roberts, 1997; Sheffield, 1995). These processes represent different levels of ecological influence (see chapter 4). The media are probably part of the exosystem (i.e., factors that affect the child but are not necessarily part of the child's daily, direct interactions). Sexual harassment and violence, on the other hand, are perpetrated by people in the child's microsystem, such as siblings, stepfathers, coaches, and classmates. Thus, feminist theory in general and objectification theory in particular emphasize the importance of change at various levels of the ecological system.

Self-Objectification

Some media images of men are not particularly realistic either. Many are unusually muscular, including the action figures with which young boys play and the professional wrestlers who are enormously popular with adolescent boys and young men (Pope, Olivardia, Gruber, & Borowiecki, 1999; Pope et al., 2000). As noted previously, boys are aware of these images and even internalize them (Smolak, Levine, & Thompson, 2001). Yet, boys are less affected than girls who are exposed to analogous images, in part because the number, consistency, and strength of messages vary by gender (Smolak & Levine, 2001b). However, it is also very likely that girls feel more pressure to achieve the media beauty ideals because of self-objectification.

Self-objectification means the gaze of others is internalized such that women think about and judge their own attractiveness as sexual objects (Fredrickson & Roberts, 1997). This process is often facilitated by the use of mirrors, which grant a form of external perspective (Cash, 1997). Women, and even girls, know they should be sexy. But being sexy has its costs. Women live with the threat of rape as well as with the normative experience of being sexually harassed. Middle and high school girls, much more frequently than boys, report feeling self-conscious and embarrassed by sexual harassment; girls are also much more likely to change their behavior in response to sexual harassment (American Association of University Women, 2001). The fact that the victim, not the perpetrator, changes her behavior underscores who has higher status in this situation and thus who has the responsibility for sustained self-monitoring.

Women also understand, even as children and adolescents, the importance of being thin to their future social and economic success. Women who are obese earn 40% less over their lifetimes than normal weight women do, after controlling for age, education, health, professional status, and marital status (Fat is a financial issue, 2000). Heavier women are less likely to get dates and get married (see Fredrickson & Roberts, 1997, and Rothblum, 1994, for reviews). It is reasonable, then, that women come to see attractiveness as important to their future success. For women, beauty is power, opening doors financially and socially. How central this equation is to a girl's self-definition will depend on her experiences, including the presence of protective factors that counteract some of the objectification. It is important to emphasize that "women's experience is variable, proximally caused, and context dependent" (Fredrickson & Roberts, 1997, p. 381).

Self-objectification leads to self-monitoring or self-surveillance. A girl will watch her body for signs that she is becoming too fat, too flabby, or generally less attractive. This may be why one study found that boys' body esteem and weight loss attempts rely more on direct encouragement from others to lose weight, whereas girls respond to parental and peer modeling and discussion of weight and shape (Vincent & McCabe, 2000). The girls, who are already self-monitoring, respond to very subtle pressure while the boys, who are not self-monitoring, react only when someone else evaluates their bodies and tells them to lose weight.

Using the two psychometrically sound measures of self-objectification that have been developed (McKinley & Hyde, 1996; Noll & Fredrickson, 1998), researchers have indeed found support for the hypotheses based on objectification theory. The theory has been used to predict age-related decreases in self-objectification, group differences in self-objectification (e.g., dancers vs. nondancers; Tiggemann & Slater, 2001), and effects of experimental manipulation of self-monitoring. For example, as predicted, trying on a bathing suit so focused women on their bodies that they actually performed more poorly on math problems than women who had not tried on swimsuits or than men (Fredrickson, Roberts, Noll, Quinn, & Twenge, 1998). All of these studies have involved adult women as participants. A recent study with first through fifth grade children suggests that girls and boys do recognize objectified images of women and men as desirable, and that girls, more than boys, take these to heart to develop self-related attitudes (Murnen et al., 2003).

Effects of Self-Objectification

In their formulation of objectification theory, Fredrickson and Roberts (1997) proposed that self-objectification has many negative effects on women. Women who self-monitor experience not just appearance anxiety, but also body shame, characteristics psychologists have associated with women since the time of Freud. Because women are focused on self-conscious surveillance of their external appearance, they also have less psychic energy to spend on internal states. Consequently, women are less in tune with and less trusting of needs and feeling arising from their own bodies. This process also renders women less able to attend to other problems. This argument is consistent with findings of poor interoceptive awareness among eating disorders clients (Garner, 1991) as well as with discussions of loss of voice and dis-embodiment among adolescent girls (Brown & Gilligan, 1992; Piran, 2002). Focusing on external appearance also interferes with women's ability to experience "flow," that is, optimal experiences of embodiment and effective performance that are an important source of fulfillment. All of this culminates in women experiencing certain types of psychopathology, most notably, unipolar depression, sexual dysfunction, eating problems, and eating disorders (Fredrickson & Roberts, 1997; McKinley, 2002).

Research has indeed found that self-objectification and self-surveillance are related to body image and eating problems (Fredrickson et al., 1998; McKinley, 1998, 1999; Tiggemann & Lynch, 2001; Tiggemann & Slater, 2001; see also Cash, 1996, 1997). Internalization of the thin ideal, which may be seen as at least an indirect measure of self-objectification, is one of the best predictors of body esteem and eating problems (Stice, 2002; Thompson & Stice, 2001). Furthermore, factors that are hypothesized to lead to self-objectification, most notably sexual harassment and exposure to media images, have also been found to be related to body image and eating problems (Groesz et al., 2002;

Harned, 2000; Larkin et al., 1999; Murnen & Smolak, 2000; Murnen et al., 2003; Smolak & Murnen, 2004).

Researchers in the field of early childhood education have long known about the "wash-out effect." If you put young, disadvantaged children in high quality child care for a year or two, they make meaningful cognitive, linguistic, and social gains. However, if they return to an environment that continues to disadvantage them educationally, financially, and socially, the gains are lost. Feminists make a similar suggestion about eating disorders prevention. Prevention programs aimed only at changing the attitudes of individual girls may temporarily reduce body dissatisfaction or plans to diet (see chapter 9 for documentation and discussion of this "program participation effect"). But returning girls to an environment in which they continue to be objectified will likely counteract those gains, pushing the girls back to high, but normative, levels of body dissatisfaction and eating problems. Thus, feminist theory argues that prevention programs need to focus on a critique and transformation of the environment. To do this, methods of program development and delivery need to change. We address these methodological issues before presenting a model feminist prevention program.

ISSUES IN PROGRAM DEVELOPMENT AND DELIVERY

Feminists have long critiqued the research methodology traditionally used in psychology and other sciences. One goal of traditional psychological research, based on the philosophical tradition of logical positivism, is to be as context-free as possible. Presumably, this enables the researcher to generate psychological principles with general, even universal, applicability. The "gold standard" for such research is the laboratory experiment, in which the researcher can, at least in theory, control all "extraneous" variables, that is, anything other than the independent variable that is being manipulated. One reason we typically need research to "translate" laboratory findings into applied research is because the former lacks ecological validity.

Some feminists argue that this decontextualized approach reflects masculine values of independence over relatedness, logic and laws over emotional understanding in specific situations, and observability over intuition or self-knowledge. Within this traditional, decontextualized approach, the researcher stands outside of the research, detached from the participants; he or she is an expert who oversees the generation of hypotheses and the interpretation of quantitative data. Feminist researchers adopt an expanded model of research that gives the participants a more central role in generating ideas and explanations. Expertise lies in the participants, who are more familiar with their own lives, feelings, and experiences than is the researcher. In this approach the researcher is no longer a detached expert, instructing lower status "subjects" and interpreting their experiences. Instead, he or she must make connections with the participants in order to relate to and otherwise understand their lived experiences.

To credit research participants with this knowledge is a first step in giving them "voice" (Gilligan, 1982). This is particularly important because feminist researchers view many of the extant measures of behavior as reflecting a male bias. This is evident in the field of eating disorders in several ways. For example, much of the research starts with the assumption that eating disorders are individual pathologies rather than adjustments to toxic societal roles and demeaning, stressful experiences. Moreover, the individual variables that researchers and therapists often focus on, such as family cohesion or self-esteem, are not the ecological ones that girls and women tend to bring up when asked about the sources of their body shame or eating problems. Girls and women tend to talk about the lack of respect for their bodies that they routinely encounter, often in the form of sexual harassment or sexual abuse (Larkin et al., 1999; Piran, 2001, 2002; Wooley, 1994). Consistent with objectification theory and with the ecological perspective discussed in chapter 4, the methodology of feminist prevention programs presumes that poor body esteem and eating problems are rooted in the societal conceptualization and treatment of women's bodies.

A common goal of prevention work is to take basic research generated from a model (such as social cognitive theory), use it to select appropriate variables, and then design an intervention program (see chapter 1). As noted in chapter 7, many critics of prevention efforts have, in fact, argued that we do not yet know enough about the risk factors and processes involved in the development of eating problems to design effective prevention programs. This, they suggest, is why so few programs have been successful. Feminists such as Piran (1995, 2001), Steiner-Adair (1994), Friedman (1999, 2000, 2003), and Smolak and Murnen (2001, 2004) offer an alternate explanation. They argue that prevention programs based on the social cognitive or cognitive-behavioral models have addressed the wrong variables in the wrong manner because these programs have failed to recognize the societal, gendered (in the sense of female lived experiences) nature of the problem. There are, then, at least two issues to be considered in terms of methods for establishing a prevention "program." The first is to share with the participants the role of expert, allowing them to voice and clarify their own concerns. The second is to use these concerns—and not solely a predetermined curriculum or lesson plan with fixed and generalized content—as the basis of the prevention or intervention program, even if, as is typically the case, that means challenging authority and making fundamental changes in the girls' immediate environment.

Voice

The concept of "voice" was popularized in psychology by Gilligan (1982). Using interview techniques and qualitative data analysis (see Brown & Gilligan, 1992, and Taylor, Gilligan, & Sullivan, 1995, for an explanation), Gilligan and her colleagues found that adolescent girls were so invested in maintaining relatedness and relationships that they gradually lost their ability to express and even recognize their own opinions. This lack of expression was not simply indicative of shyness or nonassertiveness. Instead, the girls were losing touch with what they actually felt or thought. Multiple social influences made it clear to them that "nice" girls do not express their own opinions. Rather, "good" girls try to have friends, get along at school, and generally conform to the image of girls as pretty, passive, and nurturing.

Nowhere is this message clearer than in terms of sexual harassment (Stein, 1999). When faced with sexual harassment, girls who "speak up" are frequently told by friends or family to "ignore" it. The harassment is often excused or minimized as "just boys being boys." Even when girls do seek help from a teacher or principal, the result is often that the harassment does not stop and may even worsen (Stein, 1999). Schools tend either to downplay harassment, saying they cannot do much because of the lack of witnesses or corroboration, or to overreact, disciplining rather than educating boys even for relatively small infractions. The lack of education concerning harassment, in turn, means that the offending boy is more likely to receive social support and attention for being "wrongly" punished, leaving the girl ostracized. Both under- and overreaction teach girls that it is better to suffer the indignities, and even the dangers, of violations to their own bodies and personal space, than to speak up and turn their relational world into chaos and isolation. Once you can no longer speak up to protect your own body, what can you speak up about?

Once more, society's treatment of girls as primarily a body affects girls' self-definition and behavior. The objectification of women contributes to a belittling of their opinions and ideas, which in turn becomes a silencing of the self. Research suggests that college women's level of voice, as measured by two different scales, is related to eating problems. This is not true of college men (Smolak & Munstertieger, 2002). An interview study with high school girls (Steiner-Adair, 1986) also pointed to lack of voice as contributing to eating problems.

Therefore, a major goal in feminist prevention programs is to help girls reclaim their voices. Several prominent feminists in our field argue that one powerful way to do this is to through group discussions that are reminiscent of the consciousness-raising groups of the 1960s and 1970s. The girls are encouraged to describe their feelings and experiences and to express their opinions. There is a trained facilitator, who must be open to substantial input from the girls themselves in guiding the discussion. Granting girls this level of authority is a more difficult task than it might seem. Most adults assume an expert position when talking with girls, and this status disparity will be salient in a prevention program initiated by adults. Consequently, the facilitator needs to be aware of and careful with her own knowledge and biases about what is important in understanding body image and eating disorders in the particular context, for example, a school in Boston or in Tucson. An awareness of how power and status can be simultaneously misleading and silencing, coupled with an overt respect for the girls' lived experiences and their voices, helps the facilitator to generate respectful dialogues with the girls. This attitude also helps the group leader to manage her frustration during times when the girls "just don't see" the factors that the adult expert "knows" are likely to be influencing body image, eating, and weight management in various ways. The facilitator makes many important contributions to the group and, hopefully, to the girls as individuals. But, for voice to be reinstated and reinforced, girls need to feel they are being heard and thus being taken seriously.

These group discussions can validate a girl's experiences. This helps her feel less alone in what she experiences and in the things she wants to see changed, and enables her to believe that change is possible. Of course, validation can occur only if the girls are supportive of one another. Consequently, part of the facilitator's role is to model and otherwise encourage a supportive atmosphere. Sometimes, preexisting relationships among the girls or a school's atmosphere make this impossible (Friedman, 1999). In general, however, girls are willing to support and help each other in these groups.

Neither group cohesion nor the willingness of individual girls to speak up and speak out develops overnight. It typically takes several sessions for girls to feel sufficiently comfortable with the facilitator and with the group before they will get to the core issues in their lives (Piran, 1999a). Again, girls have been taught, both directly and indirectly, not to talk about certain things, including sexual harassment and unrealistic social demands for thinness. They have already learned the perspective emphasized in the training of many mental health professionals: Negative body image and eating problems are private, *individual* problems encased in anxiety and shame. As noted, society has built a variety of supports for silencing girls. Therefore, the discussion group needs to constitute itself as a new society, a place that is different from everywhere else the girls have been, a place where girls can speak up and be heard about anything and everything.

Time and patience are part of the process of helping the girls to construct a new microsystem (see chapter 4) that will give them enough small but positive experiences with voice to counteract their previous experiences of being silenced. Patience is part of the aforementioned respect the facilitator shows the girls, thereby proving to them that their feelings and desires for change will be taken very seriously. Another part of this process is the facilitator's determination and skill in serving as an advocate for the changes the girls believe are important.

Lived Experience and the Selection of Proximal Goals for Prevention

Most commonly, eating disorders prevention programs try to reduce internalization of a thin ideal, increase acceptance of a range of body types, decrease weight concerns and calorie-restrictive dieting, and improve body esteem. These are reasonable goals given the research on risk factors for the development of eating disorders (see chapter 5).

In feminist prevention programs the intervention variables are not entirely determined prior to the program, and in some instances they may not be predetermined at all. Feminist programs, like more traditional social cognitive programs, do provide information about nutrition, exercise, pubertal development, mass media, teasing, weightist prejudices, and other variables that tend to influence body esteem and eating problems. In some programs, such as *Full of Ourselves: Advancing Girl Power, Health, and Leadership* (Steiner-Adair et al., 2002), provision of information is built into numerous activities that are part of a curriculum (see also Neumark-Sztainer, Sherwood, Coller, & Hannan, 2000). In Piran's (1995) feminist program (discussed in the next section), there is no curriculum or preestablished set of "lessons" whatsoever, because relational dialogue is the foundation for construction of the key issues and relevant information. In either case, feminist prevention programs make an effort to provide information that satisfies two basic criteria. First, the information is relevant to the girls' interests and lived experience. Second, knowledge that emerges from dialogues between the specialist's expertise and the girls' articulation of what they are going through can be translated into plans for personal and group action to change unhealthy sociocultural contexts.

The variables addressed by feminist prevention programs are determined to some degree by the participating girls, based on their particular experiences in the school or whatever the context of prevention might be. The facilitator, whether she is the program designer or a trained staff member, must be prepared to help the girls elaborate and follow up on their context-specific concerns and ideas. For example, in one school the factor that strongly influences body image and eating problems might be sexual harassment, whereas in another school it might be racism or competition with males for the staff's attention (Piran, 1999c). Regardless of the girls' specific concerns, helping them to analyze the key issues in their lives and to take constructive action requires the facilitator to be an advocate for the girls. The facilitator may need, for example, to go to school administrators to ask for changes in school policy. Or she may need to help the girls arrange for a meeting with a local retailer whose advertising policies objectify and exploit women, to help them prepare their presentation, and to accompany them to the meeting. All this means that the facilitator must have substantial support from, for example, the school administration or other organizations in the community (see chapter 15). Not surprisingly, such support is not always easy to arrange and requires its own forms of advocacy and intervention in the girls' ecology. But support from powerful adults in the girls' immediate environment is imperative for the success of a feminist approach. The girls need to know that their concerns are taken seriously by at least one adult who has the skill and courage to act on their behalf as well as with them (Piran, 1999b, 1999c, 2001).

Thus, providing girls with a forum may in and of itself result in some improvements in body image and eating problems. Activities and opportunities that increase girls' voice may decrease eating problems. But it is also very important for the facilitator to act on the girls' ideas and to support their efforts toward action. For voice to be reinstated, and for objectification to be eliminated, the girls need to feel that they are being listened to, being heard, and being taken seriously.

A FEMINIST PROGRAM

To summarize briefly, the feminist model of prevention emphasizes the importance of gender role, objectification, and loss of voice in the development of the spectrum of negative body image and disordered eating for girls and women. According to this model, the antidote to these toxic influences consists of opportunities for positive experiences "in" one's body (i.e., for "embodiment"), for establishment of voice, and for an assertive, effective presence ("substance") in the world that is not defined by appearance. These opportunities are created through relational dialogues in a setting that respects females, through activism and advocacy by the girls in order to improve their own and other people's body image and eating, and through advocacy and mentoring by the group facilitator. Based on these components, we refer to this approach as the feminist-empowerment-relational (FER) model (see Levine & Piran, 2001, 2004; Striegel-Moore & Steiner-Adair, 1998).

As of December 2004, only a handful of prevention programs have been developed and applied from an FER perspective. *Full of Ourselves*, developed by Steiner-Adair et al. (2002) at the Harvard Eating Disorders Center, is reviewed in chapter 9. Two media literacy programs (also curriculum-based) also incorporate key features of the FER model. *Free to be Me* (Neumark-Sztainer et al., 2000) and *GO GIRLS!*™ (Levine, Piran, & Stoddard, 1999) are reviewed in chapter 13.

Sandra Friedman, a Canadian therapist and prevention specialist, has designed a feminist program, but it has not been formally evaluated. *Just for Girls* (Friedman, 1999, 2000) uses open groups in which an adult woman helps middle school girls to "decode the language of fat" by discussing negative experiences concerning their bodies. These conversations foster a critical perspective for understanding why young adolescent girls are sometimes hit by the "grungies," which are negative, isolating feelings about the self. Clarification of these feelings through sharing and discussion enables the girls to learn how to deal effectively with them, mainly through communicating and connecting with other girls. Thus, *Just for Girls* uses feminist methods to provide young adolescent girls with a safe and supportive environment in which to critique their environment and thereby find and express their voices in regard to very significant aspects of their lives.

The Ballet School Study

In a series of papers, Niva Piran of the University of Toronto described her feminist prevention work in a residential school that trains elite students ages 10 to 18 to be world-class ballet dancers (Piran, 1998, 1999a, 1999b, 1999c, 2001). Although Piran prefers now to call hers a "relational empowerment" (Levine & Piran, 2001) or "critical social perspectives" approach (Piran, 2002; see also Levine & Piran, 2004), this intervention embodies FER principles in two major ways. First, Piran carefully and patiently established trusting, supportive, and respectful relationships with the staff and students. These relationships became the foundation for dialogues that enabled Piran and the "stakeholders" (administration, staff, and students) to activate key processes for improving the students' experiences within the school contexts (see chapters 10 & 12). Second, unlike almost all other prevention programs (see chapter 13), Piran's intervention actually changed the environments and daily experiences of the ballet students. Piran was certainly an important agent of change, but part of her impact was her ability to get adults in the students' environment to take responsibility for their role as socialization agents in the development of positive body image and healthy eating behavior in adolescent girls and boys.

Piran has written and spoken extensively about her work. Consequently, the following is a distillation of her approach (for other summaries see also Levine & Piran, 2001; Levine & Smolak, 2002). Piran's model is summarized in Table 8.1.

Key Change Processes. There are four important processes operating in Piran's relational-empowerment program. The first, as discussed previously, is *Facilitator Advocacy*. In her role of consultant to the ballet school, Piran was able to meet with both administrators and

TABLE 8.1
Key Components and Change Processes in Piran's Ballet School Study

Factor	Content Themes	Mechanisms for Learning
Connection-Relation-Dialogue &	*Ownership of the Body* • who dictates food choices? • who dictates appearance? • objectification (e.g., harassment and sexualization) • disruption of privacy and of natural processes such as menstruation	+ Sharing and communicating in a safe, respectful atmosphere + Listening carefully and thinking reflectively and critically + Understanding and feeling how shared experiences are influenced by context
Consciousness-Raising and Critical Knowledge	*Prejudicial Treatment* • weightism • sexism • race & ethnicity *Social Construction of Women* • women and power • body functions • control and compliance • voice, assertion, and anger • boy–girl relationships and responses to success and failure *Weight and Shape Concerns* • body mass, strength, and substance • teasing • dieting and success in ballet	+ Facilitator–student dialogues that conclude with proposed solutions to specific problems (e.g., a curriculum that emphasizes health and safety for dancers) + Facilitator input, including knowledge, questions, and techniques for stimulating constructive group processes

Environmental Changes (based on content themes from dialogues and consciousness-raising)	*Within the Groups* • Girls' norms and actions in regard to peer relations *School-Wide* • Girls' norms and actions in regard to peer relations • Norms and actions in regard to girl–boy relations • Girl–staff relationships • School policies, norms, and programs • Staffing • Physical setting	+ Student-guided changes + Facilitator advocacy + Facilitator–student–staff dialogues and relationships + Students support for each other while advocating for real change
Facilitator Advocacy	• Context-specific, systemic approach • Focus on the students and staff as the real source of potential changes in the environment that will improve health *and* performance • Focus on gender, prejudice, and inequity in the domain of the body, and how they contribute to negative body image and eating problems	+ Solid, respectful relationships with staff and students + Education of staff and students, in part through consciousness-raising in relational settings + Serving as model for positive body image, critical consciousness, and strong, embodied woman + Collaboration with students to advocate for the environmental changes they feel are necessary and fair

Note. This table is based on information contained in Piran (2001).

staff. She agreed to take the consulting position only if the administration was willing to follow through with reasonable, well-substantiated requests for change that would be made not only by Piran, but also by the ballet students themselves. As an advocate for a critical perspective—and for change—in regard to the school (and not the psychology of individual students per se), Piran laid the foundation for an ecological perspective, as well as for herself as a mentor and healthy role model.

The second critical process is *Knowledge-Through-Dialogue*. Piran met 2 to 10 times per year with age- and gender-segregated groups of adolescents. Consistent with the FER model, Piran assumes that the most important factors shaping gender roles, body image, and eating attitudes and behaviors are specific to the context of the adolescents' lives, in this case the ballet school. Furthermore, she assumes that a primary source of expertise about the nature and operation of those factors is the students themselves. Consequently, one goal of the discussion groups (a goal articulated by the girls themselves) was to create a space—the only such space in the students' lives—of respect and trust in which they could (re)learn to voice their "lived experiences" in regard to the body. It is very important to note that for the girls the topics of these discussions, although they touched on media, drive for thinness, and fear of fat (see chapter 5), revolved around feeling lost and out of control in a female body that was exposed, powerless, and devalued (Piran, 2001). As expected on the basis of Piran's (1995) theory, this knowledge, constructed from dialogues within the group, changed from shared private feelings (e.g., of anxiety, shame, anger) about body dissatisfaction to a consensual group understanding of, and discontent with, contextual factors such as gender inequity and sexual harassment. The girls' construction and voicing of context-specific knowledge—coupled with Piran's expertise, accurate empathy, and advocacy—created a new context in which "*internal struggles with body weight and shape were re-examined and reframed as informative clues for social change*" (Piran, 1999a, p. 80; italics in the original).

The third critical process is *Within-Group Transformation*. As they came to understand openly and fully the negative emotional impact of unfair school policies and of objectification by some teachers and staff, the students also forced each other to acknowledge the ways in which they colluded in these unhealthy influences on body image and gender role identity. Voicing the truths in their lives involved an acknowledgment of the power of contexts, and this, in turn, led students to adopt healthier values, norms, and practices within the groups.

Advocacy for change within the groups was an important developmental step toward the final key change process: *Ecological Activism*. In the FER model, a critically important extension of *knowing* and *voicing* what is going on is knowing *what needs to be done*. Building on Piran's status as an advocate for systemic change, students were encouraged to use the authority reinforced in the discussion groups to "speak up" and "speak out" to the administration in order to initiate the changes necessary for making their school a place that fosters positive body image, healthy eating, and better dancers. Such changes included (a) training males about what is required to be a safe, respectful partner in *pas-de-deux* classes; (b) developing a school-wide code of ethics about sexual harassment; and (c) removing a teacher from the staff because of his continually disrespectful behavior toward girls' bodies. Ecological activism helps complete the process of transforming the body from a place of confused, silent shame to a site of forceful, constructive action. It also establishes a developmental cycle of dialogue, reflection, and action (Piran, 2001).

Outcome Evaluation. Piran's (1999a) evaluation of the ballet school intervention did not include an experimental–control comparison because the school's combination of ballet and academics in a residential setting is unique. Rather, the eating attitudes and behaviors of all female students ages 12 to 18 were surveyed at baseline (1987; $N = 68$), 4 years later ($N = 65$), and 9 years later ($N = 65$). Prior to the intervention, this highly competitive ballet school was definitely an environment that fostered a spectrum of eating problems and disorders (Garner & Garfinkel, 1980; Piran, 1999a). Although this is not a longitudinal or sequential cohort design, over time and across the three different cohorts of girls, the prevalence of AN dropped tenfold to just 1%, while there were no new cases of BN. In addition, although these elite ballet students remained very concerned about sugar and fat consumption, the rates of binge eating, self-induced vomiting, laxative use, restrictive dieting, and fasting and skipping meals all dropped significantly. Moreover, for girls ages 15 through 18, the percentage scoring above the high-risk mark of 20 on the Eating Attitudes Test fell from nearly 50% in 1987 to around 17% in 1991, where it remained in 1996. The comparable figures for the younger girls (13% to 9% to around 5%) also suggested that the program was having the desired effects. Not surprisingly, these reductions in eating problems were accompanied by improvements in body image for both age groups.

Piran (1999a) acknowledges that the lack of a comparison group means these findings must be interpreted cautiously. Nevertheless, the multifaceted evidence of a prevention effect, coupled with the continuing status of the ballet world as a breeding ground for eating disorders (Piran, 1999b; see Tiggemann & Slater, 2001, for a review), strongly suggests that her FER approach is deserving of serious attention. In this regard, extensive field notes and other qualitative data support the hypothesized processes of prevention as they emerged from cycles of relationship, dialogue, reflection, and action to change individual behavior, group norms, and, most important, the ballet school environment (Piran, 2001).

SUMMARY: PROTOTYPICAL FEATURES OF FEMINIST PROGRAMS

Table 8.2 lists eight prototypical features of the feminist-empowerment-relational model. In the next chapter we rate each of the prevention programs being evaluated as to how many of these eight features it con-

TABLE 8.2
Prototypical Elements in the Feminist-Empowerment-Relational Approach to Prevention

1. Critical analysis of the gendered issues (e.g., objectification, identity, power, opportunity, etc.) contributing to negative body image and disordered eating.
2. Opportunities for dialogue about the meaning and social construction of gender (in)equity, adolescent development, and ethnicity [shared element with NSVS model].
3. Situating "knowledge," program goals, and motivation for change to a meaningful degree in the lived experience and analytical abilities of participants, not in "lessons" from experts.
4. Construction of safe "spaces" for dialogue and relationship development in order to give voice to knowledge and to develop strategies for activism.
5. Dialogues with various "stakeholders" in the system (e.g., the school) to ensure that a variety of participants are involved in clarifying the issues and creating positive changes [shared element with NSVS model].
6. Emphasis on the transformation of knowledge and relationships into community-oriented actions that make the body a site of active, constructive change (not a locus of private anxiety and shame).
7. Mentoring by an adult woman who serves as a group facilitator and a forceful advocate for systemic change, in part through coordination of dialogue between students, educators, and parents.
8. Creating healthier peer norms, school policies, teacher behavior, and community practices [shared element with NSVS model and with SCT theory, if not practice].

tains. Recently, Piran has placed her feminist prevention work, along with objectification theory and other feminist discourse about body image and disordered eating (see, e.g., Bordo, 1993; Larkin et al., 1999; Smolak & Murnen, 2001, 2004; Steiner-Adair, 1986), under the broader rubric of a "Critical Social Perspectives" (CSP) approach to prevention (Piran, 2001, 2002; see also Levine & Piran, 2004). Although Piran's new model may ultimately subsume various approaches within the social cognitive (e.g., Stice's work) and Non-Specific Vulnerability-Stressor paradigms (O'Dea's work), for the moment we see it as a *feminist*-CSP model because it involves a female-centered, critical analysis of gender-related factors (e.g., objectification, harassment, sexual violence) that the other models do not address. Piran's approach is not the only or necessarily the most effective feminist program for preventing eating problems, but the major aspects of the feminist-CSP perspective constitute a good summary of the basic features of the feminist-empowerment-relational model.

Culture, Body Image, and Disembodiment

Feminist theorists begin with the assumption that people who occupy higher status positions in a society seek to define and control the bodies of those in lower status positions. This chapter has used several feminist theories, particularly objectification theory and sexual terrorism theory, as well as research, including work by Smolak, Murnen, Piran, Fredrickson, and Steiner-Adair, to show how girls' and women's bodies have been defined and controlled in ways that contribute to eating disorders. Feminist prevention programs, like other prevention programs, challenge those definitions of what women's bodies should be. However, the feminist programs also explicitly seek to alter the power structure that *controls* definitions of the female body and put that power in the hands of girls and women.

The research reviewed in this chapter and previous chapters (e.g., chapter 5) consistently demonstrates that socially approved inequities (e.g., gender-role expectations, weightism and other prejudices, harassment, and objectification) disconnect girls and women from authentic understanding, appreciation, control, and expression of their bodies. Piran (2002) refers to this psychological disconnection as *disrupted embodiment* (or *disembodiment*), rather than body image disturbance. "Disembodiment" captures the unstable, unhealthy experience of feeling neither in control of, nor in tune with, one's body as a source of pleasure, nurturance, confidence, and strength. The disembodied person self-consciously "sees" and "treats" her own body as a flawed (imperfect), unreliable, and malleable "object" (vs. embodied subjectivity), while ignoring, rejecting, and silencing feelings connected to the body's own wisdom (Fredrickson & Roberts, 1997; McKinley, 2002). Thus, disembodiment incorporates "loss of voice" with regard to hunger, desires, feelings, and other experiences directly connected to the body. A focus on critical analysis of contexts that "disembody" women connects the topics of body image and eating problems to other phenomena on the spectrum of violation of body ownership, whether it be "normative discontent" at the milder end or self-mutilation, AN, BN, post-traumatic stress disorder, borderline personality disorder, or dissociative identity disorder at the extreme end.

Relationships, Dialogue, and Knowledge

More than any other model, the feminist-CSP model emphasizes the complexity and diversity of the ecological factors that influence embodiment and healthy eating. These include forces that operate broadly across multiple environments, such as media messages and peer teasing that glorify slenderness while stigmatizing body fat and fat people. The feminist-CSP model also highlights the role of broad structures of power, privilege, and control that function—sometimes openly, sometimes insidiously—along the dimensions of gender, race, socioeconomic status, sexual orientation, and other factors. And there are the specific ways these forces operate in a particular context, intertwined with factors unique to that environment. This means that prevention efforts will be guided by universal, feminist theories about social effects and resistance, but carefully tailored to the most important specific factors operating in the setting(s) of the intervention(s).

Piran's feminist-CSP model argues that the site of knowledge about these context-specific factors should be the girls or young women themselves, not the theory-driven experience of an "outside" expert. We agree with her contention that prevention specialists need to create safe and respectful opportunities for girls to give voice to their context-dependent experiences. However, we believe that experts, including Piran, need to continue doing and applying basic, nomothetic research in etiology and prevention. The general principles and the storehouse of broadly applicable experiences that emerge from this work will be vitally important in two ways. First, women and men committed to feminist models of prevention are entitled, if not obligated, to use research to analyze what they perceive as social-political factors shaping health and illness in girls and boys. We need not wait for girls to raise a problem before we address it. Second, the knowledge from basic, nomothetic research will be useful to adult experts in their roles as mentors for girls, as authoritative participants in dialogues with the girls, and as advocates for change. The dialogue between the adult facilitator and the girls in a feminist prevention program will be strengthened by expertise that relies in part on general principles. A critical social perspective requires a blend of the general and the specific.

Critical Knowledge Becomes Transformative Action

Clarifying "what is going on" and "how that makes girls feel in and about their bodies" sets the stage for a strong sense of what is unjust, what needs to be changed, and how that might be effectively and ethically be accomplished. Ideally, a discourse of resistance is constructed as group members move from silence, lack of voice, and private shame and disembodiment to shared and public critical knowledge about contextual influences. As a group facilitator and as an advocate-model for change, the feminist leader encourages participants to work on transforming the ways in which they take care of their own bodies, the ways in which they relate to each other in the group, and, ultimately the contexts in which they live. Feminist-CSP approaches are unique in *requiring* environmental changes as an integral component of individual and group change; this exemplifies the well-known feminist principle: "The personal is the political." This constellation of environmental, group, and personal transformations encourages girls to have experiences that stimulate a strong sense of substance, power, agency, connection, and meaning. These experiences are the foundation of embodiment, the antithesis of negative body image and disordered eating.

Challenges

Resistance. Those who seek to institute a program based on the feminist-empowerment-relational model may find that schools, parents, and some students are resistant. Many people remain reluctant to embrace feminist or other critical ideas, viewing them as radical, anti-beauty, and antimale. As emphasized in chapter 3, it is particularly important to design programs so that male students, teachers, and administrators do not feel attacked; otherwise they may undermine the program (Stein, 1999). Gender roles have important costs for boys. Thus, a truly systemic approach must recognize the restrictions and negative consequences of contexts affecting male gender roles.

Time, Skill, and Scope. Compared to many of the other programs considered in this book, the feminist approach is more time-consuming and may require a broader range of knowledge and skills. In many private and public school systems, the classroom teachers and staff would find it difficult, if not impossible, to accommodate a program as extensive as Piran's or Steiner-Adair et al.'s (2002; see chapter 9) without substantial support from the administration and parents (Smolak, Harris, Levine, & Shisslak, 2001). This means that the program could be instituted in school only after considerable effort and skillful work by the project's director, the facilitator, and their supporters in the community (see chapter 15). At present, it is unclear how long the background process requires, how long the groups need to meet for the program to be effective, or how much access to staff and administrators is necessary. Nevertheless, there is precedent for this type of intensive, collaborative intervention in the literature on the prevention of substance abuse (see chapters 10 through 12). McVey, Tweed, and Blackmore (2004) recently implemented an intensive, ecological eating problems prevention program for public middle schools. In chapter 12 we describe this 8-month project, which combines elements of all three major models, including critical analysis of media messages and facilitated discussions for adolescent girls only.

Alternatively, a more focused feminist intervention could be used. School personnel, directed by a resource coordinator (see chapter 11), could work together to make the school environment less likely to be a source of objectification and other forms of gender inequity. In this regard, Friedman (2003) has written a manual for adults seeking to change the ecology of schools so as to promote positive body image and healthy eating. Or programs such as Friedman's *Just for Girls* groups (see Appendix B) or the National Eating Disorders Association's *GO GIRLS!*™ media literacy program (see chapter 13 and Appendixes A & B) could be implemented after school, during "free" periods, or on weekends. As always, careful attention to the audience(s) and the setting is needed.

Conclusion

In conclusion, the feminist-empowerment-relational model has a great deal of promise (see also chapters 9 & 13). The theoretical framework is clear. The research base is broad, including studies of gender differences in body image and eating problems (see Smolak & Murnen, 2001, 2004), studies of objectification and sexual harassment (see, e.g., Fredrickson & Roberts, 1997; Harned, 2000; Murnen & Smolak, 2000), studies of the gendered effects of mass media (e.g., Murnen et al., 2003), and path analyses of the correlates of disembodiment (Piran, 2002). In addition, outcome evaluations of prevention programs based on the model provide some of the more promising data in the field (see, e.g., Neumark-Sztainer et al., 2000; Piran, 1999b; Steiner-Adair et al., 2002). However, the FER approach requires additional evaluation research, particularly if it is to be applied in full force to a wide range of schools. One question such research needs to address is the sequence of processes necessary to produce the desired distal changes in body image and eating problems. In particular, when do environmental changes occur and how long must girls live in the changed environments before one can accurately talk about resilience and prevention? Nonetheless, the FER approach serves to remind us and focus our attention on the clearest, least debatable statement that can be made about eating disorders: These are gendered disorders and as such are embedded in multidimensional cultural factors that shape the construction of gender. We cannot, therefore, ignore the role of gender-in-culture in the development, treatment, and prevention of eating problems and disorders.

III

REVIEW OF PREVENTION RESEARCH

9

Prevention of Body Image Disturbances and Disordered Eating: A Review of the Research

Compared to the voluminous work on the prevention of cigarette smoking and other substance use, systematic research on the prevention of body image problems and eating problems is relatively limited. Nevertheless, prevention has been the subject of recent reviews in the form of articles (Austin, 2000; Dalle Grave, 2003; Franko & Orosan-Weine, 1998; Mussell, Binford, & Fulkerson, 2000; Rosenvinge & Børresen, 1999), chapters (Levine & Piran, 2001, 2004; Levine & Smolak, 2001; McVey, 2004; Shisslak, Crago, Estes, & Gray, 1996; Smolak, 1999; Stice & Hoffman, 2004), books (Piran, Levine, & Steiner-Adair, 1999; Vandereycken & Noordenbos, 1998), databases (Pratt & Woolfenden, 2002), and meta-analyses (Littleton & Ollendick, 2003; Stice & Shaw, 2004).

The majority of prevention programs are curricula or small-group interventions for students. Consequently, they focus on changing the knowledge, beliefs, attitudes, intentions, and behaviors of individual students. Many of the literature reviews concur that such programs are likely to increase knowledge, to have a temporary positive effect on a few beliefs and attitudes, and to have little effect—and certainly little sustained effect—on disordered eating behavior. Rosenvinge and Børresen (1999) offer a particularly negative conclusion, one that is echoed by many who are critical or skeptical of prevention: "Apart from the increasing of knowledge, there is no evidence that primary prevention programmes provide changes in eating attitudes and behaviours, and some authors even suggest that primary prevention may actually do more harm than good" (p. 8). This chapter examines these conclusions through a comprehensive review of published and unpublished research on the effects of primary (universal and selective) and secondary (targeted) preventive interventions conducted prior to August 2004.

WHAT CONSTITUTES A "PREVENTION OUTCOME STUDY"?

We categorized prevention outcome studies into universal-selective (primary) and targeted (secondary). As already noted, many interventions are classroom curricula designed for general use with elementary, middle school, and high school students. Using the nomenclature and the continuum of prevention proposed by Mrazek and Haggerty (1994; see chapter 1), this type of curricular intervention lies somewhere between universal (supported by public policy and intended for large groups within the general public) and selective (focused on older preadolescent and adolescent girls as a nonsymptomatic but high-risk population) prevention. Therefore, for technical accuracy, we refer to general classroom curricula and other interventions with this type of "audience" as a "universal-selective" form of primary prevention. The status of these interventions on the continuum of prevention is complicated by the fact that a significant minority of adolescent girls in regular classroom settings will already have a negative body image and features of disordered eating (Smolak, 1996, 1999).

The specific criteria for designating a study as universal-selective prevention were (after Austin, 2000, p. 1259):

- The title and introduction of the manuscript (but not necessarily the program itself) make clear an intention to try to prevent eating problems and/or eating disorders.

- The program was delivered en masse, and therefore without significant tailoring, to a mixture of individuals in general (e.g., boys and girls ages 10–11), nonsymptomatic individuals at risk (e.g., 11-year-old girls in the later stages of pubertal weight gain), and individuals with eating problems (e.g., 10- and 11-year-old girls who are already "dieting" because of weight concerns).

- The study reports empirical results pertaining to changes in risk or resilience factors, or to signs and symptoms of eating problems/eating disorders.

Our review distinguishes universal-selective (primary) from "targeted" or "indicated" prevention (or in older parlance, "secondary" prevention; see chapter 1). Recall that in targeted prevention (Mrazek & Haggerty, 1994) the audience does yet not "have" the full-blown problem (e.g., BN or EDNOS), but they have been identified as being "at risk" because of the presence of clear precursors (e.g., negative body image or chronic dieting). The potential participants are already suffering, so the intervention is not a form of primary (universal or selective) prevention; however, as negative body image, for example, is a risk factor for eating disorders (see chapter 5), the intervention does constitute *targeted* prevention for eating disorders. A prototypical example of targeted (secondary) prevention is a manualized cognitive-behavioral program to help improve body image in young college women who are seeking help for their body-image problems (see, e.g., Rosen, Saltzberg, & Srebnik, 1989). In some studies of targeted prevention for eating problems, participants are prescreened and invited to participate (e.g., Kaminski & McNamara, 1996), whereas in others the participants respond to general announcements recruiting people who are concerned about their body image or wish to improve their body image (e.g., Franko, 1998).

ORGANIZING THE PREVENTION OUTCOME RESEARCH: UNIVERSAL-SELECTIVE PROGRAMS

The Tables

Studies of universal-selective prevention were compiled through searches of databases (e.g., PsychInfo, Medline), cataloging of references from previous review articles (e.g., Austin, 2000; Levine & Piran, 2004), and personal contacts with researchers in the field. As of August 2004, we have gathered 90 published and unpublished studies (of 67 different programs, as presented in 84 manuscripts) of the universal prevention of negative body and/or eating problems. Twelve studies (e.g., Neumark-Sztainer et al., 2000) address "media literacy," so they are reviewed in chapter 13. Wade, Davidson, and O'Dea (2003) compared a control group to O'Dea's prevention program (see chapter 7) and to a media literacy program. This study is included in Tables 9.2 and 13.1, but it was counted as only one study and included in the statistics that follow. Another study (Chally, 1998) was included in Austin's (2000) review but excluded here because participants are high school teachers.

The principal features and outcomes of the remaining 78 studies, grouped according to the school level of the target audience, are summarized in Tables 9.1 through 9.4. Each prevention program was rated as to how many distinct elements of the following models it contained: disease-specific social cognitive model (DISC, maximum = first seven features in Table 6.1); the Non-Specific Vulnerability-Stressor model (NSVS, maximum = first two features in Table 7.2); and the feminist-empowerment-relational model (FER, maximum = first seven features in Table 8.1). Each program was also rated as to whether it did or did not include an *emphasis* on each of three superordinate factors that we believe are very important for prevention: developmental psychopathology (chapter 4), gender (chapter 8), and attempts to change the ecology of the participants, not just the individual participants (chapters 4 & 12).

Of the 78 studies in Tables 9.1 through 9.4, the first study was published in 1986 (Porter, Morrell, & Moriarty, 1986), and 56 (~72%) were published in or after 1998. Of the 78, 60 (77%) are experimental or quasiexperimental with a no-intervention or minimal intervention comparison group. "Quasiexperimental" means that the comparison students were from a similar grouping (e.g., a similar classroom) but were not randomly assigned to that group. The early developmental level of this field is revealed by the fact that only 14 (18%) of the studies used some type of random assignment to an experimental or control condition, coupled with a follow-up period of at least 3 months. Of these, all but four were published or conducted after 1998.

The tables are designed to distinguish between studies while revealing general trends in their characteristics and outcomes. Before considering any conclusions, it is also necessary to acknowledge that the social cognitive (i.e., both the SCT and CBT approaches; see chapter 6), Non-Specific Vulnerability-Stressor (NSVS; see chapter 7), and feminist-empowerment-relational (FER; see chapter 8) prevention models and resulting prevention efforts share a number of features:

- emphasis on understanding the nature and determinants of body image
- discouraging calorie-restrictive dieting
- awareness of the sociocultural and developmental rationale for prevention of negative body image, eating problems, and eating disorders

- cultural "literacy" training to help students understand, critique, and resist unhealthy messages from the mass media and other "sociocultural influences"
- instruction in critical thinking about gender and adolescent development as these influence norms for—and feelings about—weight, shape, and attractiveness
- creation of more supportive environments—with healthier norms and fewer stressors—by improving the attitudes and behaviors of peers and significant adults.

ELEMENTARY SCHOOL

Smolak is the leading advocate for prevention work with children (ages 6–11) who have not yet made the transition into puberty or into middle school (Smolak, 1999; Smolak & Levine, 1994a, 1996; Smolak et al., 1998b). To date there have been 11 evaluations of interventions with this age group (see Table 9.1). Seven have included a comparison group, but none has used randomization to groups, and only one has included a follow-up assessment.

Follow-Up Studies

We constructed a 10-lesson curriculum for girls and boys ages 9 through 11 (Smolak et al., 1998a, 1998b). The "Eating Smart/Eating for Me" curriculum (ESEM; Levine, Smolak, Schermer, & Etling, 1995) was delivered by regular fourth- and fifth-grade classroom teachers, who received 2 hours of training. Control participants from the same schools received the state-mandated nutrition and physical education. Based on the social cognitive and developmental models, ESEM provides information, classroom exercises, and homework assignments that promote healthy eating and exercising, positive body image, and skepticism about calorie-restrictive dieting. A substantial component emphasizes tolerance of and appreciation for diversity in weight and shape. This includes an attempt to create individual values and group norms that define teasing as definitely harmful and clearly unacceptable. Parents of children in the curriculum condition received nine newsletters paralleling the children's lessons, as well as a final newsletter on the nature and identification of eating problems.

The ESEM program produced some significant but modest short-term gains in knowledge. Yet, with the exception of a positive change in

TABLE 9.1
Studies of Universal Prevention in Elementary School Children

Study	Program	Design	RA	Gender	Devel	Ecol	SC	NSVS	FER	K	A	B	PPE	Comment
Controlled														
Richman (1993): 180 CAN m & f (M = 10.4)	8 units 1–2 hrs each	PP	N	N	N	N	5	1	0	Y	Y	N	NA	Trends in behavioral improvement masked by reductions in controls.
Smolak et al. (1998b) 102 US m, 120 f ages 9–10	10 units 1 hour each	PP	N	N	Y	Y	5	0	0	Y	N	N	NA	Attention to teasing & weightism. Negative effect on body esteem for girls.
Smolak et al. (1998a) 102 US m, 120 f ages 10-11	10 units 1 hour each	PP	N	N	Y	Y	5	0	0	Y	N	N	NA	Attention to teasing & weightism. Only 1 attitude change.
Hewlings (2000): US f, ages 8–10	8 units	PP	Y	?	?	N	?	?	0	Y	N	N	NA	Doctoral thesis using SC theory.
Irving (2000): 81 US m, 116 f, ages 6–11	30–40 min puppet show & discussion	modified Solomon 4-group	N	N	Y	N	2	1	0	Y	Y	N	NA	Emphasis on negative impact of teasing & pressure to diet, plus social support.
Smolak & Levine (2001a); 248 US m, 252 f, ages 11–13	10 units 60 min ea	RM (24 mos)	[e.g., 20 pre-only vs. 25 post-only girls ages 10–11]		Y	Y	5	0	0	Y	Y	Y	Y	2-yr follow-up of Smolak et al. (1998a, 1998b) with a third group as control for spillover effects.
Kater et al. (2002) 209 US m, 206 f ages 9–13	10 units 45–50 min	PP	N	Y	Y	Y	5	1	0	Y	Y	nm	NA	Some work with parents.

Uncontrolled

Huon et al. (1997) 100 AUS f (*M* = 10.8)	6 units 1 hour ea	PP	NA	Y	Y	N	3	1	1	N	Y	nm	NA	Significant improvements for high-risk participants.
Coller et al. (1999) 22 US f, ages 10–12	6 units 90 min ea	PP	NA	Y	Y	Y	3	0	1	nm	N	N	NA	Program for Girl Scouts; some work with parents.
Kater et al. (2000) 105 US m, 117 f ages 9–12	10 units 45–50 min	PP	NA	Y	Y	Y	5	1	0	Y	Y	nm	NA	Same program as Kater et al. (2002); some work with parents.
DeBate & Thompson (2003); 322 US f (*M* = 10)	24 sessions 1 hour ea	PP	NA	Y	Y	Y	3	2	2	nm	Y	Y	NA	Pilot evaluation of Girls on the Run program to develop fitness, character, & positive body image.

Notes.
1. Age refers to age at the onset of the intervention.
2. Design: PP = Pre–post; RM = Repeated Measures (with length of follow-up in months in parentheses).
3. RA: random assignment by school, class, or participant.
4. Gender: Gendered nature of body image, eating, weight management was one focus.
5. Devel: Development (e.g., in adolescence) was one focus.
6. Ecology: Intervention had at least one ecological component.
7. SC: How many elements of social cognitive approach (SCT or CBT) were present (see Table 6.1).
8. NSVS: How many elements of nonspecific vulnerability-stressor approach were present (see Table 7.2).
9. FER: How many elements of feminist-empowerment-relational approach were present (see Table 8.2).
10. K = significant improvement in knowledge; A = improvement in attitude; B = improvement in behavior; nm = not measured; Y = yes, on at least one variable; N = no for all of the dependent variables.
11. PPE: program participation effect; pre–post significant improvement, but not maintained at follow-up.
12. ? = unknown; information not available at the time of writing.

the tendency of fifth graders to reduce their prejudicial assumptions about fat people, there were no significant effects on attitudes and behaviors. The 2-year longitudinal follow-up (Smolak & Levine, 2001a) compared experimental and control participants (now ages 11–13), along with a new control group of young adolescents from schools not included in the original study. Compared to this new control group, experimental participants were more knowledgeable, had higher body esteem, and used fewer unhealthy weight-management techniques. Scores of the original control group were intermediate, raising the possibility that the sociocultural impact of the original curriculum may have "spilled over" and influenced control participants within the same elementary schools (see McVey & Davis, 2002, and Outwater, 1990, for a similar phenomenon involving middle school students).

Pre–Post Evaluations

Uncontrolled. Coller, Neumark-Sztainer, Bulfer, and Engebretson (1999) developed a program of six 90-minute sessions for Girl Scouts ages 10 to 12 and their parents. The girls were engaged by the activities (concerning, e.g., body image, media, unhealthy dieting, and hereditary determinants of weight and shape), but the program produced minimal changes in eating attitudes and behaviors. More promising results for self-esteem, body size satisfaction, and eating attitudes and behaviors were reported recently by DeBate and Thompson (2003) in their pilot evaluation of *Girls on the Run* (see www.girlsontherun.org). This intensive program (two 1-hour sessions per week for 12 weeks) is designed to improve self-esteem, build character, and improve body image by combining running with many engaging activities, including community service.

Huon, Roncolato, Ritchie, and Braganza (1997) also evaluated six weekly 60-minute lessons designed to help Australian girls ages 10 to 11 understand how peers, media, and physical development influence body image and dietary practices. Unlike Coller et al. (1999), this program emphasized how a narrow construction of gender and beauty, reinforced by different sources, creates many problems. At posttest and 6-month follow-up there was a significant improvement in overall eating attitudes and behaviors. But there were no mean improvements in nutritional knowledge, body satisfaction, or drive for thinness. Individual change scores showed that some children benefited significantly from the program, whereas some deteriorated. In general, girls with the poorest body image and the highest drive for thinness showed the greatest improvements.

Controlled. In addition to Smolak et al.'s research, there have been four controlled evaluations, each using some variation of a pre–post design. A doctoral dissertation by Hewlings (2000) reported an increase in knowledge but no other significant effects of an eight-unit social cognitive intervention for girls ages 8 to 10. The other three controlled studies produced encouraging results. Richman (1993) evaluated the effectiveness of six 1- to 2-hour lessons for fifth- and sixth-grade Canadian students. Following a social cognitive model, the lessons addressed healthy and disordered eating, the relationship between body size and self-esteem, and ways to resist social pressures to be thin. Compared to controls at a different school, students receiving the curriculum learned more about the topics and had greater body satisfaction. They also had lower scores on the ChEAT (see Appendix E), but this effect was masked by an unanticipated improvement in the control group.

Irving (2000) evaluated the Puppet Program developed by EDAP, Inc. (now the National Eating Disorders Association; see Appendix A). Separate scripts and group discussions for Grades K–2 (ages 5–7) and Grades 3–5 (ages 8–11) address several of the messages also featured in the ESEM curriculum (Levine et al., 1995), for example, the natural diversity of weights and shapes, and the hurtful and unacceptable effects of weight- and shape-related teasing. According to Irving's evaluation of a subset of girls ages 11 to 12, this 45-minute puppet program increased the acceptability of a diversity of weights and shapes. Uncontrolled evaluation suggested that even a short exposure to the puppet program helps elementary school-age children learn that teasing is wrong.

Promising Recent Research

Kathy Kater (1998), a Minneapolis psychotherapist, has developed a 10-lesson curriculum entitled *Healthy Body Images: Teaching Kids to Eat, and Love Their Bodies, Too!* (see also Kater, 2004). The target audience is boys and girls ages 9 to 12. In addition to components of the social cognitive model, there are also strong elements of the NSVS perspective. One group of lessons helps children understand what they *cannot and should not try to control*, such as the developmental changes of puberty, and the impact of genetics on size and shape. A second set focuses on what children *can control*, for example, development of a multifaceted identity, and selection of realistic, encouraging role models. The final set of lessons develops resilience to unhealthy sociocultural messages about thinness and weight management, and includes material on the history of cultural attitudes concerning body image.

In an uncontrolled evaluation, Kater, Rohwer, and Levine (2000) found positive pre-to-post-program changes in knowledge of curricular material, acceptance of diversity in shape and weight, positive body esteem, and rejection of the slender ideal. A second evaluation with 390 boys and girls ages 9 to 11 found equally promising results (Kater, Rohwer, & Londre, 2002). Relative to controls, who showed no changes, children receiving *Healthy Body Images* reported many improvements in knowledge, body satisfaction, critical thinking about media, intentions to diet, and healthy choices related to nutrition and exercising.

Conclusion

The necessary studies have not been done yet to determine whether or not elementary school prevention efforts, to paraphrase Rosevinge and Børresen (1999), result in long-term, health-promoting changes in relevant eating attitudes and behaviors (Levine & Smolak, 2001; Littleton & Ollendick, 2003; Smolak, 1999). This lack of research should not be confused with negative outcomes. The majority of studies of elementary school children have produced positive changes in the relevant knowledge and attitudes of students. Moreover, longitudinal evaluation of the ESEM program (Smolak & Levine, 2001a) suggests the potential for preventive behavioral effects during the early adolescent transition. The exciting work of Kater and colleagues should be expanded to include components of other promising programs. Notable among these are the impact of gender on body image and health (Huon et al., 1997); the natural—and desirable—diversity of weights and shapes; the need to define weight/shape-related teasing as harmful and to establish policies and norms against it (Irving, 2000; Smolak et al., 1998a, 1998b); and the combination of physical competence and community service featured in *Girls on the Run* (DeBate & Thompson, 2003).

MIDDLE SCHOOL

Many eating disorders begin in adolescence. Consequently, a large number of prevention programs have been created for youth ages 11 to 14 (see Table 9.2). To date there have been 30 evaluations of interventions with middle school children. Twenty (67%) have included a com-

TABLE 9.2
Studies of Universal Prevention in Middle School Children

Study	Program	Design	RA	Gender	Devel	Ecol	SC	NSVS	FER	K	A	B	PPE	Comment
Controlled—Follow-up														
Outwater (1990); 25 US m, 25 f ages 11–12	10 units 45 min ea	RM (1 mo)	N	Y	Y	N	3	1	0	nm	N	N	N	Body image and self-esteem improved in both conditions.
Killen et al. (1993); 931 US f, ages 11–13	18 units 50 min ea	RM (7, 14, 24)	Y	N	Y	N	5	0	0	Y	N	N	N	Body image not addressed; trend toward effects for high-risk participants.
Moreno & Thelen (1993)—2 studies; 104 & 115 US f, M = 13.7	6.5-min video plus 30-min discussion	RM (1 mo)	N	N	N	N	4	0	0	Y	Y	nm	N	Effects declined from post to fu; attrition was a problem.
Richman (1997); 297 CAN m, 307 f; M = 11	6 units 60–120 min ea	RM (6 mo)	N	N	N	N	5	1	0	Y	N	N	Y	Pre-post sig treatment effects for body esteem & ChEAT dieting.
O'Dea & Abraham (2000); 170 AUS f ages 11.1–14.5	9 units 50–80 min ea	RM (12 mo)	Y	Y	N	Y	2	2	2	nm	Y	N	Y	Self-esteem based approach; sustained improvement in body esteem for HR participants.
Stewart et al. (2001) 752 UK f, M = 13.4	6 units 45 min ea	RM (6 mo)	N	N	Y	N	7	2	0	Y	N	N	Y	Intervention has many positive effects at posttest.
Varnado-Sullivan et al. (2001); 157 US f, 130 m, ages 11–13	3 units 49 min ea	mult basel School 1 (fu = 10.5 weeks) School 2 (fu = 3 weeks)	N	Y	Y	Y	3	1	2	nm nm	Y N	N N	nm nm	No effects for males; participation in parent program was very low.
Baranowski & Hetherington (2001); 29 SCOT f, ages 11–12	5 units 90 min ea	RM (6 mo)	N	N	N	N	4	1	0	nm	N	N	nm	Undesirable treatment effect on dietary restraint at posttest.
Dalle Grave et al. (2001); 61 ITAL f, 45 m, M = 11.6	6 units 120 min ea at 6-mo fu: two 120-min booster sessions	RM (6, 12 mo)	Y	N	Y	N	5	1	1	Y	N	N	Y	Authors feel a "spillover" effect may be operating.
McVey & Davis (2002) 263 CAN f, M = 10.9	6 units 55 min ea	RM (6, 12 mo)	Y	Y	N	N	6	2	0	nm	N	N	N	"Life skills promotion approach."

(Continued)

TABLE 9.2
(Continued)

Study	Program	Design	RA	Gender	Devel	Ecol	SC	NSVS	FER	K	A	B	PPE	Comment
Withers et al. (2002) 218 AUS f, M = 13.0	22-min video no discuss	RM (1 mo)	N	Y	Y	N	6	0	0	Y	N	nm	Y	Extends Heinze et al. (2000).
Steiner-Adair et al. (2002); 411 US f M = 12.6	8 units 45–90 min ea	RM (6 mo)	Y & N	Y	Y	N	5	2	4	Y	Y	N	N	Participants designed & delivered 1–3 sessions for 9–11-yr-old girls.
Wade et al. (2003a) 53 AUS m, 33 f, M = 13.42	5 units 50 min ea	RM (3 mo) Self-esteem Media Lit	Y	Y N	N N	N Y	1 1	2 0	1 2	nm nm	N N	N N	N Y	Control versus short versions of O'Dea & Abraham (2000) and GO GIRLS! media literacy.
McVey et al.(2003a) 206 CAN f, M = 12.5	10 units 60 min ea	RM (3 mo)	N	Y	N	N	6	2	1	nm	Y	Y	na	Prevention effect for body esteem (wt), dieting, & bulimic behavior; GirlTalk peer support groups.
McVey et al. (2003b) 270 CAN f, M = 12.3	10 units 60 min ea	RM (3 mo)	N	Y	N	N	6	2	1	nm	N	N	N	Failure to replicate preventive effect of GirlTalk peer support.
McVey, Davis, et al. (2004) 258 CAN f, M = 11.2	6 units 55 min ea	RM (6, 12 mo)	Y	Y	N	Y	6	2	0	nm	N	N*	Y	3-hr parent workshop, but <20% attend; at 12-mo fu body image scores lower for IG than control.
McVey, Tweed, & Blackmore (2004) 784 CAN f, 665 m; M = 11.7	10 units 60 min ea; throughout school year	RM (6 mo)	Y	Y	Y	Y	6	2	1	NM	Y	N	Y	Multidimensional ecological program focusing on students, parents, and teachers, with some changes in school environment.
Tilgner et al. (2004) 677 AUS f, M = 13.1	22-min video & discussion [same video as in Heinze et al., 2000]	RM (1 mo)	Y	Y	Y	N	6	0	0	Y	N	nm	Y	No differences between video alone, video plus elaborative discussion, or video plus discussion of production values.

190

Study	Intervention	Design											Notes
Withers & Wertheim (2004); 187 AUS f	22-min video & discussion [same video as in Heinze et al., 2000; controls were two conditions from Withers et al., 2002]	RM (1, 3 mo)	Y	Y	Y	N	6	0	0	Y	Y	nm	Y	Complicated results, but no differences between video alone group and video plus either verbal or written or control elaboration.

Pre to Post (C = controlled; NC = no control) or Follow-up but No Control (RM-NC)

Study	Intervention	Design											Notes
Porter et al. (1986) 25 CAN m, 19 f, ages 9–16, M = 11.9	half-day program	NC	na	N	N	N	4	2	0	nm	Y	nm	Y	ED video, experiential workshops in art, music, dance; drive for thinness decreased in HR group.
Moriarty et al. (1990) 144 CAN m, 321 f, ages 11–14	5 units 66 min ea	C	N	N	Y	N	3	1	0	Y	Y	nm	na	EDI data collected but not reported.
Schuman et al. (1994) 102 US f, ages 11–12	16 units 45 min ea	C	N	N	Y	N	7	0	0	Y	Y	Y?	na	No multivariate effect for behavior change; univar effect for dieting.
Carter et al. (1997) 50 UK f, ages 13–14	8 units 45 min ea	RM-NC	na	N	Y	N	7	2	0	Y	N	N	Y	Significant pre-post decline in EAT & EDE-Q scores, but return to baseline at 6-mo follow-up.
Villena & Castillo (1999); 2,109 SPAN f, ages 12–15	1 unit 75 min	RM-NC (1, 3 mo)	na	Y	N	Y	4	1	1	nm	Y	nm	na	Cognitive-behavioral groups + information for parents.
Piran (1999a); 45, 35, & 40 CAN f, M = 13.0	6 units, 60 min ea + booster	3 cohort survey: 1987, 1991, 1996	na	Y	Y	Y	3	2	7	Y	Y	Y	N	Residential, world-class ballet school; intensive work w/staff.
Heinze et al. (2000) 103 AUS f, M = 12.5	24-min video no discuss	NC	Y	Y	Y	N	6	0	0	Y	Y	nm	na	See Withers et al. (2002); video is didactic; status of presenter in video does not matter.
Phelps et al. (2000) 530 US f, ages 11–15	6 units	C	N	N	Y	N	5	1	0	nm	N	N	na	Program emphasizes physical competence and other life skills.

(Continued)

TABLE 9.2
(Continued)

Study	Program	Design	RA	Gender	Devel	Ecol	SC	NSVS	FER	K	A	B	PPE	Comment
Austin et al. (2002); 484 US f, ages 12–14	32 core units over 2 yrs	C	Y	N	N	Y	1	0	0	nm	nm	Y	na	Planet Health obesity prevention program. Ecological approach includes PE and special efforts to reduce TV viewing.
Pasqualoni et al. (2002); 28 ITAL f, 24 m, M = 13.6	6 units 120 min ea	NC	Y	N	Y	N	5	1	1	Y	Y	Y	Y	Open trial of the program evaluated by Dalle Grave et al. (2001); see above.

Notes.
1. Age refers to age at the onset of the intervention.
2. Design: PP = Pre–post; RM = Repeated Measures (with length of follow-up in months in parentheses).
3. RA: random assignment by school, class, or participant.
4. Gender: Gendered nature of body image, eating, weight management was one focus.
5. Devel: Development (e.g., in adolescence) was one focus.
6. Ecology: Intervention had at least one ecological component.
7. SC: How many elements of disease-specific social cognitive approach were present (see Table 6.1).
8. NSVS: How many elements of nonspecific vulnerability-stressor approach were present (see Table 7.2).
9. FER: How many elements of feminist-empowerment-relational approach were present (see Table 8.2).
10. K = significant improvement in knowledge; A = improvement in attitude; B = improvement in behavior; nm = not measured; Y = yes, on at least one variable; N = no for all of the dependent variables.
11. PPE: program participation effect; pre–post significant improvement, but not maintained at follow-up.

parison group and at least a 1-month follow-up. Of that subset, seven (23% of the middle school studies) have arranged for some type of random assignment to experimental or control conditions, plus at least a 6-month follow-up assessment.

Controlled Evaluations With At Least 6-Month Follow-up

Negative Results. A very important study was conducted by Killen, Taylor, and colleagues at Stanford University (Killen, 1996; Killen et al., 1993). The 18 lessons, derived explicitly from Bandura's social cognitive model, produced only modest increases in knowledge and no short- or long-term changes in attitudes or behaviors. The researchers do believe, however, that low statistical power obscured the program's positive impact on students with weight concerns. At 2-year follow-up, the effect size for change in weight concerns for high-risk students in the intervention versus control groups was approximately .50 (Killen, 1996; C. Barr Taylor, personal communications, December 15, 1998, and April 25, 2003).

Another important negative outcome emerged from a Canadian study recently reported by McVey and Davis (2002). Their curricular program, *Every Body Is a Somebody* (Seaver et al., 1997), offers six 1-hour lessons for 11–12-year-old girls beginning the transition into adolescence. It combines features of the social cognitive and developmental models with the NSVS model's emphasis on positive self-esteem and stress management. In a controlled and randomized (by school) study, there were no significant between-group differences in body satisfaction and eating attitudes. Demand characteristics, or the positive effect of a standard health curriculum with some overlap in content, may have been operating: The experimental and control groups both demonstrated improvements at the 12-month follow-up. A recent quasiexperimental evaluation of a small-scale social cognitive program for sixth-grade girls (ages 11–12) in Scotland also had little effect; in fact, the comparison group who received information about healthy eating showed a greater reduction in dieting (Baranowski & Hetherington, 2001).

The Program Participation Effect. Stewart, Carter, Fairburn, and colleagues, working in Great Britain, conducted two longitudinal evaluations of a six-lesson program based on Stewart's (1998) cognitive-behavioral model (see chapter 6), as well as several aspects of the NSVS model. In both instances there were disappointing but intriguing results for girls ages 13 to 14. In the first study (Carter, Stewart, Dunn, & Fairburn, 1997), which was uncontrolled, the program produced significant posttest improvements in knowledge and in eating problems, as measured by EDE-Q and EAT scores. At 6-month follow-up, however, the mean scores had reverted to baseline. In the second study (Stewart et al., 2001) there was a lasting increase in knowledge. And for the experimental group, but not the control group, there were significant pre-to-post decreases in various dependent measures, including shape concerns, EDE-Q, and EAT scores. Yet, once again, at the 6-month follow-up, scores on all these variables reverted to baseline.

Let us call this pattern of results—modest or even substantial posttest improvements in knowledge, attitudes, and/or behaviors while the program is ongoing, coupled with no long-term effects except perhaps for knowledge—the *program participation effect* or PPE. The PPE seen in the two studies by Stewart and colleagues in the United Kingdom has been found in four other studies of young adolescents: (a) Steiner-Adair et al.'s (2002) FER program for U.S. girls; (b) Richman's (1997) six-unit social cognitive program for Canadian youth; (c) a six-unit, 12-hour cognitive-behavioral program (with an additional 4 hours of booster sessions at 6-month follow-up) for Italian youth (Dalle Grave, de Luca, & Campello, 2001); and (d) a second evaluation of *Every Body Is a Somebody* (McVey, Davis, Tweed, & Shaw, 2004). This last study is a powerful demonstration of the importance of a comparison group and a longer follow-up. Although there were no between-group effects for eating attitudes, both groups showed significant improvement from pretest to 6-month follow-up. At posttest McVey, Davis, et al.'s (2004) program produced the predicted benefits in body satisfaction, dieting, and global self-esteem. The latter was maintained at 6-month follow-up, but by the 12-month follow-up the comparison group's self-esteem had risen very significantly from posttest to match the higher, stable level attained by the experimental group. Moreover, the experimental group's body satisfaction had declined by the 12-month follow-up, whereas the comparison group's rose sharply from the 6-month to 12-month follow-up, nearly matching the PPE attained by the experimental group.

Other Controlled Evaluations

Positive Outcomes. Moreno and Thelen (1993) conducted two quasiexperimental studies of a social cognitive intervention for U.S. girls ages 12 to 14. This "one-shot" program consisted of a 6.5-minute video in which two actors portray sisters who discuss the negative effects of dietary restraint, bingeing, and purging, and the benefits of understanding and resisting unhealthy sociocultural attitudes about thinness. After the video there was a 30-minute class discussion facilitated by a graduate student. Although the implications of this research are tempered by problems with participant attrition, both studies found that at 1-month follow-up the experimental group had fewer weight concerns, and more knowledge and more negative attitudes about calorie-restrictive dieting and about purging.

These positive findings are supported, to a degree, by a programmatic series of prevention studies by Wertheim and colleagues in Australia. These researchers are trying to understand prevention effects in terms of several different theories of attitude change, including McGuire's social influence theory, which segments persuasion processes into presenter characteristics, message channel (format or mode), content, and characteristics of the receiver or audience. In the first, uncontrolled study Heinze, Wertheim, and Kashima (2000) developed a 24-minute videotape that covered almost all features of the social cognitive model, for example, biological determinants of size and shape, natural weight gain during puberty, sociocultural influences on appearance and body image, and harmful consequences of dieting and emotional eating. Regardless of whether the information was conveyed by an expert or a peer or a recovered peer, at the posttest immediately after viewing (with no discussion), this video resulted in more knowledge about dieting, a reduced disparity between current and ideal shape, fewer aspirations to diet, and less concern about pubertal weight gain. There was no effect for body dissatisfaction as measured by the EDI. The positive effects of this brief videotape were, in general, more prominent for girls ages 12 and 13 (Grade 7) than for girls ages 15 and 16 (Grade 10). In general, the subsequent studies with Grade 7 and Grade 8 girls indicate that (a) the videotape has a strong immediate effect in increasing knowledge and reducing drive for thinness and intention to diet; (b) the increase in knowledge and the reduction in drive for thinness *may* be sustained for several weeks to several months; and (c) somewhat surprisingly, various forms of elaboration or discussion for 30–45 minutes do not appear to enhance the effect of the videotape (Tilgner, Wertheim, & Paxton, 2004; Withers, Twigg, Wertheim, & Paxton; 2002; Withers & Wertheim, 2004; E. H. Wertheim, personal communication, July 8, 2004). Overall, the findings of Wertheim, Withers, and colleagues support those of Moreno and Thelen (1993) in pointing to the value of *di-*

dactic, consciousness-raising information derived from the social cognitive and feminist-empowerment-relational model as one important element in prevention with middle school students (see also Strong, 2000, reviewed in chapter 13). This issue is discussed in more detail in the next chapter.

As shown in Table 9.2, some support for the social cognitive model is also provided by two controlled studies of multilesson programs in the United States (Schuman, Contento, Graber, & Brooks-Gunn, 1994; Varnado-Sullivan et al., 2001) and by an uncontrolled Italian study. Pasqualoni, Ginetti, Guardini, Sartirana, and Dalle Grave (2002) found that the 12-hour social cognitive program devised and assessed by Dalle Grave et al. (2001) significantly increased knowledge and reduced EAT scores at posttest. Hopefully, further research currently being conducted by Dalle Grave and colleagues (R. Dalle Grave, personal communication, March 9, 2003) will disconfirm that the positive findings of Pasqualoni et al. (2002) are only a replication of the PPE reported by Dalle Grave et al. (2001).

Negative Outcomes. Not all social cognitive programs with no or brief follow-up have been successful. Interestingly, two unsuccessful interventions were delivered to boys and girls together, and both arranged for experimental and comparison classes in the same school. Outwater's (1990) dissertation used a quasiexperimental design with a 1-month follow-up to evaluate a program for 11–12-year-old U.S. boys and girls. The 10 lessons were based primarily on the social cognitive model (A. Outwater, personal communication, April 6, 1998). There was no prevention effect, as body image and self-esteem scores improved significantly for experimental and comparison students, regardless of gender.

A program developed by Phelps et al. (1999) combined social cognitive components with two NSVS elements: the importance of self-efficacy and an internal locus of control in regard to one's overall health and fitness; and the advantages of physical strength and stamina attained from healthy eating and exercising (see also Phelps, Sapia, Nathanson, & Nelson, 2000). As was the case in Outwater's (1990) study, girls receiving the six lessons showed a pre-to-post increase in body satisfaction, coupled with decreases in EDI drive for thinness and in intent to use unhealthy weight-management techniques. However, these changes did not produce a statistically significant experimental effect because girls in the comparison group also improved (L. Phelps, personal communication, June 18, 2002). Thus, in both studies there may have been a "spillover" effect of program material and/or the demand characteristics of participation in a study (cf. Smolak & Levine, 2001a). As was the case for Varnado-Sullivan et al. (2001) and Outwater (1990), Phelps et al. found that their program had little effect on males.

Promising Results

Social Cognitive Theory. *Planet Health* is an intensive school-based *obesity* prevention program for youth ages 11 to 13 (Grades 6 and 7; Gortmaker et al., 1999; see also Austin, Field, Wiecha, Peterson, & Gortmaker, 2005). The specific goals of this social cognitive intervention are to limit TV viewing, to increase moderate and vigorous activity, to increase consumption of fruits and vegetables, and to reduce intake of high-fat foods. Although there is a focus on changing the cognitive and behavioral skills of individual students, the approach is expressly ecological and population-based. Supported by teacher training and teacher input, the curriculum is infused into multiple classes (e.g., math, language arts, science), requiring a variety of skills and approaches to learning. There are 16 core lessons per year, plus a large number of physical education activities and a special 2-week campaign to reduce TV viewing at home.

Ten schools from four communities in the Boston area were randomly assigned to receive *Planet Health* or to serve as controls. Of the nearly 1,300 students assessed at baseline and 2 years later, approximately 28% were obese. After 2 years in place, the program was successful in reducing the *prevalence* of obesity in girls, probably through a reduction of obesity among a subset of girls who were obese at baseline. However, there was no prevention effect over the course of the study. That is, there was no difference at 2 years in the *incidence* of obesity for girls who were not obese at baseline (Gortmaker et al., 1999, Table 2, p. 415). There were no significant effects on obesity for boys. Although girls participating in *Planet Health* did reduce their overall energy intake while increasing consumption of fruits and vegetables, regression analysis indicated that obesity reduction was mediated, not by these desired changes, but by reduction in TV viewing.

The *Planet Health* researchers also evaluated the program's impact on two types of disordered weight control behaviors: purging and diet pill use in the past 30 days (Austin, Field, & Gortmaker, 2002; see also Austin et al., 2004). Among the 186 girls who were not dieting or eating disordered at baseline, only one (0.5%) who participated in *Planet Health* reported purging or using diet pills 2 years later, as compared to nine (5.6%) of 162 in the control condition. This yields a preventive fraction ([incidence$_{control}$ − incidence$_{experimental}$]/incidence$_{control}$) of .91, suggesting that approximately 91% of the new cases of disordered eating among the nondieting girls could have been prevented by *Planet Health* (Austin et al., 2002, 2005; S. B. Austin, personal communication, July 15, 2004). The program was not helpful in reducing the number of new cases (during the study period) of purging and diet pill use among girls who were dieting at baseline. Nevertheless, for all the girls available at follow-up, regardless of initial dieting status, the preventive fraction was .59.

Feminist-Empowerment-Relational Model. Chapters 7 and 8, respectively, review very promising research in Australia by O'Dea and Abraham (2000) and in Canada by Piran (1998, 1999a, 2001). Although their models differ in important respects, these programs share significant features of the FER model described in chapter 8 (see Table 8.2). This overlap is based in large part on O'Dea's and Piran's shared endorsement of the World Health Organization's concept of Health Promoting Schools (O'Dea & Maloney, 2000; Piran, 1999b; see chapter 15).

The FER model is also a significant part of the *Full of Ourselves* program for girls ages 12 to 14, developed by the Harvard Eating Disorder Center with consultation from Dr. Piran (Steiner-Adair et al., 2002). This curriculum consists of 70 activities, organized into eight units delivered across 2–4 months. *Full of Ourselves* helps girls become more assertive and more supportive of each other as they learn about weight- and shape-related prejudice and as they practice critical evaluation of various cultural messages pertaining to gender, beauty, weight, and eating. As the name implies, girls are explicitly encouraged to have a sense of self and substance in the world. This includes taking active leadership roles in social justice issues concerning body image (Steiner-Adair, 1994). The girls are given the opportunity to work closely with trained adult mentors and to serve as mentors themselves for girls ages 9 to 11.

Steiner-Adair et al. (2002) conducted a controlled evaluation, with a 6-month follow-up, of *Full of Ourselves*. Twenty-four schools in the Northeast participated; there was a plan to institute the program in Tulsa, Oklahoma, as well, but this had to be abandoned. Overall, the results in the Northeast are among the most positive to date for middle school girls. Program participants showed a sustained increase in knowledge about weightism, mass media, and health. Moreover, as predicted, they also had sustained improvements in body satisfaction. Although there were no significant effects on weight management *behavior* (including use of dieting as a means of coping with stress) or physical activity, there was a PPE for global self-esteem, negative self-talk about the body, and internalization of the slender beauty ideal.

Everybody is Somebody has recently been modified to involve some of the relational aspects of the FER model (McVey, Lieberman, Voorberg, Wardrope, & Blackmore, 2003a). Canadian public health nurses, who have ongoing contact with schools, received 3 hours of training and ongoing supervision in the conduct of *GirlTalk* peer support groups. These groups were held in school for girls ages 12 to 14. This version of McVey et al.'s program increased body esteem from pre-to-posttest and, more impressively, from posttest to 3-month follow-up. In addition, there were significant pre-to-follow-up reductions in dieting behavior for the experimental group; for the control group, dieting was unchanged, while bulimic behavior worsened. It should be noted that a recent replication of the *GirlTalk* program was not successful (McVey, Lieberman, Voorberg, Wardrope, Blackmore, & Tweed, 2003b).

Conclusions

The studies by Killen et al. (1993; Killen, 1996) and McVey and Davis (2002) were well-designed, had a clear foundation in the social cognitive model, and were implemented by researchers with considerable experience in prevention and health promotion. The negative results of these studies must reduce our faith in the standard social cognitive approach with adolescents ages 11 to 14. Nevertheless, the results of 10 studies (see Table 9.2) suggest that lessons based on the social cognitive model, sometimes incorporating elements of the NSVS model, can produce short-term positive effects not only on knowledge, but also on attitudes, intentions, and behaviors. These findings in turn suggest that elements of the social cognitive approach (e.g., understanding of pubertal development and critical evaluation of cultural messages about thinness and diversity) can serve as the foundation for programs that incorporate social cognitive elements with an emphasis on developmental theory (see chapter 4) and on critical social perspectives such as the FER model (Levine & Piran, 2001, 2004; Levine & Smolak, 2002). This idea is developed more fully in the final chapter of this book.

HIGH SCHOOL

There have been 20 evaluations of preventive interventions with high school students (ages 14 to 18; see Table 9.3). Six (30% of the high school interventions) included a comparison group and at least a 1-month follow-up. Of that subset, only one (5% of the total) has some type of random assignment to experimental or control conditions, as well as at least a 6-month follow-up assessment. Two others (10%) have used random assignment and a 2- or 3-month follow-up.

Controlled Evaluations With At Least 2-Month Follow-up

Negative or Limited Results. Paxton (1993) evaluated a social cognitive program for Australian girls ages 14 and 15. The five units (90 minutes each) covered, for example, biopsychosocial determinants of weight and shape, and the ways in which eating is influenced by emotional and physical needs. At 11-month follow-up there were no significant effects on body dissatisfaction, drive for thinness, eating behavior, and weight management. Buddeberg-Fischer and colleagues in Switzerland also found negative results in a well-designed study of a prevention program with substantial elements of the social cognitive and NSVS models, including an ecological perspective for the high school setting (Buddeberg-Fischer, Klaghofer, Gnam, & Buddeberg, 1998; see also Buddeberg-Fischer, Klaghofer, Reed, & Buddeberg, 2000; Buddeberg-Fischer & Reed, 2001). As was the case for McVey and Davis' (2002) study (with 6- and 12-month follow-ups) of Canadian adolescents, absence of a prevention effect in Buddeberg-Fischer et al.'s (1998) study was attributable to improvement by both experimental and control students from pretest to 3-month follow-up.

Weiss' (2001) dissertation evaluated the *Making Choices* program for Australian girls ages 14 to 15. The program was carefully constructed over several years and through considerable pilot work. Four units (100 minutes each) intentionally integrated elements of all three prevention models (see Table 9.3), as well as some attention to parents and peers. Regardless, at 3-month follow-up sustained changes were evident only on several EDI variables for the high-risk group. In fact, low-risk girls receiving the program reported decreases in their body satisfaction while their feelings of susceptibility to eating disorder increased.

TABLE 9.3
Studies of Universal Prevention in High School Students

Study	Program	Design	RA	Gender	Devel	Ecol	DISC	NSVS	FER	K	A	B	PPE	Comment
Controlled—Follow-up														
Paxton (1993); 136 AUS f, $M = 14.1$	5 units 90 min ea	RM (11 mo)	N	N	N	N	4	0	0	nm	N	N	nm	Focus: nutrition, dieting, emotions & eating, determinants of size.
Neumark-Sztainer et al. (1995); 341 Jewish ISRAELI f, $M = 15.3$	10 units 60 min ea	RM (6, 24 mo)	Y/N	Y	Y	N	7	0	2	N	N	N	Y	Emphasis on nutrition and healthy eating.
Buddeberg-Fischer et al. (1998); 109 SWISS m, 205 f; $M = 16.1$	3 units 90 min ea	RM (3 mo)	Y	Y	Y	N	4	0	2	nm	N	N	nm	Classes had M of 30% students at risk (EAT > 10).
Santonastaso et al. 1999; 265 ITAL f, $M = 16.1$	4 units 120 min ea	RM (12 mo)	N	N	Y	N	3	0	0	nm	Y	Y	nm	Low-risk girls (EAT < 30) had lower body dissatisfaction + less increase in bulimic beh/attitudes.
Shepard (2000); 88 US m, 65 f, $M \sim 14.5$	5 units 50 min ea	RM (2 mo)	N	Y	N	N	5	0	1	Y	N	N	Y	Conducted by peer educators.
Weiss (2001); 173 AUS f, $M = 15.1$	4 units 100 min ea	RM (3 mo)	Y	Y	Y	Y	7	2	2	Y	N	N	N	Low-risk girls had decreased body satisfaction at follow-up; HR girls appeared to benefit from program.
Pre to Post (C = controlled; NC = no control) or Follow-up but No Control (RM-NC)														
Jerome (1987, 1991); 32 US m, 43 f; $M=16.5$	26-min video & review	RM-NC	N	Y	N	N	2	0	0	Y	N	N	N	Sig pre-to-follow-up deterioration in restraint & body satisfaction.
Jerome (1991); 58 US m, 51 f; $M = 15.07$	26-min video & discussion	PP-C	Y	Y	N	N	2	0	0	Y	N	N	na	Students seeing film did indicate a reduced intent to diet.
Rosen (1989); 100 US m & f, ages 14–18	8 units 45 min ea	PP-C	Y	N	Y	N	4	0	0	Y	nm	N	na	Cognitive-behav focus: positive body image & wt management.

(Continued)

TABLE 9.3
(Continued)

Study	Program	Design	RA	Gender	Devel	Ecol	DISC	NSVS	FER	K	A	B	PPE	Comment
Moriarty et al. (1990); ~223 CAN f; $M \sim 15.3$	10 units 60–70 min ea	PP-C	N	N	Y	N	6	1	0	Y	Y	nm	na	Worked w/faculty, staff, students to increase knowledge.
Shisslak et al. (1990) 153 US f, ages 15–16	8 units	Post only C	N	Y	N	Y	3	0	0	Y	nm	nm	na	
Nichter et al. (1999); 22 US f, ages 14–18	5 workshops 16.5 hrs total	RM-NC	na	Y	N	N	3	1	2	Y	Y	Y	na	Intentional mix of Caucasian, Hispanic, & African American.
Piran (1999a); 23, 30, & 25 CAN f, $M = 16.1$	2–6 units, 1 hr ea + boosters	3 waves	N	Y	Y	Y	3	2	7	Y	Y	Y	na	Residential, competitive, elite ballet school.
Phelps et al. (2000); 312 US f, ages 14–16	6 units	Post only C	Y	N	Y	N	5	1	0	nm	Y	N	na	
Heinze et al. (2000); 88 AUS f, $M = 15.8$	24-min video no discuss	NC	Y	Y	Y	N	6	0	0	Y	Y	nm	na	Didactic video; status of presenter does not matter; effects less than for girls in 7th grade.
Rocco et al. (2001); 80 ITAL f, $M = 16.1$	9 units 120 min ea	PP-C	N	N	Y	N	6	0	2	nm	N	N	na	Some evidence for negative effect of intervention.
Kelton-Locke (2001); 365 US f & m, ages 14–15	60-min presentation	PP-C	N	Y	N	Y	4	0	2	Y	nm	nm	na	The Body Positive's Prevention Program.
Wiseman et al. (2001) 138 ITAL f, 56 US f, ages 15–16	6 units	PP-C	Y	?	?	N		1		nm	N	N	na	Didactic lectures: self-esteem, body image, nutrition, ED.

| Abascal et al. (2002); 106 US f, ages 15–16 | 8-week interactive software | PP-NC HR-HM LR-HM | Y nm nm | N Y Y | N Y N | N na na | 6 | 1 | 0 | nm nm | Y Y | Y N | na na | Replication/extension of Abascal et al. (2004); low motivation groups did not benefit. |
| Abascal et al. (2004) 78 US f, $M = 15.3$ | 8-week interactive software | PP-NC HR-HM LR-LM Mixed | Y | N N N | N N N | N na na | 6 | 1 | 0 | | Y Y Y | Y Y Y | N N Y | H = high; L = low; R = risk; M = motivation; HR participants in both groups improved more; only HR in mixed had improved restraint scores. |

Notes.
1. Age refers to age at the onset of the intervention.
2. Design: PP = Pre–post; RM = Repeated Measures (with length of follow-up in months in parentheses).
3. RA: random assignment by school, class, or participant.
4. Gender: Gendered nature of body image, eating, weight management was one focus.
5. Devel: Development (e.g., in adolescence) was one focus.
6. Ecology: Intervention had at least one ecological component.
7. SC: How many elements of disease-specific social cognitive approach were present (see Table 6.1).
8. NSVS: How many elements of nonspecific vulnerability-stressor approach were present (see Table 7.2).
9. FER: How many elements of feminist-empowerment-relational approach were present (see Table 8.2).
10. K = significant improvement in knowledge; A = improvement in attitude; B = improvement in behavior; nm = not measured; Y = yes, on at least one variable; N = no for all of the dependent variables.
11. PPE: program participation effect; pre–post significant improvement, but not maintained at follow-up.

In another doctoral dissertation, Shepard (2000), at the University of Oregon, also reported disappointing results. Her five-unit program (*Body and Soul*) incorporated almost all the social cognitive elements. It was conducted by peer educators who had participated in an intensive 2-day training session. Although there were sustained improvements in knowledge, the only significant effect emerging from the many attitudinal and behavioral variables examined posttest and at a 2-month follow-up was a PPE for internalization of the slender beauty ideal. Four other controlled studies of high school students, all based on the social cognitive model, yielded no significant pre-to-postprogram effects (Jerome, 1987, in the United States; Rocco, Ciano, & Balestrieri, 2001, in Italy; Rosen, 1989, in the United States; Wiseman, Sunday, Bortollotti, & Halmi, 2001, in the United States and in Italy).

Positive Results. Three controlled studies applying the social cognitive model and varying degrees of the NSVS model have produced some positive pre-to-postprogram changes (see Table 9.3). The empirical changes were limited, however, to drive for thinness (Wiseman et al., 2001, in Italy), or to attitudes about sociocultural factors (Moriarty, Shore, & Maxim, 1990, in Canada; Phelps et al., 2000, in the United States) and to intentions to diet (Phelps et al., 2000).

Two studies with longer follow-up periods yielded much more support for the preventive effects of a social cognitive program for older adolescents. *The Weigh to Eat!* program for Israeli girls ages 15 to 16 (Neumark-Sztainer et al., 1995) was described in detail in chapter 6. Its positive findings for a social cognitive program were replicated by Santonastaso et al. (1999), who randomly assigned 16-year-old Italian girls (by classes) to a comparison condition or to participation in four 2-hour presentations and group discussions. At 1-year follow-up there was a significant preventive effect for the body dissatisfaction and bulimic behavior of "low-risk" participants. There was no prevention effect for high-risk participants, and no effect for either risk group on drive for thinness.

Conclusions

Based on the many studies conducted with girls ages 14 to 16, it is certainly *possible* to use the social cognitive model to create attitudinal and behavioral prevention effects that can be sustained for 6 to 12 months (Neumark-Sztainer et al., 1995; Santonastaso et al., 1999; see also

Nichter et al., 1999). Recall that Piran's (1999a) uncontrolled but extensive and longitudinal application of the FER model to elite ballet students ages 14 to 18 was very successful (see chapter 8). It is, in some respects, the most promising program. However, given the modest effects of the four studies with pre–post designs—and more important, given that eight studies in five different countries produced virtually no significant effects for attitudes and behavior—it is clear that high school students are a very difficult audience for universal-selective prevention (but not for targeted prevention; see Stice & Shaw, 2004). In fact, an abbreviated version of O'Dea's NSVS program *Everybody's Different* (see chapter 7), which had very encouraging outcomes in middle school students, produced null results when applied to 9th-grade Australian boys and girls (Wade, Davidson, & O'Dea, 2003). Similarly, the prevention videotape evaluated by Werteim, Withers, and colleagues (see, e.g., Heinze et al., 2000) had a greater effect on the knowledge and attitudes of 7th-grade (ages 12–13) Australian girls than 10th-grade girls (ages 15–16).

OLDER ADOLESCENTS AND YOUNG ADULTS

Excluding media literacy programs (see chapter 13), there are 17 evaluations of interventions for older adolescents or young adults who have not been recruited on the basis of high scores on body dissatisfaction or eating problems (see Table 9.4). Nine (53%) included a comparison group and at least a 1-month follow-up. However, only one (6%) included random assignment and a 6-month follow-up assessment. Three others used random assignment and a 3-month follow-up.

One-Shot Programs

Due to limitations on resources, many colleges in the United States offer one-time ("one-shot") programs. In addition to prevention of negative body image and disordered eating, these presentations are designed to be an initial step (case identification and self-referral) in targeted prevention or treatment. The best-known study of this type was conducted by Mann et al. (1997). Groups of 10 to 20 women in their first year at Stanford University spent 90 minutes with two high-profile students who were recovering from an eating disorder. These peer educators presented their personal narratives and factual information about eating disorders. Although methodology, attrition, and ethics make this

TABLE 9.4
Studies of Universal Prevention in College Students and Young Adults

Study	Program	Design	RA	Gender	Devel	EcoI	DISC	NSVS	FER	K	A	B	PPE	Comment
Controlled—Follow-up														
Gurney (1997); 244 US college f	30-min video	PP-C (~2 mo)	Y	N	N	N	2	0	0	nm	N	N	na	Intervention and control video on good nutrition had minimal effects.
Mann et al. (1997); 329 US f, ages 18–19	90-min pres by 2 ED patients	RM (3 mo)	N	N	N	N	1	0	0	nm	N	N	N	Negative effect at posttest; no effects from pre-to-FU for $n = 379$.
Winzelberg et al. (1998); 45 US f, $M = 19.7$	8-week interactive software	RM (3 mo)	Y	N	N	N	6	0	0	N	Y	N	N	*Student Bodies* program; includes e-mail support group. Program fidelity was low.
Martz & Bazzini (1999, Study 1); 114 US f, $M = 19.0$	1-hour	Solomon 4-group (1 mo)	Y	Y	N	N	3	0	0	nm	Y	Y	na	Didactic peer education; authors note effects are "small" and "minimal."
Martz & Bazzini (1999, Study 2); 77 US f, $M = 19.0$	1-hour	Pre-Fu (1 mo)	Y	Y	N	N	4	0	0	nm	N	Y	na	Psychologist conducted intervention; intervention yields less dieting *but* less body esteem.
Winzelberg et al. (2000); 44 US f, $M = 20$	8-week interactive software	RM (3 mo)	Y	N	N	N	6	1	0	nm	Y	Y	na	*Student Bodies* plus element of social support; compliance still an issue.
Celio et al. (2000); 76 US f, $M = 19.6$	8-week interactive software	RM (6 mos)	Y	Y	Y	N	6	1	0	nm	Y	Y	na	*Student Bodies* vs. *Body Traps* (see Springer et al., 1999); participants had high body dissatisfaction.
Nicolino et al. (2001); 85 US f, $M = 18.9$	2-hour group session	Pre-Fu (1 mo)	Y	N	N	N	2	1	0	nm	N	N	na	Cognitive-behavioral intervention by Martz and colleagues.
Franko et al. (2004); 240 f, $M = 18.2$	2 sessions 60 min ea: interactive software	RM (3 mos)	Y	Y	Y	N	7	2	0	Y	Y	Y	N	120 HR & 120 LR students received *Food, Mood, & Attitude* CD-ROM program. Moderate to strong effects for HR students.
Pre to Post (C = controlled; NC = no control) or Follow-up but No Control (RM-NC)														
Nebel (1995); 203 US f, $M = 19.6$	5 workshops 20–30 min ea	PP-C	N	Y	N	N	3	2	0	N	N	Y	na	Didactic program for sororities; attrition was a problem.

Study	Design	Duration	Gender	Devel	Ecology	SC	NSVS	FER	K	A	B	PPE	Notes
Martz et al. (1997); 36 US f, M = 20	PP-C	1 month	Y	N	N	N	Y	na	na	N	N	N	na	Peer leaders in sororities trained to promote ED awareness and non-dieting approach to eating; attrition was large.
Springer et al. (1999); 41 US f, M = 19.5	PP-C	10-wk course 120 min/wk	N	Y	N	Y	N	6	0	2	nm	Y	Y	na	*Body Traps* class at Stanford; see Celio et al. (2000).
Phelps et al. (2000); 63 US f, ages 18-25	PP-C	4 sessions 90 min ea	N	N	N	Y	N	5	1	0	nm	Y	Y	na	Didactic material plus discussion in sorority; q & a with recovered person.
Spiller (2000); 43 US f, ages 18-20	PP-C	3 workshops 60 min ea	N	Y	N	N	N	5	0	3	nm	Y	N	na	Feminist-nondieting program for sororities; attrition is a problem.
Abood & Black (2000) 70 US f college athletes (Div I), M = 19	PP-C	8-week 60 min ea	Y	N	N	N	N	3	2	0	Y	Y	nm	na	"Health education intervention" focusing promoting health for enhanced athletic performance.
Mutterperl & Sanderson (2002); 107 US f, M = 18.1	RM-NC Healthy eating Norm misperception	1 session 10 min [4-page brochure]	Y	N N	N N	N N	N N	1 1	0 0	0 0	nm	N	N	N	Accurate norm information helped young women who had initially tended not to internalize the slender beauty ideal.
Sanderson & Holloway (2003); 112 US f, M = 18.8	RM-NC Healthy eating Disordered eat. (3 mos)	1 session 45 min	Y	N	N	N	N	3 1	0 0	0 0	nm	N	N	N	Young women with initial high drive for thinness were harmed by focus on disordered eating.

Notes.
1. Age refers to age at the onset of the intervention.
2. Design: PP = Pre-post; RM = Repeated Measures (with length of follow-up in months in parentheses).
3. RA: random assignment by school, class, or participant.
4. Gender: Gendered nature of body image, eating, weight management was one focus.
5. Devel: Development (e.g., in adolescence) was one focus.
6. Ecology: Intervention had at least one ecological component.
7. SC: How many elements of social cognitive approach were present (see Table 6.1).
8. NSVS: How many elements of nonspecific vulnerability-stressor approach were present (see Table 7.2).
9. FER: How many elements of feminist-empowerment-relational approach were present (see Table 8.2).
10. K = significant improvement in knowledge; A = improvement in attitude; B = improvement in behavior; nm = not measured; Y = yes, on at least one variable; N = no for all of the dependent variables.
11. PPE: program participation effect; pre-post significant improvement, but not maintained at follow-up.

study controversial (Cohn & Maine, 1998, vs. Carter, Stewart, & Fairburn, 1998; Mann & Burgard, 1998), such an intervention appears to be ineffective and potentially harmful, that is, iatrogenic (Mann et al., 1997). More recently, three studies by Martz and colleagues and two by Sanderson and colleagues (reviewed next) demonstrated that even a carefully designed 1-hour presentation is not particularly helpful, and may raise self-consciousness about body image in ways that are iatrogenic (Martz & Bazzini, 1999; Nicolino, Martz, & Curtin, 2001). Gurney's (1997) doctoral study evaluated a one-shot intervention that combined didactic information about body image, self-esteem, nutrition, and exercise with discussions of media influences on body image. Compared to a placebo video on good nutrition, this intervention also had no meaningful effects at an assessment 7 weeks later.

Like Wertheim, Paxton, and associates in Australia, Catherine Sanderson and her colleagues in the United States have applied a social psychological perspective to understanding the interaction between the specific features of an educational message and the characteristics of the audience. Sanderson and Holloway (2003) compared two types of 45-minute educational programs for first-year college women. One type focused on the nature and effects of eating disorders, as well as the process of recovery. The second set of messages addressed healthy eating and exercising, how the construction of unrealistic media images of beauty affects women's body image, and how eating comes to be linked with various emotions and external cues. At 3-month follow-up, neither set of messages was more effective in terms of body size estimates and drive for thinness. Moreover, the findings contradicted the expected positive effects of message relevance for different audiences. The healthy eating condition did not have a more beneficial effect on women with a low drive for thinness, whereas the eating disorders condition had several different *negative* effects on those young women who initially had a high drive for thinness. In fact, if anything, the women with a low drive for thinness responded more positively to the eating disorders information.

Mutterperl and Sanderson (2002) had first-year college women read a brief brochure that challenged their misguided tendency to see restrained eating and frequent exercising as the norm among college women. Compared to reading about healthy eating in a college environment, this one-shot effort to combat norm misperception had no general effects on either internalization of the slender beauty ideal or disordered eating. However, as predicted, correction of norm misperception did have positive associations (albeit very small) with higher ideal body weight and lower disordered eating at 3-month follow-up for young women who already had low internalization scores. This finding suggests that correct information about actual social norms at college may indeed help young women who tend not to compare themselves to media images of the slender beauty ideal. The importance of norms is considered in more detail in chapter 10. In general, Sanderson's research suggests that the interaction between message and audience characteristics is deserving of future research (see chapter 15).

Longer Controlled Evaluations

Perhaps a longer, more intensive program would be more effective for young adults. Surprisingly, with the exception of the work of Taylor and colleagues at Stanford University, only a few have been evaluated, most of which are preliminary ("pilot") studies (Irving, Levine, & Piran, 2003). Nebel's (1995) dissertation assessed a selective (but not targeted; see chapter 1) prevention program consisting of five 20–30-minute psychoeducational sessions for young women in a high-risk setting: sororities. Presentations combined information and exercises based on the social cognitive model with two aspects of the NSVS approach: stress management and improving self-image. Although there were no experimental versus control effects for knowledge (e.g., of nutrition), body dissatisfaction, or drive for thinness, the intervention produced lower scores on the bulimia and ineffectiveness subscales of the EDI. Martz, Graves, and Sturgis (1997) took a different approach by training selected woman in sororities to use posters, buttons, education, and their own behavior to discourage dieting and to emphasize healthy eating and exercising. This more ecological form of selective prevention produced no meaningful changes in participants, including the peer leaders, who received 6 hours of training for prevention and for identification and referral of disordered eating. Attrition was a major problem in the Nebel (1995) and Martz et al. (1997) studies.

More encouraging results were found in three other recent studies of selective prevention, two of which incorporated FER elements in working with young sorority members. Phelps et al. (1999, 2000) evaluated a version of the program (described earlier) developed for middle and high school students. At posttest, four 75-minute sessions, including a question and answer period with a woman who has recovered from an eating disorder (cf. Mann et al., 1997), reduced current use of unhealthy weight-management techniques, decreased body dissatisfaction, and increased physical self-esteem. Spiller's (2000) doctoral thesis was an uncontrolled evaluation of three weekly 1-hour workshops emphasizing "feminist collaborative tenets." Although attrition was high (37%), immediately following the program there were encouraging increases in knowledge and decreases in drive for thinness and likelihood of dieting. Finally, in a well-designed study, Abood and Black (2000) evaluated an 8-hour educational program for female college athletes (Division I). These researchers found that nutrition education to enhance athletic performance, coupled with exercises to improve self-esteem and stress management, helped these young women to improve body satisfaction, reduce drive for thinness, maintain their self-esteem (relative to decreases in the control group), and increase their nutrition knowledge.

Promising Directions: *Student Bodies*

Stanford University's long-term investment in developing a computer-assisted psychoeducational program (CAPP) for college women has been described in detail elsewhere (Celio, Winzelberg, Dev, & Taylor, 2002; Taylor, Winzelberg, & Celio, 2001; Zabinski, Celio, Jacobs, Manwaring, & Wilfley, 2003; see Table 9.4). The 8-week intervention, *Student Bodies,* is designed to reduce body dissatisfaction and "weight concerns" (Killen, 1996; Taylor et al., 2001).

Based on the social cognitive and cognitive-behavioral models (see chapter 6), participants receive multimedia "psychoeducation" about body image, the development and consequences of eating disorders, cultural determinants of beauty, and healthy nutrition and exercise. Some of the important information provided in *Student Bodies* is contained in a curriculum entitled *Body Traps*. Springer, Winzelberg, Perkins, and Taylor (1999) first implemented *Body Traps* as a 10-week Stanford seminar for credit. Readings, reaction papers, and discussions emphasized *content* from the social cognitive model, as well as both content and the *critical social perspective* featured in the FER model (see chapter 8). Springer et al. (1999) found that a nonrandomized control group changed very little over the duration of the course, whereas seminar participants reported improved body satisfaction, fewer bulimic symptoms, a lower drive for thinness, and reduced weight and shape concerns.

In *Student Bodies* the relevant information from *Body Traps* is reinforced by cognitive-behavioral exercises (see, e.g., Cash, 1996, 1997), three moderated face-to-face discussion sessions, weekly readings and short critical analyses, and computer-based changes designed to increase connection between the participants. Celio et al. (2000) found that, compared to a wait-list control, women randomly assigned to receive this version had (at 3-month follow-up) significantly improved attitudes and behaviors with regard to weight, shape, and eating (see also Taylor et al., 2001). Women assigned to the *Body Traps* class had scores intermediate to the control and *Student Bodies* conditions, but also had a higher rate of attrition than occurred in the latter.

The Stanford researchers use advertisements and presentations to recruit women "with a desire to improve body image satisfaction" (Winzelberg et al., 2000, p. 347). This could apply to the vast majority of women college students, but, not surprisingly, the young women participating in the CAPP studies tend at pretest to have high levels of body dissatisfaction and weight concerns (Celio et al., 2002; see also Bearman, Stice, & Chase, 2003, for a description of the high body dissatisfaction scores of young women responding to an invitation to participate in a program "aimed at helping females [in college] improve their body image" [p. 280]). We acknowledge that those with eating disorders and/or purging behaviors are screened out, and that, technically, this research does not target those with high levels of body dissatisfaction and weight concerns. Nevertheless, characterization of *Student Bodies* (Celio et al., 2000; Winzelberg et al., 1998, 2000) as "universal prevention" or even "selective" prevention (high risk but not symptomatic; see chapter 1) is debatable.

This important issue is discussed in detail in chapter 14. However, it is worth mentioning at this point that the distinction between low-risk and at-risk college students appears to be important in considering the benefits of CAPP. Recently, Inflexxion, Inc., in Newton, Massachusetts (see Appendix B), developed an interactive, psychoeduational CD-ROM program called *Food, Mood, and Attitude* (Franko, 2004; Franko et al., 2004). This 2-hour (two-session) program engages female college students in playing the role of a peer counselor who enters the virtual worlds of three other young women who have various issues with eating, weight, and body image. Each of the three has a "scrapbook" that provides the program user with pscyhoeducational information and interactive tools, based on the principles of cognitive-behavioral theory (see chapter 6), Stice's (2001a) dual-pathway model, and interpersonal theory. In a randomized, controlled trial, Franko et al. (2004) found that at 3-month follow-up *Food, Mood, and Attitude* had a moderately strong positive effect (partial eta^2s = .50–.70) in helping at-risk young women in their first year of college to increase their knowledge and to decrease their internalization of the slender beauty ideal. In addition, the at-risk young women (who had some symptoms of disordered eating) who participated in the program had modest decreases (partial eta^2s = .25–.30) in weight and shape concerns, as well as in restrained eating. Low-risk women who received the program demonstrated an increase in awareness and knowledge, while the effects for attitudes and behavior were nonsignificant.

One advantage of CAPP is that it permits some tailoring of the program to the individual participant's needs. This creates the potential for combining universal and targeted prevention in a school setting (Abascal, Brown, Winzelberg, Dev, & Taylor, 2004; Abascal, Bruning, Winzelberg, Dev, & Taylor, 2002; Taylor, Cameron, Newman, & Junge, 2002). Abascal and her colleagues at Stanford assessed the impact of *Student Bodies* on students ages 15 to 16 at an all-girls private school. In the first study (Abascal et al., 2004), two classes of students were divided into high-risk/high motivation or low-risk/low motivation groups. In a third class all participants completed the curriculum as one "mixed group." All three groups either improved or remained the same on the EDE-Q or EDI subscales; although there was evidence for broader positive effects in the two groups with high-risk participants, there were no significant between-group differences from pre- to postprogram. In the second study (Abascal et al., 2002) a different set of students ages 15 to 16 at the same school were assigned to four groups formed from a cross of high–low risk and high–low motivation. Although all groups benefited, girls with high motivation showed the greatest pre-to-post improvements in body image and eating measures. Once again, the broadest improvements and most positive feelings about the program were demonstrated by high-risk girls with the high motivation to change. These findings add to the construct validity of the *Student Bodies* program, while indicating a need for further development in programming for students with lower motivation.

Conclusions

It is clear that one-shot didactic presentations of information about eating disorders are ineffective. Furthermore, multisession but short-term interventions based solely on the SCT and/or CBT models (see chapter 6) are also likely to be ineffective as prevention. The study by Phelps et al. (1999, 2000) suggests that a combination of the social cognitive and NSVS models, with an emphasis on women's hardiness, may be effective in the short run. However, longitudinal data are lacking, and research with younger populations supports the proposition that the Phelps et al.'s positive outcome is probably a program participation effect. Perhaps by ages 18 to 24, so many young women have internalized the slender beauty ideal, have at least moderate levels of weight and shape concern, have significant doubts about their own beauty and desirability, and have some experience with dieting, that "prevention" of these components of eating problems is futile, if not illogical (see, e.g., Drewnowski, Yee, Kurth, & Krahn, 1994; Mintz & Betz, 1988). Yet, young adulthood remains a risk period for the *onset* of eating problems and eating disorders (Smolak & Levine, 1996). Perhaps the solution is the development of prevention programs that combine universal and targeted features (see also chapter 14). *Student Bodies*, the most promising development of this sort, is notable for its combination of the following: psychoeducation in a variety of areas derived from the social cognitive and FER areas; individualized programming based on the SCT and CBT models; and social support.

TARGETED PREVENTION

As described earlier, some interventions are definitely "targeted" (e.g., Franko et al., 2004; see chapter 1). Their goal is to prevent development of full-blown disorders in women who are at great risk because they are "chronic dieters" and/or because they already have elevated scores on measures of negative body image or eating disorder symptomatology. Stice is prominent among those who argue that targeted prevention is more effective than universal prevention (see, e.g., Stice et al., 2001; Stice & Hoffman, 2004; Stice & Shaw, 2004). The following sections discuss promising developments in this area. For more comprehensive reviews, the reader is referred to Cash and Hrabrosky (2004) and Stice and Shaw (2004). Portions of our review of targeted programs are based on Irving et al. (2003).

Women With Negative Body Image

Cognitive-Behavioral Therapy. In general, young women with negative body image suffer from social anxiety, depressive symptoms, and unhealthy forms of eating and weight management. Thus, many clinical researchers, led by James Rosen and Thomas Cash, have developed cognitive-behavioral therapies (CBT; see chapter 6) to improve body image and thereby prevent eating disorders. Cash's widely used CBT program includes (a) psychoeducation about body image; (b) guided exercises for assessing and challenging unhealthy cognitions and for developing more positive, adaptive beliefs and thoughts about appearance; and (c) training in skills for mastering the situations that generate body-image anxiety and unproductive behaviors such as avoidance (Cash, 1997). In a series of controlled and uncontrolled outcomes studies, both Cash and Rosen and their colleagues have found that, over 3-to-6-month follow-up periods, this type of program causes meaningful improvements in various important components of body image, as well as in self-esteem and social confidence (Cash & Hrabosky, 2004; Cash & Strachan, 2002).

CBT is a promising form of targeted prevention because it is relatively brief (1–3 months) and can be applied equally effectively in an individual, group, or self-help format. For example, Bearman et al. (2003) constructed a CBT program to prevent bulimic pathology and depression in young female college students with "body image concerns." The four 1-hour sessions, conducted for small groups of women, focused on basic principles (e.g., identifying and challenging negative thoughts pertaining to body image) from the work of Cash and Rosen. At 3-month follow-up (but not at 6-month follow-up) Bearman et al. (2003) found that this form of brief, focused CBT produced significant improvements (relative to the control group and to baseline) in negative affect, depressive symptoms, and bulimic symptoms. At 3- and 6-month follow-up there was also a treatment effect for body dissatisfaction. Moreover, as predicted, multiple regression analyses revealed that the positive changes in negative affect, depressive symptoms, and bulimic pathology were partially or fully mediated by improvements in body satisfaction. This program is a positive step in the direction of targeted prevention, and we anticipate that further research with extended follow-up periods will determine whether or not CBT can truly prevent eating disorders, dysfunctional eating attitudes and behaviors, and depression.

Dissonance-Based Programs. Three further studies by Stice, Chase, and colleagues indicate that a "dissonance-based" program can reduce risk factors and symptoms in college women with "elevated body image concerns" (Stice, Mazotti, Weibel, & Agras, 2000; Stice et al., 2001; Stice, Trost, & Chase, 2003; see also Mann et al., 1999). The intervention consisted of three 1-hour sessions in which small groups of participants, working with a clinical psychologist (or graduate student), create a "body acceptance program" ostensibly for high school girls. Thus, participants act contrary to their previously held internalization of the slender beauty ideal by publicly articulating a critical social perspective that culminates in a respect for diverse body weight and shapes. Based on the SCT approach, topics critically analyzed by the group include origins and effects of the thin ideal, how it is perpetuated, and who benefits. Participants also completed body acceptance exercises, as well as a counterattitudinal role-play and counterattitudinal essay in which they provided reasons for challenging the thin ideal.

In the first study (Stice, Mazotti, et al., 2000), at 1-month follow-up the dissonance program was more successful than a no-intervention control in reducing thin-ideal internalization, body dissatisfaction, and bulimic symptoms. In the second study (Stice et al., 2001), this intervention and a healthy weight-management control condition both produced similar positive results at 1-month follow-up. The dissonance program more quickly reduced the crucial risk factors of thin-ideal internalization and body dissatisfaction.

Stice et al. (2003) conducted a more rigorous longitudinal test of the dissonance model of prevention. High school and college students were randomly assigned to the dissonance treatment, the healthy weight-management condition, or a wait-list control. The healthy weight-management group received information and behavior modification techniques to help them eat a "balanced diet," engage in "regular moderate exercising," and distinguish between "ineffective and effective dieting" (p. 14). The key group × time interactions for the main dependent variables (e.g., internalization of slender beauty ideal) were not significant. Keeping this negative result in mind, analysis of changes within the treatment groups indicated that at 6-month follow-up the dissonance group had a sustained reduction in their internalization of the thin ideal, but the effects for the other measures dissipated after the program (between posttest and the 1-month follow-up; body dissatisfaction) or at 6-month follow-up (negative affect and bulimic behavior). If anything, the healthy weight intervention resulted in longer term improvements in negative affect and bulimic symptoms. More research is needed to clarify the active ingredients of both interventions (and perhaps to combine them), to determine how to increase facilitators' fidelity to the program (this was a problem in this third study), and to create the conditions for a sustained effect in all risk factors, including body dissatisfaction.

Clinical Psychoeducation. Franko (1998) invited University of Massachusetts students to participate in a workshop "if they were troubled by their eating habits or had body image concerns" (p. 32). The program consisted of eight 90-minute group sessions in which 10 women meeting this criterion (without having an eating disorder) participated in didactic presentations, discussion, and in-session and homework activities. The curriculum was based on a combination of the SCT and CBT approaches, as the group's work focused on the nature of healthy eating and healthy weight management, dysfunctional beliefs about weight and shape, and the importance of identity and life skills in resisting the negative impact of cultural ideals of thinness on women. Franko's (1998) program was not particularly effective. Global body image improved, but there were no experimental versus control treatment effects for body dissatisfaction, drive for thinness, bulimic symptoms, and weight concerns.

One subgroup at risk for eating problems is girls with insulin-dependent (Type 1) diabetes mellitus (IDDM; Nielsen, 2002). Olmsted and colleagues at Toronto General Hospital randomly assigned 85 adolescent girls with IDDM to receive either six 90-minute sessions of group psychoeducation, or IDDM treatment as usual with no psychoeducation (Olmsted, Daneman, Rydall, Lawson, & Rodin, 2002). The topics in the psychoeducation were derived from both the SCT approach and the developmental model (with a focus on the challenges of puberty), and then tailored to the special challenges that diabetes poses for body image, eating attitudes, healthy eating, family dynamics, and so forth. Screening ensured that all participants reported high levels of body dissatisfaction, drive for thinness, or disturbed eating attitudes and behaviors. Girls age 14 or less were in one group, while the older girls were in another. At 6-month follow-up there were significant reductions in body dissatisfaction, drive for thinness, dietary restraint, and eating concerns. Although this was encouraging, the authors note that these findings may be of limited clinical significance because there were no improvements in metabolic control or binge eating. Moreover, of the 130 girls initially identified as candidates for the program, only 85 (~65.5%) expressed an initial interest, and only 36 (~28%) completed the psychoeducational program.

Computer-Assisted Psychoeducation Program (CAPP). Zabinski, Pung, et al. (2001) assessed the effects of the *Student Bodies* CAPP on young female undergraduates in San Diego, California. At 2.5-month follow-up the program participants reported no change in drive for thinness, but modest improvements in body satisfaction and in weight and shape concerns. For undetermined reasons, the comparison group also improved, so there were no significant group × time interactions. Nevertheless, the researchers argue that this study supports the efficacy of the *Students Bodies* CAPP for targeted prevention because the interaction effect sizes for body dissatisfaction, EDI drive for thinness, and overall EDE-Q scores were moderate to large, ranging from .36 to .53 (see Franko et al., 2004, as previously described). Zabinski et al. (2001) acknowledge that more research is needed because the behavioral effects of the CAPP were limited.

Classroom Psychoeducation. Stice and Ragan (2001) reported the quasiexperimental evaluation of an eating disorders seminar for students in their third and fourth years of undergraduate study at the University of Texas. Although described in the article as an "intensive psychoeducational intervention" (p. 159), the course was advertised and conducted as a university class. Although participants reported low levels of eating disorder symptoms, this is a form of targeted prevention because as a group the students who signed up had moderate to high levels of body dissatisfaction and dieting behavior. Didactic presentations and group discussion were used to cover the nature, epidemiology, etiology, and prevention of disordered eating; there was also attention to obesity, nutrition, and healthy weight management. Consistent with the positive effects of the Stanford *Body Traps* curriculum (Springer et al., 1999; see Table 9.4), Stice and Ragan (2001) found that, compared to matched control participants from other university psychology courses, the students reported (at the conclusion of the eating disorders class) significant reductions in internalization of the thin beauty ideal, body dissatisfaction, dieting, and eating disorder symptoms. The design did not include a follow-up.

Women With Chronic Dieting and Subclinical Eating Disorders

Cognitive-Behavioral Psychoeducation. Kaminski and McNamara (1996) screened 315 young female undergraduates at an American university. Twenty-nine (9.2%) were identified who, although they did not have BN, were considered "at risk" for a serious eating disorder because they had high scores on a measure of eating disorder symptomatology and at least two other correlates (e.g., high perfectionism, low body esteem). These at-risk women were then randomly assigned to a no-treatment control or a cognitive-behavioral group. Two female graduate students led eight weekly 90-minute group sessions based on a combination of CBT and NSVS elements. At 1-month follow-up the intervention group demonstrated significant improvements in weight management behavior, body satisfaction, self-esteem, and fear of negative evaluation (Kaminski & McNamara, 1996).

In her dissertation research Chase (2000) delivered a modified version of Kaminski and McNamara's (1996) program to groups of women at the University of Texas who "exhibited elevated levels of preoccupation with body weight and shape and unhealthful dieting behaviors and did not meet diagnostic criteria for an eating disorder" (p. 48). The results supported the utility of brief cognitive-behavioral groups in teaching young women how to challenge sociocultural pressures and to correct maladaptive schema concerning weight and shape. Compared to a placebo-group control, participants demonstrated (at 1-month follow-up) increased knowledge about program components and reductions in dieting behavior, body dissatisfaction and weight concerns, and anxiety.

The studies by Kaminski and McNamara (1996) and by Chase (2000; see also Foster, 2003) are promising. Their findings are also consistent with the body of literature suggesting that certain (as yet unspecified) features of CBT are helpful for college women with negative body image and a history of dieting (Cash & Hrabosky, 2004). However, the relevance of this research to more heterogeneous community samples of adult women needs to be demonstrated. In a study of one such sample, Smith, Wolfe, and Laframboise (2001) conducted a controlled evaluation of CBT's effects on the body dissatisfaction of normal-weight women who were obligatory or nonobligatory exercisers. Obligatory exercisers have been shown to have high levels of weight concerns and obsessionality. The women (M age = 36.7, range = 17–69) were selected from a sample of volunteers with high levels of body dissatisfaction in Albuquerque, New Mexico. The treatment, based closely on Cash's work (see, e.g., Cash, 1996, 1997), was delivered by clinical psychology graduate students to groups of 6 to 10 women in eight 90-minute sessions. Results, including attrition at 2-month follow-up, revealed a program participation effect, that is, no sustained positive effect of the CBT treatment.

The **Freedom From Dieting** *Program.* In the only other randomized controlled study to use a community sample, Higgins and Gray (1998) evaluated *Freedom From Dieting*. Participants were 82 adult women (M age = 44.4, range = 24–67 years) recruited from the community via mass media. All participants were overweight or obese dieters (mean BMI = 31.4) who did not have an eating disorder. *Freedom From Dieting* consists of didactic presentations, group discussions, and activities. The program combines elements of the SCT (e.g., resisting cultural pressures to diet) and NSVS (e.g., coping more effectively with stress) approaches. Two components of special theoretical significance are (a) shifting feelings of self-worth from a weight-based standard to goals based on acknowledging and meeting all of one's basic needs; and (b) replacing chronic dieting with "natural eating"—being aware of and responding to the body's naturally occurring signals of hunger and satiety (as opposed to eating in response to emotional or situational triggers). Positive modeling was provided by former chronic dieters who had become successful "natural eaters." Following completion of the six 2-hour sessions, engagement with participants was maintained by two review sessions and two newsletters.

The findings of this project were very positive. At posttest, compared to a control condition, *Freedom From Dieting* produced reductions in restrained eating and in eating triggered by emotions and external factors, reductions in body shape concern, and increased self-esteem. Reductions in body shape concerns were maintained at 6- and 12-month follow-up. Moreover, further reductions in unhealthy eating attitudes and increases in self-esteem were observed at 6- and 12-month follow-up.

DOES PREVENTION WORK?

We begin our summary by critically evaluating the Rosenvinge and Børresen (1999) statement quoted early in this chapter: "Apart from the increasing of knowledge, there is no evidence that primary prevention programmes provide changes in eating attitudes and behaviours, and some authors even suggest that primary prevention may actually do more harm than good" (p. 8).

Universal Prevention: Limited Evidence or Limited Research?

One must distinguish the contention that there is very limited evidence for prevention from the fact that there is limited high-quality research on prevention. The 78 universal-selective studies reviewed include 12 (~15.5%) unpublished theses or dissertations. Furthermore, only 13 universal studies (or ~16.5% of the 78) to date would meet the minimal criteria for a "high quality experimental evaluation" used by Tobler et al. (2000): random assignment, 4 or more hours of program time, and a follow-up period of at least 3 months. By contrast, Tobler et al. (2000) identified 207 *controlled* studies of school-based drug prevention as of 1998, almost all of which were designed for non-high-risk students ages 11 to 18. Of that sample, 93 (45%) were categorized as high quality.

Does Universal Prevention Change Only Knowledge?

The answer to this question is a resounding "no." Our review leaves no doubt that many universal-selective prevention programs produce changes in affective, attitudinal, and motivational variables. Based on our review, this is particularly true in the following instances: (a) programs for children ages 6 to 11 (although Stice & Shaw, 2004, disagree); (b) programs for youth ages 12 to 14 that include significant aspects of the FER model (see chapter 8, Table 8.1); and (c) the *Student Bodies* computer-assisted psychoeducation program for college students. In their recent meta-analysis of controlled outcome studies, Stice and Shaw (2004) found small but statistically significant prevention effects *at follow-up* for internalization of the slender beauty ideal ($n = 10$ studies, $r = +.09$; range $= .00-+.18$) and for body dissatisfaction ($n = 22$, $r = +.06$, range $= +.05-+.21$).

Does Universal Prevention Result in Sustained Changes, Particularly in Behavior?

The answer to this question is complicated. Far too few studies have arranged for extensive follow-up periods *and* measures of eating pathology (Stice & Hoffman, 2004; Stice & Shaw, 2004). Furthermore, many studies have produced a program participation effect for attitudinal and/or behavioral variables, which does indeed suggest a lack of power to produce sustained changes. Specifically, out of 22 universal-selective prevention studies (in the United States, the United Kingdom, Canada, Italy, and Australia) that reported data for postprogram and follow-up effects, 11 (50%) demonstrated this phenomenon. Although the robustness of the program participation effect raises the possibility that follow-up interventions ("booster sessions") would be useful, we argue in chapters 10, 12, and 15 that this phenomenon points directly to the need for ecological interventions.

Nevertheless, even with the many challenges clearly inherent in producing sustained prevention effects, it important to acknowledge that researchers have demonstrated longer term (6–12 months) prevention effects in the eating attitudes and behaviors of:

- elementary school students (Smolak & Levine, 2001a—social cognitive and developmental models)
- middle school students (Austin et al., 2005—SCT approach; O'Dea & Abraham, 2000—NSVS model; Piran, 1999a—FER model)
- high school students (Neumark-Sztainer et al., 1995—SCT approach; Piran, 1999a; Santonastaso et al., 1999—social cognitive and developmental models).

Stice and Shaw's (2004) meta-analysis supports this conclusion to a degree. They evaluated universal programs incorporating a control group and a follow-up period. Even using a very conservative process of substituting an effect size of zero for reported statistical nonsignificance, the composite effect sizes of universal programs were small but significantly greater than zero for dieting ($n = 20$ studies, $r = +.05$, range = .00–+.20) and for eating pathology ($n = 15$, $r = +.07$, range = .00–+.17).

Does Universal Prevention Do More Harm Than Good?

Around the time prevention research began, Garner (1985) argued that such efforts in schools or in the mass media may inadvertently glamorize disordered eating, teach unhealthy weight management techniques, and otherwise create the negative effects they seek to prevent. *Iatrogenesis* remains a concern of those evaluating curriculum-based prevention (Carter, Stewart, Dunn, & Fairburn, 1997; O'Dea, 2000; Piran, 1995).

Stice's recent reviews of controlled outcome studies find no evidence for iatrogenesis (Stice & Hoffman, 2004; Stice & Shaw, 2004). Our review finds relatively little evidence of negative effects, but does suggest, as discussed further in chapter 10, that iatrogenesis does occur and is therefore an important matter (see negative program effects in Baranowski & Hetherington, 2001; Martz & Bazzini, 1999, Study 2; Sanderson & Holloway, 2003; Smolak et al., 1998b; Weiss, 2001). For example, in Smolak et al.'s (1998b) research, body esteem improved over the course of the pre-to-post assessment for all conditions except fourth-grade girls receiving the ESEM curriculum. This troubling outcome recalls Huon et al.'s (1997) finding that program content *may*, for at least a significant minority of the girls, intensify or create negative feelings about their bodies.

It has been known for a long time that both psychotherapy and pharmacotherapy can produce a "deterioration effect" in a minority of patients (Bergin & Lambert, 1978). Yet no one is suggesting that these interventions be abandoned. Rather, the emphasis is on improvement of programming (see chapter 10) and on careful attention to research ethics.

Shouldn't We Focus on Targeted Prevention Because It Works?

A critical or even cynical view of universal-selective (primary) prevention implies either that prevention be abandoned or that efforts be concentrated on targeted prevention. We reject both conclusions, but we acknowledge that research with college students and, in a few instances, with high school students strongly suggests that multisession, intensive targeted prevention programs can be modestly effective (see, e.g., Cash & Hrabosky, 2004; Taylor et al., 2001). The variety of such effective programs is broad. It encompasses CBT, dissonance reduction, and CAPP. Moreover, a *Freedom From Dieting* (Higgins & Gray, 1998) program was preventive for significantly overweight women with a history of chronic dieting, while behavioral strategies to maintain a 1,200-calorie per day weight loss diet prevented bulimic pathology in nonoverweight or moderately overweight young women (Presnell & Stice, 2003).

It may well be the case, also, that targeted programs are more powerful than universal-selective programs. Stice and Shaw (2004) found that the effect sizes at follow-up for targeted programs were small to moderate for internalization of the slender beauty ideal ($n = 7$; $r \sim +.21$; range $= +.08-+.44$), body dissatisfaction ($n = 15$; $r = +.25$; range $= +.11-+.56$), dieting ($n = 12$; $r = +.24$; range $= +.09-+.47$), and eating pathology ($n = 13$; $r = +.22$; range = .00–+.37). However, our review of the outcome literature for targeted prevention indicates that this approach has the same major problem facing claims about universal-selective prevention: lack of high quality studies producing multidimensional and meaningful positive effects on mediators and on eating pathology over a meaningfully long-term follow-up (see also Cash & Hrabosky, 2004). The issue of targeted prevention is considered in more detail in chapter 14.

In conclusion, the data simply do not support the pessimism contained in Rosenvinge and Børresen's (1999) analysis of universal-selective prevention. The data do, however, strongly suggest that our current prevention efforts need to be substantially improved. Three candidates for improvement are (a) the content of programs; (b) the need for a more critical social perspective (see chapter 8); and (c), in a related vein, more attention to ecology rather than simply to refinement of curriculum (see chapters 12 and 15). We find it particularly noteworthy that only 12 (~20%) of the 61 different universal-selective programs that have been evaluated contained at least one clear element of an ecological approach, and this was typically a minimal feature such as brief training of teachers or information for parents. In fact, the only eating disorders prevention program to date other than Piran's to include an explicit multidimensional ecological approach is a very recent study by McVey, Tweed, and Blackmore (2004; see Table 9.2). This program is discussed in some detail in chapter 12. In the next chapter we consider how our efforts to improve in the three realms listed here can be informed by theory and research concerning prevention of cigarette smoking and other substance use.

IV

PREVENTION RESEARCH: LESSONS FROM THE FIELD

10

Lessons From the Field I: Curriculum and Program Development

Those committed to preventing negative body image and disordered eating face a basic challenge that is all too familiar to researchers involved in school-based substance abuse prevention (Hansen, 1992): How can one reconcile (a) the theory and sometimes successful practice of prevention; (b) the very modest effectiveness or ineffectiveness of most prevention efforts; (c) the pragmatic concerns of teachers, administrators, parents, and funding sources; and (d) the multicultural nature of modern societies? To address these questions, this chapter is divided into three parts. Theory and research concerning prevention of substance abuse are 25 years ahead of parallel work in the eating disorders field, so the first part considers important lessons from substance abuse prevention that could potentially improve prevention of eating problems. The second part uses those lessons and the prevention outcome literature reviewed in chapter 9 to examine some general issues in the content of prevention programs. The final part offers specific suggestions for program content as a function of age and developmental level of the target audience. Specific suggestions for a multidimensional ecological approach that links school-based prevention to community-based prevention are offered in the concluding chapter of this book.

SIX LESSONS FROM SCHOOL-BASED PREVENTION OF SUBSTANCE USE IN EARLY ADOLESCENCE

Lesson 1: School as the Basis of Prevention

The vast majority of eating disorders prevention efforts are psychoeducational programs, delivered in school classrooms (see chapters 9 & 13). Prevention specialists (e.g., Hansen, 1992) have long noted that school-based interventions make good sense for universal, selective, and targeted prevention. School provides relatively easy access to large numbers of children and adolescents. It also provides some access to their parents. Eating disorders curricula need not be as highly specialized as they sound to overburdened administrators and teachers. Learning about weight/shape concerns and disordered eating can be integrated with other educational goals (see Table 10.4) such as proper nutrition, social studies, the sciences, tolerance and even appreciation of diversity, citizenship in a democracy (see chapter 13), and various forms of critical thinking, including research skills. Children and adolescents spend a substantial amount of their time in school, so curricular programs that are carefully tied to teacher training, to community support of school policies (e.g., against teasing), and to other changes in the school ecology might well have multiple positive effects on students (Pentz, 2000).

Lesson 2: Prevention Can Work, But Effects Are Limited and Conclusions Complicated

The Database. Our discussion draws heavily from the work of Hansen (1992), Botvin (2000; Botvin & Griffin, 2002), and Tobler et al. (2000). Hansen (1992) reviewed 41 curricula whose outcome evaluations were published between 1980 and 1992, and that were designed to prevent use of two or more substances. Tobler et al. (2000) conducted a sophisticated meta-analysis of 207 universal or selective prevention studies published between 1978 and 1998. All studies involved youth ages 10 to 18, and all were experimental or quasiexperimental. Of the total, 45% were considered "high quality" because they used random assignment to conditions, had a minimum of 4 hours of program participation, had a follow-up period of at least 3 months, and adjusted for pretest levels of the dependent variable(s).

Findings and Implications. School-based programs for young adolescents can prevent initiation and escalation of tobacco, alcohol, and other drug use. However, because many variables can dilute the impact of universal prevention, the expected magnitude of effect sizes for multifaceted social interventions will be small (.10–.30; Tobler et al., 2000). Moreover, each of the different approaches, including information dissemination and affective education, has some demonstrated successes, and many failures are attributable to severe methodological shortcomings: bias in the selection of experimental and control conditions; inadequate statistical power to detect reasonable changes in the key dependent measures; and low fidelity of program delivery. All this suggests that attempts to demonstrate that one approach is necessary or sufficient are futile (Hansen, 1992; Tobler et al., 2000).

Lesson 3: Information Dissemination, Values Clarification, and Affective Education Have Limited and Riskier Effects

Information-based programs educate students about the nature of drugs, negative consequences of drug use, and the processes by which people become drug abusers. Some programs offer this material to guide rational decision making, whereas other programs seek to frighten participants into avoiding use. In some programs the teacher presents the information, whereas other interventions try to heighten credibility by using doctors, therapists, or recovered addicts. *Values clarification* programs use group discussions and workbooks to help students clarify and consolidate personal values (e.g., being a good friend, being able to participate in sports) that are incompatible with drug use and abuse. The salience of these values is considered a fundamental aspect of making healthy choices. *Affective education* has similar goals, but uses experiential games and other classroom activities to foster greater appreciation and respect for the self and others in realms antithetical to drug use.

Limited and Inconsistent Effects. Tobler et al.'s (2000) meta-analysis indicated that the weighted effect size for 18 knowledge-only programs and 14 knowledge + affective programs was a statistically insignificant .05. Hansen's (1992) review is more optimistic but also offers a warning. Although nearly a third of the behavioral results from informational, values-based, and affective programs conducted during the

1980s were positive, another 25% to 30% of these programs had the negative, undesirable effect of increasing either drug use or positive attitudes toward drug use.

Lesson 4: Resistance Skills Are an Important Part of Competence Enhancement

Resistance Skills. Richard Evans (1976; cited in Botvin & Griffin, 2002) was a pioneer in teaching youth to understand and resist social psychological factors that lead them to begin smoking cigarettes. Evans' approach assumes that, although most adolescents do not wish to smoke cigarettes, drink alcohol, or use other drugs, they lack the necessary information (e.g., about the relatively low prevalence of use among young adolescents), the skills, and the confidence (efficacy expectation) to resist prodrug messages from parents, peers, and mass media. Consequently, Evans sought to "inoculate" students by exposing them to weak prosmoking messages from peers and media (the "antigen") and then teaching them resistance skills, including how to generate their own counterarguments (the "antibodies"). Thus inoculated, students were then exposed to increasingly stronger promotions and pressures, which they practiced resisting.

Over the years the emphasis has shifted from inoculation to teaching specific skills for developing a critical awareness of prodrug media messages and for recognizing and avoiding high-risk situations with peers (Botvin, 2000; Botvin & Griffin, 2002; Donaldson et al., 1996). These "social influence" programs usually retain Evans' focus on clarifying the normative expectation that most adolescents do not smoke cigarettes or use other drugs, and on reinforcing this norm with public pledges not to use tobacco, alcohol, and other drugs. According to Donaldson et al. (1996), resistance skills training without normative education may be harmful because it inadvertently reinforces a proposition that legitimizes drug use: "You really have to watch out for social influences because so many people are using drugs."

Inconsistent and Limited Effectiveness. Meta-analyses and other types of reviews indicate that social influence programs tend to have a more robust positive effect on knowledge, attitudes, and behavior than do information dissemination and other non-skill-based interventions. They are also less risky, but they are not without potential negative effects, as noted by Donaldson et al. (1996). Hansen (1992) analyzed 15 outcome evaluations of 12 social influence programs published between 1980 and 1990. Sixty-three percent had a positive behavioral effect, 26% had no significant effect, and 11% increased drug use. Botvin's literature review concluded that, compared to control conditions, resistance skills programs for young adolescents reduce smoking initiation by 30% to 50%. These effects tend to last several years, but gradually decay throughout high school (Botvin, 2000; Botvin & Griffin, 2002). Tobler et al. (2000) found that the weighted effect size for 82 social influence programs (~39.5% of their sample of studies) was positive but small (.12, with 99% CI = .10–.15; high quality studies = .14).

Lesson 5: Multifaceted Competence Enhancement Is More Effective Than Resistance Skills Alone

Life Skills and Resistance Skills. Another set of programs assumes that some adolescents want or need to use tobacco and other drugs in order to deal with low self-esteem, social anxiety, and distress caused by poor coping skills. According to this perspective, prevention of substance use by young adolescents will be facilitated by establishing norms for avoiding use and by enhancing student competence in not only resisting drug use, but also in personal and social areas called *life skills* (Botvin & Griffin, 2002).

Example: Life Skills Training. The best-known and most thoroughly evaluated approach to competence enhancement is Botvin's *Life Skills Training* (LST) program for students ages 11 to 13 (Grades 6 or 7; Botvin, 1996). The program consists of 15 to 17 lessons (45 minutes each) in Grade 7 (or Grade 6), 10 "booster" sessions in Grade 8 (or 7), and 5 more lessons in Grade 9 (or 8). LST is designed to achieve three specific goals: (a) provide students with information about healthy norms and social values in regard to avoiding drug use, and about the immediate, negative physiological consequences of smoking; (b) teach skills for resisting specific peer and media pressures to use drugs; and (c) help students develop generic life skills such as decision making, problem solving, stress management, media literacy, assertion, effective communication, and self-management (goal setting, self-monitoring, and self-reinforcement). Teaching techniques include demonstration, guided group discussion, a small amount of lecturing, and various cognitive-behavioral techniques (see chapter 6).

Numerous long-term evaluations of LST strongly support several conclusions (Botvin, 1996, 2000; Botvin & Griffin, 2002). First, the program produces 40% to 80% reductions in the initiation of tobacco use by seventh graders. Second, these prevention effects are durable. One large-scale study revealed lower smoking and less alcohol and marijuana use relative to controls at the end of the 12th grade. This finding supports the contention that prevention is attributable to acquisition (or consolidation) of skills and healthy norms, but the specific processes mediating the long-term prevention effects of LST are not yet known. Third, consistent with the theory of competence enhancement, LST produces prevention effects for tobacco, alcohol, marijuana, and other drug use. Fourth (and on the other hand), competence enhancement is not sufficient without specific skills for resisting drug use and without development of norms that discourage drug use (see Donaldson et al., 1996). Fifth, fidelity of program delivery and of participant exposure is very important: The more programming received, the greater the probability of prevention. Finally, whether they be regular classroom teachers, older peers, or health professionals, the people who deliver the program need to be committed to prevention in general and to the particulars of LST; they also need to be enthusiastic, willing to serve as a positive role model, and experienced. Initial experience is typically in the form of a 1- to 2-day training workshop.

Increased Effectiveness and Reduced Risk. LST is not unique in its very positive prevention effects. Hansen (1992) concluded that the best *behavioral* outcomes are indeed produced by comprehensive, competence enhancement programming. Across 17 studies of 7 different programs, 72% had positive behavioral outcomes, 28% were neutral, and none were negative. Forty-seven (~23%) of the programs in Tobler et al.'s (2000) meta-analysis were comprehensive. The weighted effect size for these programs was .17 (99% CI = .13–.21) for all the studies and for the 30 considered high quality.

Lesson 6: Interactive Delivery Is Important

Effective programs for teaching resistance skills and/or multiple competencies tend to be guided by teacher manuals and student workbooks offering structured lessons based on previous theory and research (Botvin & Griffin, 2002; Perry, 1999). This reflects their roots in the social cognitive and cognitive-behavioral paradigms (see chapter 6). Regardless of whether these programs are delivered by mental health professionals, classroom teachers, or peer educators, *interactive* lessons are much more effective than didactic, noninteractive interventions relying on lectures and films. It is important for programs to be delivered in an engaging fashion via peer discussion, role playing, interactive games, and structured group activities and homework assignments. Tobler et al.'s (2000) calculations suggest a maximum effect size of .28 for an interactive, multifaceted competence enhancement program for prevention of tobacco use delivered to 100 students in 5 classrooms. This means a 34% reduction in the percentage of eighth graders using tobacco in the past 30 days. The meta-analysis by Stice and Shaw (2004) revealed that eating disorder prevention programs with an interactive format were more effective than those with a purely didactic format.

ECOLOGICAL APPROACHES TO STRENGTHENING SCHOOL-BASED PREVENTION

Rationale

Many programs featuring resistance skill training and competence enhancement have limited long-term effects, that is, limited durability. And even the most successful programs such as LST need to be improved (Botvin & Griffin, 2002). As noted throughout this book, limited prevention effects are probably due to lack of attention to significant factors in the ecology of children and adolescents, notably the school environment, parents, the community, and mass media (Botvin & Griffin, 2002; Perry, 1999). In this regard, a recent large-scale study of a nationally representative sample of 8th, 10th, and 12th graders showed that, over and above students' personal approval or disapproval of substance use, the general level of approval in the school climate contributed to prediction of substance use (Kumar, O'Malley, Johnston, Schulenberg, & Bachman, 2002). Social influence models of drug prevention focus on changing proximal predictors of substance use such as normative expectations, peer influence, and internalization of pro-use media messages. Competence enhancement approaches extend this approach to include lack of life skills as one source of motives for drug use. All of these proximal predictors are deeply embedded in sociocultural factors, so an ecological perspective is a logical source of potential support for more constructive knowledge, attitudes, and behavior (Flay, 2000; Perry, 1999; see chapters 4 & 12).

Superior Effectiveness of Ecological Approaches: Tobler et al.'s Meta-Analysis

Tobler et al.'s (2000) meta-analysis identified only 9 (4.3% of 207) programs for "system-wide" changes. These constituted the most effective form of intervention. The weighted effect size was .27 (99% CI = .21–.33), including an effect size of .22 for the three high-quality studies. Moreover, comparison of the three major types of interactive programs indicated that, as components are added, the predicted effect increases. Comprehensive programs combining life skills with resistance skills are more effective than social influence programs. Similarly, system-wide programs that include skills training but expand the focus of prevention to family and community are more effective than comprehensive programs. In all, Tobler et al.'s (2000) meta-analysis strongly supports an ecological approach to prevention.

Flay's Review: Schools, Parents, and Media

Brian Flay (2000), an expert on the causes and prevention of adolescent substance abuse, provides a more nuanced review of substance abuse programs that combine social influence or comprehensive curricula with one or two types of ecological changes.

Students, Teachers, and Parents. In general, holistic changes within a school setting—in drug policies, teacher training, teaching practices, and incorporation of LST into the general curriculum—have proven difficult to implement. When such changes are possible, they tend to have mixed or negligible outcomes in regard to substance use and abuse. One promising development, however, is the Adolescent Transitions Program, which offers universal, selective, and targeted interventions for families of middle school students (Dishion & Kavanagh, 2000). A key structure in the program is a Family Resource Room that promotes effective communication (e.g., about homework) between the school and the family. The Resource Room also provides information to families about effective parenting and prevention of substance use. At school, students receive a 6-hour curriculum offering life skills, goal-setting for academic success, and peaceful conflict resolution. In conjunction, parents work with children to complete homework assignments. The entire process is facilitated by weekly newsletters that help parents to reinforce healthy norms and practices for teenagers (cf.

Smolak et al., 1998a, 1998b). The Adolescent Transitions Program is effective in retarding the growth of deviant peer relationships, antisocial behavior, and substance use across the middle school years (Dishion & Kavanagh, 2000).

Curriculum and Media Campaigns. In independent trials, prevention specialists such as Flay, Jason, and Murray have integrated social influence curricula with carefully constructed media campaigns, only to find very limited or no significant effects on initiation of cigarette smoking (Flay, 2000). There has been one notable success. Flynn, Worden, and colleagues in Vermont (see, e.g., Flynn et al., 1994) combined school-based resistance skill training with frequent radio, cable TV, and broadcast TV "spots." The key to this program's effectiveness is probably its careful planning of the media campaign. This effort provided a wide variety of engaging messages that address normative expectations, the advantages of not smoking, strategic use of refusal skills, tobacco industry motives, and attitudinal and behavioral alternatives to tobacco use. The combination resulted in much more effective prevention of cigarette smoking by 9- to 12-year-olds at 2-year follow-up than did the school intervention alone.

Community-Based Programs

Reviews by Flay (2000) and Perry (1999) indicate that an effective ecological approach to prevention needs to integrate school-based interventions with well-coordinated efforts to structure and reinforce the *community* as a set of environments supporting healthy behaviors (see chapters 4 & 7).

Project Star. The Midwestern Prevention Project ("Project Star") has been in operation in 50 American middle and junior high schools since 1984 (Pentz et al., 1989). It integrates social influence curricula in the schools with mobilization of parents, who review and support relevant school policies, serve as healthy role models, and learn to communicate more effectively with adolescents about developmental challenges and alternatives to substance use. Program developers also organize and train community leaders, including representatives of the mass media. Community leaders help arrange fairly extensive news coverage of the project, as well as numerous educational "events" on television, radio, and in the newspapers. At the 1-year follow-up, program participants were less likely to be using cigarettes, alcohol, and marijuana than were comparison students, and the net increase in substance use in intervention schools was 50% less. Over 3 years of follow-up, Project Star was fairly successful in preventing or delaying initiation (for several years) of cigarette smoking and marijuana use by 11- to 14-year-old boys and girls from both high- and low-risk categories.

Project SixTeen. In the early 1990s, a group from the prestigious Oregon Research Institute implemented an ecological intervention for preventing adolescent tobacco use in middle school and high school adolescents (Biglan, Ary, Smolkowski, Duncan, & Black, 2000). Nine small Oregon communities, located far enough apart to prevent program contamination, were randomly assigned to receive a school plus community (CP) program, while nine other disconnected small communities received only a school-based (SBO) intervention delivered by teachers with 2 to 3 hours of training. The school-based intervention received by both groups had a total of 9 five-session units (i.e., 45 sessions) across Grades 6 through 12, with at least one unit each year. In middle school this consisted of focused social learning activities to develop refusal skills and public commitment not to smoke, whereas in high school information and activities were integrated into health, social studies, biology, and English courses. In CP cities a paid coordinator worked with adult and youth volunteers to develop and implement the four key components of "Project SixTeen": (a) multimodal media advocacy to reach community leaders and adults in general; (b) a variety of youth antitobacco activities such as T-shirt give-aways and sidewalk art; (c) family communications activities, including provision of normative information on tobacco use and on parents' attitudes toward smoking; and (d) mobilization of the business community to reduce tobacco sales to minors.

Assessment was conducted five times over a 4-year period. The sophisticated multivariate analysis for nested cross-sectional designs indicated a true prevention effect 1 year after the CP programs were in place and 1 year after the project ended: Smoking prevalence in seventh and ninth graders increased significantly for SBO students, while it remained the same in the CP condition. The effect size for the SBO–CP difference in covariate-adjusted prevalence was quite striking, $d = 1.03$. Analysis of mediators indicated that, as intended, programming in the CP communities intensified awareness of prevention efforts and negative attitudes toward smoking, whereas in the SBO cities youth reported more friends smoking and more peer deviance. Project SixTeen demonstrates that an ecological program integrating media, parents, and the business community with a school-based intervention has much greater potential for a sustained prevention effect than does a school-based program alone, at least for rural communities with limited ethnic diversity (Biglan et al., 2000).

Community Organizing and Policy Change

Policy Change. Project Star and Project SixTeen point to the importance of policy in an extended ecological approach to prevention. Policy refers to agreed-on public practices such as establishment of organizations for community activism and advocacy, funds for youth development, enforcement of laws governing the availability and use of tobacco and alcohol, and institutionalizing the school system's commitment to prevention. Pentz (2000), a leader of Project Star, documented the effectiveness of both programmatic and regulatory policy changes in community-based prevention. However, a recent study of random samples of public and private schools in the United States ($N = 2,648$) indicated that only 4% had policies and practices regarding drug use prevention in middle schools that could be considered even to approximate Pentz's recommendations that communities support a comprehensive combination of school policy, curriculum development, teacher training, parent involvement, and program assessment (Wenter et al., 2002).

Communities That Care. There is a lot of unexplored territory between actual practices and best practices in extensive ecological approaches to substance abuse prevention. Lest this journey seem like true science fiction, readers are referred to Hawkins et al. (2002) for a detailed presentation of the Communities That Care (CTC) initiative. Experts from the CTC organization work with business or government funding sources to help community members apply the public health model of assessing problems, establishing risk factor profiles for specific neighborhoods, mobilizing resources, developing community interventions, and evaluating the ongoing impact of these programs. The goal is participatory empowerment of communities as part of the process of tailoring interventions to local needs and practices. Although the assessment and intervention phases of the ambitious CTC program have been successfully implemented in the United States, the United Kingdom, the Netherlands, and Australia, as yet there are no controlled, randomized assessments of its outcomes. Preliminary evaluations in over 60 communities in Oregon and Washington State indicate that the program is attractive to communities and enables them, even with limited funding, to develop and implement proven interventions for specific risk and protective factors (Hawkins et al., 2002).

THE BRIDGE TO PREVENTING EATING PROBLEMS: CONCLUSIONS FROM SUBSTANCE ABUSE PREVENTION

Reviews of the literature on prevention of tobacco, alcohol, and other drug use—and reviews of those reviews (e.g., Cuijpers, 2002)—paint a picture containing many elements that emerge from our review in chapter 9 of outcome research in the prevention of negative body image and eating problems. It is not difficult to increase knowledge, and not all that hard to improve some attitudes. It is much harder to change behavior, and when programs do effect desired behavioral changes, such positive outcomes are all too often short-lived. Nevertheless, despite the fact that "*most* drug prevention have been shown to have no effects on drug use or abuse" (Cuijpers, 2002, p. 1019; italics added), and despite the many methodological challenges to demonstrating the internal and external validity of a prevention effect, there are lessons from the drug prevention arena that should be useful for prevention of negative body image and disordered eating. Table 10.1 presents the conclusions for

TABLE 10.1
Components of Effective Substance Abuse Prevention Programs

- Classroom lessons that use a variety of techniques to engage students in the processes of exchanging ideas, learning new skills, and receiving constructive criticism and encouragement from peer and adult coaches.
- Imparting the knowledge that "certainly not everybody is using (e.g., smoking)."
- Clarifying and reinforcing social norms and values that proclaim in clear and certain terms: "Relatively few peers and adults think using (e.g., smoking) is 'cool' and otherwise approve of it, and many adolescents and adults do not intend to use—indeed are committed to not using."
- Teaching students the skills to identify, critically evaluate, and resist social pressures for substance use.
- Teaching students life skills for meeting needs and coping with stress.
- Use of peer leaders strengthens short-term program effects.
- A school policy that discourages drug use and promotes teaching and peer training, parent involvement, and assessment of prevention outcomes.
- Community programming that includes organization and mobilization of mass media, parents, the business community, and leaders for youth activities such as sports and religion.

which there is strong, if not incontrovertible, empirical evidence (Cuijpers, 2002; Flay, 2000; Hansen, 1992; Hawkins et al., 2002; Tobler et al., 2000; see also Kirby, 1999, for the overlap with conclusions based on effective pregnancy prevention programs with adolescents).

DEVELOPING SCHOOL-BASED PROGRAMS FOR PREVENTING EATING PROBLEMS: GENERAL ISSUES

School-based interventions are a significant part of the community-based ecological approach to prevention of eating problems. Currently, several very good curricula are available for elementary and middle school students (see, e.g., Kater, 1998; O'Dea & Abraham, 2000; Seaver et al., 1997; see also Appendix B), but there is certainly room for improvement in their effectiveness. Furthermore, there are as yet no readily available and effective curricula for high school students and young adults.

An ecological approach to prevention strongly recommends that programs be developed in consultation with the school(s) and with the broader community (Hawkins et al., 2002; Moran & Reaman, 2002; O'Dea & Maloney, 2000; Piran, 1995). In the course of this dialogue it is likely that at least six broad issues will need to be addressed (Perry, 1999). First, the developer must identify the goals of the curriculum. This process is crucial in deciding whether a universal, targeted, or clinical program is more appropriate (see chapter 14). Second, there is ample evidence that learning life skills facilitates prevention of substance abuse (Botvin, 1996, 2000; Botvin & Griffin, 2002), but only in combination with problem-specific (e.g., reducing body image or eating problems) knowledge and skills. Thus, in defining program objectives, program designers must decide on the balance between problem-specific lessons and lessons that operate from the Non-Specific Vulnerability-Stressor model (chapter 7).

In line with this choice, the third issue is to designate an audience. Will the curriculum be for both boys and girls? Will it involve middle school or high school students? Fourth, is the prevention model underlying the program sensitive to the ethnic and racial composition of the target audience? Fifth, what learning methods will be used, and what time and resources would be required by those methods? Will there be informational lectures? Will videos be used? Will there be class discussions or projects? Interactive lessons are much more likely to be effective than didactic presentations (Cuijpers, 2002; Tobler et al., 2000; see also O'Dea & Maloney, 2000; Piran, 1995), so how will students (and perhaps their parents) be engaged in the processes of discovery, learning, and communication? The final question is: Who will deliver the program? Will it be a teacher? Will an experienced psychologist or other prevention specialist supervise the program? There is some evidence from the drug prevention literature that a combination of peer and adult educators is desirable (Botvin, 1996; Cuijpers, 2002). Returning to the third issue, if peers and/or teachers are to implement the lessons, are they indeed not part of the target audience(s) for the program?

The following two sections address two particularly important matters pertaining to the target audience for prevention.

Gender

Of the 57 prevention programs (evaluated in 72 studies reviewed in chapter 9) plus 10 media literacy programs (evaluated in 12 studies reviewed in chapter 13), 43 (~64%) have been aimed only at girls or young women. Elsewhere in this book (e.g., chapters 3 & 8) and in previous work, we have argued this is a mistake (Levine, 1994; Smolak, 1999). To elaborate, even if a program designer is interested exclusively in girls' body image and eating problems, there is no doubt that the behavior of boys and men is a relevant factor. Males engage in teasing and sexual harassment that appear to be related to development of girls' body dissatisfaction and eating problems (Eisenberg, Neumark-Sztainer, & Story, 2003; Larkin et al., 1999; Murnen & Smolak, 2000; Thompson et al., 1999). Unfortunately, some boys and men are unaware of how hurtful and dehumanizing these comments are. Many males think the girls understand that they are "just kidding" (Kowalski, 2000). Education is also needed concerning physical and sexual violence within dating relationships; this too has been found to be related to girls' eating problems (Silverman, Raj, Mucci, & Hathaway, 2001). Other environmental changes, ranging from greater respect for girls' interests and abilities to acceptance of reading assignments that focus on girls or women's achievements or lives, will also require cooperation from boys *and* their parents, as well as from male administrators and teachers (Levine, 1994).

Many of us who try to raise issues of teasing, sexual harassment, and general respect for girls encounter resistance from boys' parents and even from male and female teachers. As noted in chapter 3, some adults feel we are "blaming" the boys for girls' body image and eating problems, and they want us to know that this attribution will only alienate the boys (and them). This is a complex and delicate issue for any program to address. On one hand, we certainly do not want to lose the support of parents, teachers, and boys who want to make a positive difference in the world. On the other hand, data are accumulating that male behavior is part of the problem (Smolak & Murnen, 2001, 2004; Thompson et al., 1999). We simply cannot ignore teasing, sexual harassment, and dating violence. They are less obvious, less glamorous, and more emotional factors than mass media, but they definitely contribute to the development and reinforcement of negative body image and disordered eating (see Piran, 2001, 2002). Only *some* boys and men share in the responsibility for promoting negative body image and eating problems among girls; *all* boys and men share in the responsibility for creating healthier, safer, more respectful environments for females and for themselves (Levine, 1994; Maine, 1991, 2000; Smolak, 1999; see chapter 3).

There are several possible approaches to this issue; which one works is largely a function of the community or school within which the program is operating. One possibility is to embed messages about boys in more general messages about children. Teasing and harassment could be discussed as hurtful, undesirable behavior no matter who says it. Moreover, the many schools that proudly promote a serious academic environment, citizenship, and student leadership can emphasize each individual's responsibility for improving the social climate, even if he or she does not practice hurtful behavior. Certainly, girls are capable of being cruel to each other (Crick & Bigbee, 1998). But girls seem to be very aware of boys' comments, whereas boys seem unaware of the effects of their comments on girls. So another approach is for adults to work with the specific proposition that "boys don't intend to be hurtful; they just don't understand and we need to help them understand."

A related option is to be sure to involve adult men (Levine, 1994). These men can not only help "sell" the program to concerned parents and school officials, they can also be actively involved in presenting material to the children. Boys might be particularly receptive to messages from younger men, such as college students, as well as from respected, popular teachers, coaches, or athletes (see research by Goldberg et al., 1996, 2000). Just as middle school girls have worked with adult mentors to help older elementary school girls negotiate and change cultural messages regarding thinness (Steiner-Adair et al., 2002), high school boys might help middle school boys become more respectful of girls and women. The drug prevention literature suggests that properly trained peers can be very effective leaders in a prevention program (Botvin & Griffin, 2000; Cuijpers, 2002).

Programs for Boys. These suggestions are relevant to programs that primarily aim to reduce eating or body esteem problems in girls. Some program designers may wish to include boys' problems with body image in their prevention efforts. It has been long been evident that some boys are dissatisfied with their bodies (Cohane & Pope, 2001; Pope et al., 2000; Ricciardelli, McCabe, & Banfield, 2000; Smolak & Levine, 2001b), and that a minority of males suffers from eating disorders and eating problems (see review in chapter 3). However, until quite recently, these problems were largely ignored. There are three reasons for this. First, boys showed body image problems and eating problems at much lower levels than did girls, both in terms of frequency and severity (see chapter 3). Second, boys who were distressed about their body's appearance were typically genuinely overweight (Dornbusch et al., 1984), that is, in the top 2 or 3 deciles in terms of BMI or weight. Many researchers, then, assumed that there was a "rational" explanation for the boys' dissatisfaction. Conversely, even girls who were in the normal or below average range for BMI and weight tended to feel "too fat," so the girls' problems were viewed as more problematic and even pathological.

Finally, boys did not seem particularly motivated to do something about their body dissatisfaction. They were not likely to be on extreme calorie-restrictive diets, nor did they use extreme purging methods, as did girls (Field, Camargo, Taylor, Berkey, Frazier, et al., 1999). Exceptions to this trend, including steroid abusers or high school and college wrestlers, have drawn some attention from program designers, but they tended to be perceived as obvious extremes (e.g., sufferers of "roid rage") that obviously needed targeted or clinical intervention.

Over the past 10 years an increasing body of data indicates that we may have underestimated boys' body image problems as well as the techniques they frequently use to resolve these problems. Some of the key studies in this area were reviewed in chapter 3, so here it is necessary only to reemphasize that boys are often concerned about being too small or too thin, a trend missed by many of our body dissatisfaction measures that ask primarily about fears or concerns about being fat (Labre, 2002; Smolak & Levine, 2001b). For example, Project EAT's survey of 4,746 adolescents from urban public schools in Minnesota found that 21.6% of the boys reported trying to gain weight, as compared with 7.1% of the girls (Neumark-Sztainer, Croll, et al., 2002). Furthermore, social pressures to be more muscular and bigger may be contributing to an increase in body dissatisfaction among boys (Pope et al., 1999, 2000). These pressures, including the prominent behavior and "image" of hugely muscled entertainers (e.g., The Rock) and athletes (e.g., Mark McGwire) who serve as role models for boys, appear to be contributing to the use of steroids and food supplements by boys (see chapter 3).

These recent developments raise concerns about boys' health in terms of body image. However, it appears that prevention programs developed for use with girls are not likely to be adequate in addressing boys' problems. The drive for muscularity and bulk (also discussed in chapter 3) is not a focus of programs for girls. In addition, some variables that are associated with increased risk of body image and eating problems in girls do not show comparable relationships for boys. These include sexual harassment by the other gender (Murnen & Smolak, 2000; Smolak & Murnen, 2004) and loss of voice (Smolak & Munsterteiger, 2002). Some factors do show similar patterns of relationships, but the correlations are considerably weaker in boys than for girls (e.g., Eisenberg et al., 2003; Smolak, Levine, & Thompson, 2001). For example, in a recent study, Jones, Vigfussdottir, and Lee (2004) reported that five variables—BMI, exposure to appearance magazines, appearance-oriented conversations with friends, peer criticisms about appearance, and internalization of media ideals—accounted for nearly 50% of the variance in girls' body image dissatisfaction but just over 20% of the variance in boys' dissatisfaction. Although the risk and protective factor research that has been done with girls may provide some guidance as to how to develop models of boys' body image problems, much more research is needed concerning boys. One area that may well provide guidance is the prevention of steroid and supplement abuse in male athletes (Goldberg & Elliot, 2000; Goldberg et al., 2000). Development and outcome evaluation of the ATLAS program for preventing steroid use in high school football players is discussed in detail in chapter 13's consideration of media literacy.

Racial and Ethnic Factors in Program Development

Lessons From Drug Prevention. Tobler et al.'s (2000) meta-analysis found that minority groups benefited from high-quality prevention programs as much as, if not slightly more than, White students did, with one exception. In general, if the program was not interactive, the weighted effect size for minority students was negative, that is, noninteractive programs tended to be harmful. Thus, designers need to be sensitive to the relevance and acceptability of their prevention programs for minority youth.

Botvin and colleagues used a strategy of focus groups and expert advice to develop prevention materials tailored to African American and Hispanic youth (Botvin, 1996; Botvin & Griffin, 2002). Initially, the principal changes involved culturally sensitive language, examples, graphics, and role-play scenarios; later, the *Life Skills Training* material also drew on myths and legends embedded in the African American and Hispanic cultures. These materials were assessed through interviews with teachers and students, pilot studies, and very large-scale ($Ns = 2,500$ to $3,500$) randomized outcome evaluations. The process has produced programs for these ethnic groups that are effective at preventing cigarette smoking in the short term and across ages 12 through 15.

Community advocacy is well suited for addressing cultural and ethnic issues in prevention (Botvin & Griffin, 2002; Roosa, Dumka, Gonzales, & Knight, 2002). Prevention specialists need to acknowledge not only the traditional values of non-White cultural groups, but also the differences within diverse groups. This refers to differences within fuzzy ethnic classifications (e.g., Hispanic), and to differences caused by the dynamics of acculturation, multicultural identity development, and social context variables such as neighborhood and school composition (Roosa et al., 2002). Understanding the impact of these factors on both problem behaviors and sources of resilience is best accomplished by patient development of respectful relationships between prevention specialists and key stakeholders in the community. Long-term investment in collaborative community organizing helps a prevention program to establish credibility as it mobilizes stakeholders to develop multidimensional strategies that respect and promote cultural values. Collaborative organizing also motivates community members to participate in program implementation, in culturally sensitive evaluation, and in maintenance of the program (Roosa et al., 2002; see also Piran, 2001).

Moran and Reaman (2002) offer many examples of this prevention process in their review of substance abuse prevention programs for one minority that is at very high risk and that has a long, well-founded tradition of mistrust of the dominant culture: American Indian youth. Moran and Reaman describe a number of successful programs for a wide variety of Indian communities, including Coast Salish and Puyallup in the Pacific Northwest, Ojibwe in Wisconsin and Minnesota, and Lakota in Colorado. Some of these sophisticated ecological programs have been implemented by well-known prevention specialists such as Schinke and Gilchrist.

For reasons that remain unclear, these programs tended to be effective in preventing alcohol and marijuana (ab)use, but not cigarette smoking. Cultural components that facilitate prevention in American Indian adolescents are similar to those implemented by Botvin and colleagues in their work with African American and Hispanic adolescents. These include strong and sustained involvement of the Indian community, tailoring of program content to specific tribal knowledge and practices, building bicultural competencies, and program delivery by Indians who have an investment in the program. For example, Moran (as cited in Moran & Reaman, 2002) worked with the Indian community in Denver to develop a program that was successful at 1-year follow-up in preventing alcohol use in youth ages 9 through 13. The school curriculum combined elements of normative expectations, affective education, resistance skills, and life skills (see Hansen, 1992, as reviewed earlier). Early involvement of the community led to two key decisions. First, the program was entitled "The Seventh Generation" in order to emphasize the pivotal role of the current generation in providing a healing connection between the wisdom of the previous three generations and their own responsibility for the next three generations. Second, focus groups stimulated Moran to weave the curriculum around seven key values for Indians of the Northern Plains: harmony, respect, generosity, courage, wisdom, humility, and honesty.

Prevention of Eating Problems. It is evident that no ethnic group in the United States is immune to body image and eating problems. It is equally clear, however, that the distribution and severity of these problems varies across ethnic groups. These differences are demonstrated by the data from surveys of children and adolescents (see reviews by Douchinis et al., 2001; Smolak & Striegel-Moore, 2001). In general, Black girls have a more positive body image than do girls from other ethnic groups. Even among Blacks, however, girls have poorer body image than boys do. Blacks, Hispanics, and American Indians appear to have relatively higher rates of obesity. Some evidence suggests that binge eating occurs in all ethnic groups, while AN, which is rare anyway, is particularly unusual, although not unheard of, among Black girls. Limited evidence indicates that purging behavior may be particularly common within American Indian communities.

We need to be very cautious in using such summary statements as guidelines for developing ethnically sensitive prevention programs. First, the data are quite limited, especially for Asian and for American Indian children and adolescents. There are also inconsistencies in the findings. Furthermore, most of the available data are descriptive. Some data do indicate that the relationships between some risk factors and eating problems are similar across ethnic groups (e.g., Eisenberg et al., 2003; French et al., 1997). However, just as it is likely that causal models developed with girls will not fully capture the development of body image and eating problems among boys, it is unlikely that theories concerning the onset, maintenance, treatment, and prevention of body image and eating problems among Whites will map perfectly on the experience of ethnic minority groups, particularly if socioeconomic status and its correlates are not taken into account. In fact, even when contributing factors seem similar, it is possible that the nature of the contribution varies by ethnicity. For example, sexual harassment may be a problem for girls from various ethnic groups. But research also suggests that sexual harassment often incorporates ethnic prejudice (Larkin et al., 1999; Piran, 2001). Thus, ethnic minority girls may face double jeopardy. Conversely, inasmuch as they are taught not to permit racist behavior by others to define their own sense of self (Crocker, Luhtanen, Blaine, & Broadnax, 1994), ethnic minority girls may be less vulnerable to sexual harassment. Only additional research can answer this question.

It is also important to distinguish among ethnic minority groups. Certainly, all ethnic minority groups share certain experiences of being a minority, including prejudice and discrimination (Smolak & Striegel-Moore, 2001). For example, unlike children from the "majority" culture, ethnic minority children have to develop an identity addressing both the majority and their minority cultures and standards (Phinney, 1996). However, the precise nature of this experience will vary depending on a number of factors. Thus, Asian Americans may face the "model minority" stereotype, whereas the stereotype of African Americans is much more derogatory. Phinney and Chavera's (1995) interviews with a small sample of adolescents indicated that 81% of the African Americans, 46% of the Mexican Americans, and 28% of the Japanese Americans experienced discrimination. Children whose families are recent immigrants might face particular problems because of language and cultural differences. For example, the high school dropout rate is higher among Hispanic teens whose parents were not born in the United States (National Center for Education Statistics/U.S. Dept. of Education, undated).

Similarly, as noted in regard to American Indians, we need to acknowledge diversity within these broad ethnic groups. Hispanics may originate, for example, from Mexico, Cuba, Puerto Rico, the Dominican Republic, Central America, South America, or Spain. Although there are some commonalities across these countries, there are also many major differences—differences that may be exacerbated by the reasons for and the recency of immigration. In a recent study The McKnight Investigators (2003) found that Hispanic girls in the Tucson area had a higher rate of onset of clinical levels of eating problems than did Black or White girls. There was no such racial/ethnic difference in the sample of girls from central California. It is interesting that the California girls self-identified as primarily "Latin American," whereas the Arizona group considered themselves "Mexican" or "Mexican American." Furthermore, more of the Californians reported coming from non-English-speaking homes. Whether these differences created the variation in findings from the two sites is not known. Smolak and Striegel-Moore (2001) argued that ethnicity is really a summary variable, capturing disparities in acculturation, socioeconomic status, gender roles, immigration status, and a number of other factors.

It is an understatement to say that ethnicity is a complex factor with tangled relationships to body image and eating problems. Again, however, it is evident that all ethnic groups suffer from such problems. Given the limitations of our knowledge of risk factors as a function of ethnicity, and given the paucity of models of ethnically sensitive programs (for an exception, see Nichter et al., 1999), how might program designers proceed?

As discussed earlier, the experience of prevention specialists in the substance abuse field indicates that it is crucial to ascertain what issues the community would like to see addressed in a program (Moran & Reaman, 2002). In many ethnic minority communities it is likely that obesity and/or poor nutrition is a much greater concern than is AN or extreme dieting. In communities where both obesity and dieting-based problems are of concern, it may be important to develop a program that addresses both (Irving & Neumark-Sztainer, 2002; see chapter 3).

Next, the program needs to be presented in ways that recognize and honor the culture(s) of the community (Moran & Reaman, 2002;

Nichter et al., 1999). Nutrition lessons might emphasize what is good about the cultural group's diet, identifying foods that the children and adolescents will find familiar, accessible, and enjoyable to prepare and eat with their families. If the group speaks a language other than English, at least part of the program should integrate that language, and serious consideration should be given to arranging for bilingual people from the community to be among the prominent presenters of the program. At the very least, any letters to or meetings with parents should employ their primary language. Making sure the children's own culture is respectfully represented in the psychoeducational program should make it more relevant to the children and their families. Representation of community members in the development of the program works to ensure its integration and its maintenance in the schools (Moran & Reaman, 2002; Roosa et al., 2002).

DEVELOPING SCHOOL-BASED PROGRAMS FOR PREVENTING EATING PROBLEMS: GENERAL THEMES

Knowledge Is a Basis for Power

Our review of universal prevention research (chapter 9) indicates that, as is the case in preventing substance abuse, information or knowledge alone is insufficient for prevention and, in fact, may backfire (Hansen, 1992; Tobler et al., 2000; see Table 10.1). As is also true for prevention of substance abuse (see Hansen, 1992), a variety of different approaches offering different types of information to the same target audience have met with some success, whereas seemingly slight variations of those approaches have been ineffective. Furthermore, several successful programs such as Piran's (1999a) and O'Dea and Abraham's (2000) are founded on the principle that didactic delivery of information, no matter how well organized or clever, is either useless or harmful (see also Piran, 1995; O'Dea, 2000). This set of observations makes it daunting to offer program developers solid recommendations about the content of curriculum for the classroom (or for programs such as 4-H or the Girl Scouts).

However, the indisputable fact that information is not sufficient for preventive changes in beliefs, attitudes, and behaviors does not mean that knowledge is unnecessary to the process of prevention. In fact, even Botvin's (1996, 2000) celebrated drug prevention program acknowledges that certain types of information must complement the life skills approach. For example, information about the prevalence of use among middle school students provides the foundation for the individual belief, as well as the social norm, that middle school users of tobacco and other drugs are in the minority. In addition, a key part of *Life Skills Training* is a set of facts about the specific, immediate, and undesirable effects that tobacco, alcohol, and other drugs have on young adolescents (Botvin, 1996, 2000).

The remainder of this chapter addresses the nature of curricular content and the prospects for curriculum development in the prevention of eating problems. After presenting some themes that apply across a wide range of ages, we consider the implications of eating disorder prevention research (see chapter 9), drug abuse prevention, and developmental theory (see chapter 4) for curricular content at different ages and stages of development.

General Themes in Curricular Content

With the reminder that correspondence still does not mean causality, and that no specific set of facts will be either necessary or sufficient to produce universal-selective prevention at any age level, Table 10.2 presents the curricular components of the nine most successful universal programs containing a significant didactic element. All or almost all of these programs emphasize the conflict between physical development (e.g., weight gain during puberty) plus psychosocial development (e.g., basic needs for self-respect, a sense of control, and appreciation by others) versus a variety of unhealthy sociocultural factors (e.g., media glorification of slenderness and dieting, peer teasing about fat). This clash promotes body objectification, body dissatisfaction, calorie-restrictive dieting, and negative affect. Body dissatisfaction may be socially reinforced by gender norms and by the role of "fat talk" in peer relationships (Nichter, 2000), while in the short term, calorie-restrictive dieting may result in weight loss, compliments for improved appearance according to prevailing social standards, and a heightened sense of control. However, such dieting constitutes a "dilemma" (Bennett & Gurin, 1982; Smolak et al., 1998b) because in many instances body dissatisfaction and calorie-restrictive dieting also lead to a variety of short-term and long-term negative effects. Apparently, successful eating disorder prevention programs (see Table 10.2) are like successful drug prevention programs (see Table 10.1) in providing information that exposes the seductive psychological traps created by culture and that offers ways to

TABLE 10.2
Curricular Contents of Nine Moderately Successful Universal Prevention Programs

	Program
	Elementary	Middle School	HS	College
Content Category	1	2	3	4	5	6	7	8	9
---	---	---	---	---	---	---	---	---	---
Healthy eating	X	X		X	X	X	X		X
Healthy exercising	X	X		X		X	X		X
Positive body image	X				X		X	X	X
Physical and psychological development	X	X	X		X	X	X	X	X
Weightism	X	X	X		X				X
Analysis and resistance: sociocultural factors	X	X	X	X	X	X	X	X	X
Genetics: weight/shape	X	X			X	X			
Dieting dilemma	X	X	X			X		X	X
Eating disorders						X	X	X	X
Balanced identity and positive role models					X				
Life skills					X	X			
Activism			X		X		X		
Obesity				X	X		X		X

Note. Elementary school: 1 = Smolak & Levine (2001a); 2 = Kater et al. (2002); 3 = Neumark-Sztainer et al. (2000); Middle school: 4 = Austin et al. (2005); 5 = Steiner-Adair et al. (2002); 6 = McVey et al. (2003a); High school: 7 = Neumark-Sztainer et al. (1995); 8 = Santonastaso et al. (1999); College: 9 = Taylor et al. (2001; see also Springer et al., 1999).

resist seemingly "normal" sociocultural influences. In this regard, information about—and training in—healthy eating and exercising constitute one form of resistance (see Tables 10.1 and 10.2).

Repetition and Integration

Theory and practice suggest that students will be more likely to learn and to use this information if it is presented in an engaging, interactive fashion (Kater, 1998; O'Dea & Abraham, 2000; Tobler et al., 2000; see Table 10.1), and if it is repeated and thus reinforced in similar and different contexts (Gortmaker et al., 1999; Perry, 1999). The empirical evidence concerning "booster sessions" and "program intensity" indicates that, although neither is a major factor by itself, both can augment effective interventions such as *Life Skills Training* (Cuijpers, 2002; see also Botvin, 2000). Based on Gortmaker et al.'s (1999; see also Austin et al., 2002,

2005) work in the prevention of obesity and disordered eating (see chapter 9), and on Weissberg and colleagues' (1997) social competence approach to preventing substance abuse (see chapter 7), it appears that curricular interventions will be more successful if key "health" lessons involving information, values, and skills are integrated with other subjects that form part of state standards for education. Connections to multiple topics and subject areas have the potential to make curricular material both more manageable for school staff and an integral part of the ecology of learning (Gortmaker et al., 1999; Kater, 1998, p. ix). Table 10.3 presents ideas for integrating the aforementioned general themes in curricular content with other subjects taught in middle school; Table 10.4 does the same for content that may be important specifically for students ages 11 to 14. Weightist prejudice does not emerge as a consistently im-

TABLE 10.3
Integrating General Content With Standard Subjects:
The Example of Middle School

Information	Subjects	Sample Topic
Sociocultural factors	Social studies	Effects of propaganda on gender and health
	Health	Myths about sports, size, and success
	The arts	Collages/paintings satirizing commercials/ads pertaining to shape/weight
Physical and psychosocial development	Biology	Individual differences in weight, mass, and pubertal development: What's changeable, what's not?
	Health	Adolescent needs versus the body trap: growing up versus diets, supplements, steroids
Body dissatisfaction and dieting	Biology	Psychobiology of starvation
	Home economics	Healthy diet versus unhealthy dieting
	Mathematics	Basics of survey research and statistics: sources of negative body image at school
Resisting negative social influences	Health	Warning labels for diets
	English	Reading and writing narratives of courage and resistance in the face of social pressures
	The arts	Rap, music, and being yourself: Creating a public service announcement
Healthy eating and exercising	Health	Nutrition, immunology, and resisting illness
	Physical education	"Shake what you got": Safe and sound ways to be active every day
	Home economics	Food, fun, and other cultures

TABLE 10.4
Integrating Specific Content With Standard Subjects:
The Example of Middle School

Information	Subjects	Sample Topic
Genetics of weight and shape	Biology	Genetics of individual differences in size and shape
	Health	The clash: sociocultural factors versus biology and beauty of diversity
	Mathematics	Normal curves versus narrow definitions: The nature and cost of body dissatisfaction
Weightist prejudice	History	We shall overcome: How does prejudice arise and fall?
	English	Reading and writing stories about the cost and resistance of modern prejudices
	Home economics	Myths about fat, eating fat, and fat people
Life skills	Health	What's really eating you? Body talk isn't good coping
	The arts	Using the arts for self-expression and effective management of stress
	English or Speech & Communications	Media literacy, clear communication, and activism for citizens in a democracy

portant topic for the successful middle school programs listed in Table 10.2, but it is included as a specific topic in Table 10.4 for two reasons. As one element in appearance-related teasing and in the glorification of slenderness, it is a key ecological risk factor during the early adolescent transition (Smolak & Levine, 1996; Smolak et al., 1998b). In addition, successful elementary school programs featuring that topic have targeted students ages 9 to 11, so there is some overlap with Grade 6. All our recommendations concerning repetition and integration should be seen as guidelines for further program development and for research, rather than as empirically based conclusions.

DEVELOPING SCHOOL-BASED PROGRAMS FOR PREVENTING EATING PROBLEMS: DEVELOPMENTAL CONSIDERATIONS

Not surprisingly, the analysis in Table 10.2 also suggests that the content of effective prevention programs will vary somewhat as a function of the target age group. This is consistent with the basic principles and assumptions of a developmental approach to prevention, as listed in Ta-

CURRICULUM AND PROGRAM DEVELOPMENT   253

TABLE 10.5
Basic Principles and Assumptions of a
Developmental Approach to Prevention

- Transactions between personal vulnerabilities and psychosocial stressors shape risk for eating problems.
- Periods of transition (e.g., from childhood to adolescence) constitute periods of high risk and periods for the reorganization of people and systems in the direction of resilience.
- Parents are important sources of negative influences (risk) and positive influence (resilience) throughout childhood and adolescence, whereas peers become increasingly important in late childhood and adolescence.
- Understanding and changing the multisystemic ecology of children and adolescents is a critical element of preventing eating problems.
- Etiology and prevention of eating problems needs to be placed in the context of the relationship between gender socialization, ethnicity, and risk for (or resilience to) anxiety, depression, and other emotional issues.
- Childhood is particularly important for prevention efforts because the "thinness schema," prejudice toward fat and fat people, and social comparison processes have not been consolidated.
- Developmental psychologists can help prevention specialists develop classroom lessons and other educational experiences that are tailored to the cognitive level and interests of the target populations.

ble 10.5 (see Levine & Smolak, 2001, p. 247). We strongly believe that in order for psychoeducational programs to be maximally effective, they must be designed to be sensitive to developmental changes in all of the following: cognition, self-concept, vulnerabilities, coping mechanisms, and social supports. The next sections offer specific suggestions for tailoring material to the cognitive developmental level of the target audience. These suggestions are based on the material in chapters 5, 9, and 13, the analyses in Tables 10.1 and 10.2, and previous reviews from a developmental perspective (see, e.g., Levine & Smolak, 2001; Shisslak et al., 1996; Smolak, 1999; Smolak & Levine, 1994a, 1996, 2001b).

Preschool

There are currently no formal, published programs aimed at preventing body image or eating problems by working with a preschool audience. Yet, we know that by very early elementary school (age 5 or less) children have developed prejudices against fat people (for a review, see Smolak, 2004). Children this young also express body dissatisfaction and weight concerns, albeit at lower levels than older children do (for a review, see Smolak & Levine, 2001b). Thus, preschool-age children must be exposed to the attitudes and other social learning factors that lay the foundation for the thinness schema.

Health-promoting messages about body image and eating directed at children this age should be simple and straightforward. One might design a program, for example, about acceptance of diverse body types. Songs or picture books, such as *Shapesville* (Mills, Osborn, & Neitz, 2003), can demonstrate to young children in an engaging fashion that various shapes, such as a star or a circle, can be "successful"—and can be appreciated—in various ways (see also Zeckhausen & Boyd, 2003). Short plays or skits, modeled perhaps after NEDA's Puppet Program (Irving, 2000; see Appendix B), might be written to be presented by the children themselves. The point here is to pick fun, child-involving activities and use them to teach about body shape.

Parental and teacher involvement may be especially crucial at this age. Parents and teachers need to be educated about the detrimental effects of negative comments concerning their own or other people's body shapes (Cash, 1997; Thompson et al., 1999). Part of this education should include actively discouraging appearance-related teasing. Preschool policies for classroom behavior and for selection and training of teachers and volunteers can help adults convey to children, and reinforce for each other, that appearance-related teasing is as unacceptable as race-related teasing or gender-based harassment. Prevention specialists need to work with preschool teachers and early childhood education experts to develop various (ecological) ways to teach young children to be respectful of various body shapes. An excellent template for this effort is the set of vignettes and other teaching tools for parents and teachers in the book *Am I Fat? Helping Young Children Accept Differences in Body Size* (Ikeda & Naworski, 1992; see Appendix B).

Parents also need to understand what constitutes good nutrition and what promotes good eating and exercise patterns in preschool children. Research suggests, for example, that young children will go through "food fads" and that too much parental pressure to eat specific healthy foods, including using desserts as a bribe, is likely to produce the opposite effect (for a review, see Fisher & Birch, 2001). Parents who model healthy eating and exercise while offering children a range of healthy meals and snacks and helping them to enjoy physical activity are more likely to have children with healthy body images and eating patterns. Appendix C presents a list of resources for parents and for professionals who work with parents.

Elementary School

We have argued that elementary school is a particularly important age for prevention programs because these children's schema about body weight and shape have not consolidated yet (Smolak, 1999; Smolak & Levine, 1994a, 2001b; Smolak et al., 1998b). In other words, with children ages 5 through 11, as with preschoolers, there is an opportunity to influence directly the nature of attitudes and beliefs about body shape while they are forming, rather than having to change entrenched motives and values during middle or high school. Thus, one may be able to prevent internalization of the slender beauty ideal, or dieting to lose weight, or the integration of body dissatisfaction into self-definition. Additionally, and despite all too poignant exceptions, children ages 6 to 10 rarely are identifiable as "high risk" for eating problems (Doyle & Bryant-Waugh, 2000). Thus, a universal prevention approach seems particularly appropriate for elementary school age children (i.e., children ≤ 11 years old).

Children at this age are, of course, in classrooms every day. So one can design a full curriculum aimed at preventing eating problems. Table 10.2 indicates that information about "weightism" (the prejudice glorifying slenderness and vilifying fat and fat people) may be helpful for elementary school students (Smolak & Levine, 2001b; Smolak et al., 1999; Steiner-Adair & Vorenberg, 1999; but see Anesbury & Tiggemann, 2000). This information may be particularly useful if it is supported by policies and norms that prohibit appearance-related teasing, and by lessons about the genetic basis of individual differences in weight and shape, that is, the natural and beautiful aspects of human diversity (see Table 10.2). For children ages 9 to 11, information about psychobiology should be extended to the roles of each of the following in healthy pubertal development: acceptance of diversity, body fat, positive body image, and healthy eating and exercising.

Unfortunately, we are much clearer about the risk and protective factors operating in middle school and beyond than we are those in elementary school, particularly early elementary school. It is evident that body image is an issue for even young elementary school children, but we are not certain how they arrive at these concerns. Therefore, we should err on the side of caution in selecting topics and foci for prevention programs for these children. Perhaps the greatest implication of this caution is that information concerning eating disorders per se, including how we define obesity, should probably be omitted from elementary school programs (Smolak, 1999). If even healthy young adults can sometimes fall victim to trying extreme weight-loss behaviors after hearing about them (see chapter 9), young children are probably at even greater risk. Conversely, they may mistake healthy behavior for eating disordered behavior. For example, in administering the Children's Eating Attitudes Test (ChEAT; Maloney et al., 1989), we often encounter children who answer the question about vomiting in the affirmative because they have gotten sick after a meal. We certainly would not want children to confuse the flu with bulimia nervosa.

We have also found, both empirically and anecdotally, that discussion of body image may temporarily focus girls on their bodies (or cultural ideals) and thus actually increase body dissatisfaction in the short run (Smolak et al., 1998a; see chapter 9). This experience gives us pause in terms of discussing obesity per se with young children. It seems very likely that such discussions might increase body dissatisfaction and teasing.

As noted previously in our discussion of general themes, caution does not mean that issues of body acceptance, healthy eating, and the risks of dieting or obesity cannot be broached at all with children (see chapter 9). We are arguing that we need to contextualize these discussions so that children do not misunderstand the message. There are real constraints in terms of cognitive and self-development that need to guide our presentation of such material (Smolak, 1999). Furthermore, parents of elementary school children should be informed about eating problems (including signs of BN and AN) as well as obesity. Part of the message here should be (a) there are large individual differences across children in height and weight and eating habits, so in general the focus should be on health and fitness; and (b) children should and do gain substantial weight as they go through puberty, and for some children this weight gain predates the pubertal height spurt. With some aspects of puberty increasingly appearing during the elementary school years, particularly among Black children, parents need to be ready to support their children's concerns without assuming that their child is at risk for obesity.

Middle School

It is challenging to specify the content of curriculum for middle school students because by ages 11 to 14 many girls and boys will have internalized cultural attitudes about thin, fat, dieting, and so on, and a number will be wrestling with anxiety, dysphoria, and depression, the emotional pillars supporting disordered eating. In other words, classes will consist of students at very low or no risk, students at some risk for stepping onto the developmental pathways for eating problems, students at high risk, students with the dieting mentality and a history of weight control efforts, and a few students with disordered eating. Moreover, students who may be at low risk themselves might constitute, via teasing, for example, a source of increased risk for other students. Without minimizing this challenge (see chapter 14), we feel that drug prevention outcome studies, as well as research on risk factors for eating problems (see chapter 5) and on eating problems prevention (see chapters 9 and 13), all point to the following content areas as being especially important as supplements to the general themes.

Understanding and Appreciating Diversity. Early adolescence is a time of rapid and uneven physical change. This is accompanied by increases in self-consciousness and in attention to gender-role norms, including those concerning beauty and sexuality (Smolak & Levine, 1996). It is important for adolescents to appreciate the role of eating, exercise, and fashion in good physical and mental health. It is also very important for young adolescents to understand the genetic basis and appreciate the value of diversity in weight and shape, and to understand individual differences in the timing and process of physical development. In our experience this information is a striking revelation to many youth. As such, it sets the stage for discussions of a number of factors that contribute to positive body image and to good health in general. These include what one can and cannot control, the unfairness and stupidity of appearance-related teasing, the immediate and long-term costs of calorie-restrictive dieting, and development of a self-concept that is not tied solely to weight and shape (Kater et al., 2000, 2002; Smolak & Levine, 2001b; Smolak & Murnen, 2001).

Developing Healthy Normative Expectations. One factor addressed by many successful drug prevention programs is the misguided belief that "everyone is doing it," that is, most adolescents smoke cigarettes, drink, etc. (Botvin, 1996, 2000; Cuijpers, 2002; Donaldson et al., 1996). Information about the actual, low prevalence of drug use is part of the effort to establish or reinforce nonuse as a social norm. Currently, there are two studies of eating problems and norm (mis)perception. Sanderson, Darley, and Messinger (2002) surveyed a small, random sample of young women attending Princeton University. These women did indeed tend to perceive a campus-wide norm that differed from their own personal beliefs and attitudes by exaggerating a commitment to thinness and to exercise a means of attaining this ideal. This discrepancy was greater for older students with more exposure to campus life. Furthermore, as predicted, the degree of discrepancy between self-perception and perceived campus norms was associated with higher levels of negative body image and disordered eating. As described in chapter 9, Mutterperl and Sanderson (2002) found that a brief informational pamphlet challenging these mistaken subjective norms did prevent a rise in disordered eating for young college women who initially had not endorsed the slender beauty ideal.

These preliminary findings with a select group of students support the proposition that correction of perceived norms, long a staple of substance abuse prevention, might be incorporated into psychoeducation for prevention of eating problems. "Fat talk" (Nichter, 2000) and discontent with one's body may be indeed be widespread, but we have to be careful about using the adjective "normative," especially in creating materials for concrete operational thinkers (cf. Rodin, Silberstein, & Striegel-Moore, 1985). Negative body image may be common, but it does not mean the same thing as "distorted body image." Therefore, negative body image should not be considered normative or fashionable, because it is associated with depression and other psychological problems, especially for girls (Levine & Smolak, 2002). Moreover, "dieting" does not typically mean "calorie-restrictive dieting" and other unhealthy forms of weight control. Instead, it refers to efforts to manage one's weight by eating more fruits and vegetables, eating fewer sweets, and watching more carefully what one eats (French & Jeffrey, 1994; Nichter, 2000; Utter, Neumark-Sztainer, Wall, & Story, 2003). In fact, relatively few young adolescent girls or boys are frequently or regularly restricting their caloric intake in order to lose weight (see, e.g., Field, Camargo, Taylor, Berkey, Frazier, et al., 1999).

This type of information, reinforced by quantitative and qualitative research that students could easily learn to do in their own school, could be used to convey three important points to girls and boys. First, in large groups there are powerful social forces operating to establish and enforce social norms that are inaccurate representations of what most individuals believe and feel. This is particularly true when people are uncertain about their group status and want to fit in, such as when young adolescents enter middle school or late adolescents enter college (Sanderson et al., 2002). Second, not everyone is dieting or using other forms of weight management that, like calorie-restrictive dieting, may have a number of immediate negative consequences. If the question arises, the curriculum can also be prepared to offer the information that the subclinical and full-blown forms of disordered eating are, contrary to oft-heard claims, neither "epidemic" nor "widespread" (Hoek & van Hoeken, 2003; see also chapter 2). Far too few adolescents practice good nutrition (Berg, 2001), but this does not mean that dieting and unhealthy weight management are the social norms. Finally, negative body image is all too common, but it is not desirable, especially when one understands the limits of overemphasizing one's appearance (Cash, 1997) and the benefits of a positive body image.

Obesity. As documented in chapter 3, obesity is prevalent in children and young adolescents, and its incidence is increasing. Table 10.2 provides some evidence for the value of information about obesity, and efforts to prevent obesity, in programs seeking to prevent eating disorders (Austin et al., 2002, 2004; Steiner-Adair et al., 2002; see chapter 9). In particular, the success of the *Planet Health* obesity reduction curriculum (Gortmaker et al., 1999) in preventing unhealthy weight-management behaviors (e.g., purging and diet pills) suggests that components such as limiting TV viewing, increasing moderate and vigorous activity, and reducing consumption of high-fat foods may be particularly useful additions to general themes in health promotion for middle school students. It is crucially important to note that acknowledging obesity and taking steps to prevent it are not an endorsement of any of the following: stigmatizing obese people, glorifying slenderness, or normalizing calorie-restrictive dieting (Irving & Neumark-Sztainer, 2002; Neumark-Sztainer, 2003).

Learning Life Skills, Coping With Transition. A review of the drug prevention literature indicates that teaching nonspecific life skills may be a helpful component in curricula designed to prevent eating problems in middle school students (see Table 10.2). There are many stressors and challenges in the transition from childhood in elementary school to young adolescence in middle school (Smolak & Levine, 1996). Thus, it makes sense to teach young adolescents about the normative challenges they face and then to teach them skills—such as stress management, effective communication, and problem solving—that are useful in coping with stress. Life skills are also intended to help adolescents with normative developmental tasks, such as adjustment to physical and sexual changes, positive relationships with peers, and realistic exploration of abilities and interests (Smolak & Levine, 1996).

It is well established that one important source of effective coping with stressors is social support (Taylor, 2003). The early adolescent transition may be particularly stressful for some youth because a number of challenges occur at a time when social support from parents must be reorganized (Smolak & Levine, 1996; see chapter 4). And, given that negative body image and eating problems are particularly salient for girls, and given that developmental stressors tend to be cumulative for girls, social support is particularly important for them. Life skills training, with its emphasis on effective communication, should improve girls' ability to engage social support. Field work by Friedman (2000) and Piran (2001), and outcome research by Piran (1999b), Steiner-Adair et al. (2002), and McVey et al. (2003a) converge to demonstrate that curricula for girls ages 12 to 14 need to provide them with regular, reliable opportunities to discuss and work through their concerns in a safe, supportive group setting.

Cultural Literacy in Action. It is important that middle school students understand the clash between unhealthy sociocultural pressures and various aspects of psychobiology, including the genetics of diversity in weight and shape and the nutritional needs of growing and active bodies. It is equally important that analyses of cultural factors help girls and boys understand how weightist prejudice, sexism, and objectification unfairly constrict their ability to meet their psychosocial needs (see chapter 8). Although abstract thinking is limited in early adolescence, youth ages 11 to 14 are certainly capable of analyzing concrete instances of unhealthy sociocultural messages and taking specific individual and collective actions to challenge them. Researchers working from an FER model (see chapter 8) have demonstrated the value of developing opportunities for young adolescents to (a) clarify the source, content, and impact of negative cultural messages for girls; and (b) work together to take constructive action to replace unhealthy messages with more constructive influences (Neumark-Sztainer et al., 2000; Piran,

1999a, 1999b, 2001; Steiner-Adair et al., 2002). These messages are easily detected in the mass media (see chapter 13), but they are also readily encountered in the realm of peers, textbooks, school policies, posters in the halls, and so on.

High School

It is hard to offer much guidance in the way of recommending specific content for high school curriculum. Universal prevention is a difficult goal for work with youth ages 14 to 18 (see chapter 9). Only three prevention programs for high school students have produced evidence for a sustained prevention effect. Piran's (1999a, 1999b) FER work with male and female students at the elite Toronto Ballet school (see chapter 8) did not involve a curriculum, but the many student-initiated discussions that Piran facilitated often revolved around some of the general and specific curricular themes described thus far (Piran, personal communication, July 15, 2000). The other two effective programs, one from Italy (Santonastaso et al., 1999) and one from Israel (Neumark-Sztainer et al., 1995), had a sustained positive effect on adolescent girls who were not symptomatic at baseline. These programs had two similar components in addition to some of the general curricular themes such as knowledge and skills for resisting unhealthy sociocultural influences. Both programs provided information about developing a positive body image; conversely, both also educated students about the nature and warning signs of full-blown eating disorders. It is likely that across the high school years it becomes increasingly difficult to prevent internalization of the slender beauty ideal, body dissatisfaction, negative affectivity, and other basic risk factors. Consequently, it is possible that older students may benefit, not only from ongoing practice in cultural literacy and activism, but also from warnings about the pathways to full-blown eating disorders, coupled with cognitive-behavioral ways to improve body image (see, e.g., Cash, 1997; see also the description in chapter 9 of the cognitive-behavioral approach to body image).

College and Young Adulthood

Ages 18 to 24 constitute another transitional period in which the risk for eating disorders rises (Woodside & Garfinkel, 1992). This is one basis for educational programs at colleges and universities throughout the world. Some programs are more universal in nature (i.e., less targeted to high-risk young women), whereas other programs have been created specifically to help the many young women who, by age 20 or so, already have a negative body image and/or high scores on instruments indicating risk for eating disorders (see chapters 9 and 14). Our review in chapter 9 indicates that relatively few of the universal programs for older adolescents and young adults have been systematically evaluated. Of those that have been, the only one that has universal application and well-documented, sustained effects is Stanford University's *Student Bodies* program (Celio et al., 2000; Taylor et al., 2001). The key components of this multifaceted, interactive, computer-assisted intervention have not been elucidated, but it appears that psychoeducation is an important element (see Springer et al., 1999). Curriculum contents are an amalgam of lessons that figure prominently in our recommendations for middle school and high school, namely: (a) determinants of body image; (b) developing a positive body image; (c) the nature, causes, and consequences of eating disorders; (d) cultural influences on conceptions of beauty; and (e) healthy eating and exercising. Interestingly, content from the FER model has also been incorporated into the social cognitive model that is the basis of *Student Bodies* (see Springer et al., 1999; Taylor et al., 2001). Perhaps the life experiences of college-age women and their capacity for abstract thinking enables them to benefit substantially from readings, discussions, and critical analyses of the history of beauty standards, the nature of weightist prejudice, the relationship between disability, ability, and body image, and cultural and ethnic differences in body image (see Springer et al., 1999, p. 16; see also Franko et al., 2004). These and related topics (e.g., "men, masculinity, and the Adonis Complex"; see Pope et al., 2000) could be taught in a psychology course entitled Body Image. They could also be taught and thus elaborated within a wide variety of courses, for example, psychology of gender (Smolak & Murnen, 2004); philosophy of mind and body (Bordo, 1993); cultural or medical anthropology (Nichter, 2000); sociology of health and illness; history of fashion and design; mass communications and health; and art history.

CONCLUDING REMARKS

Reviews of prevention theory and outcomes in the fields of eating disorders and substance abuse point to several ways in which eating disorder prevention programs could be improved. This chapter considered in detail some of the major ways in which the content of curricular programs could be refined, particularly in regard to the following: (a) a critical social perspective; (b) correction of normative expectations; (c) integration of focal topics with many other aspects of the overall curricula; and (d) sensitivity to developmental needs and ethnic diversity. However, although psychoeducation via curriculum can be an important part of universal-selective prevention, it is unlikely by itself to have sustained, powerful effects (Piran, 1995). The theory and research reviewed in chapters 9 and 10 support the argument that is the foundation of chapter 4: A critically important missing element in almost all current efforts at prevention is an ecological approach. This is the subject of chapter 12. Before addressing this matter, we turn now to a fuller consideration of another very significant set of issues that emerges from a review of the prevention literature in fields of substance abuse and eating problems. Chapter 11 considers the challenge of program evaluation.

11

Lessons From the Field II: Practical Issues in Program Evaluation and Delivery

The numerous available articles, chapters, and books concerning prevention program evaluation all agree on at least two core points. First, it is essential to outline a clear theoretical model of prevention prior to developing the program or designing the intervention (e.g., Hansen, 2002; Perry, 1999; Prevention Research Steering Committee, 1993). This model facilitates identification of the variables to be assessed in the evaluation. These will include not only the outcome variables but also the components of the program assumed to affect outcome and the mediating, "proximal" variables believed to link the program and the "distal" outcome. For example, several interrelated questions of interest in an evaluation might be whether critical thinking about culture (important from a theoretical perspective; see chapters 9 and 10) was indeed taught in an engaging way (program fidelity), whether this led to a change in attitudes about the slender beauty ideal (proximal, mediating variable) at posttest, and whether this in turn can be linked to a reduced incidence of eating disordered behavior at 1-year follow-up (distal, prevention outcome).

Having identified these variables and specified their relationships, the researcher must select appropriate measures. This is the second point of agreement in the evaluation literature. These measures must have psychometric reliability and validity. They must be appropriate to the age of the participants who are the focus of the program, with some attention to changing developmental structures over the course of a longitudinal study. The measures must also consider the ethnicity and social class of the participants. There is also the important issue of whether the measures should all be self-report, as they typically are, and whether honesty is an issue in these self-reports (Hansen, 2002).

We begin this chapter with these two points in order to remind evaluation designers of their importance. People new to the prevention area are referred particularly to Perry's (1999) brief but very practical volume on designing intervention–prevention programs. We urge more experienced researchers to specify in their published work how their model and measurement decisions were made. This will facilitate the efforts of researchers seeking to compare the effectiveness of various programs, including their component parts and their delivery methods (see, e.g., chapters 9 and 10, as well as Stice & Shaw, 2004). Perhaps more important, it will assist policymakers in choosing programs that are most appropriate for their audiences.

All readers of this volume probably have at least some background in experimental design and research methods. We will not, therefore, review definitions of experimental designs or the value of a control group. Instead, the focus of this chapter is on designing prevention programs and evaluation protocols that are workable in three ways: (a) program delivery and evaluation allow the researcher to address the key research questions; (b) the programs and the evaluation protocols are acceptable to the participants; and (c) program development, program delivery, and evaluation methodology are all practical in terms of time, money, and human resources. In the first two sections of the chapter, we try to address some of these issues in a fairly general way, that is, in a way that will apply to the delivery and evaluation of a wide variety of types of programs for the prevention of eating disorders. In the third section of the chapter, we move on to what we view as a particularly difficult type of program to evaluate: a program aimed at working with and transforming various levels of environmental context along with facilitating individual development and change.

BASIC ISSUES

Everyone learns in their first research methods class that questions of causality are best addressed within an experimental design. Clearly, prevention program evaluation deals with causality: Did the program cause changes in behavior or in the risk of developing eating problems (see chapter 1)? Some researchers and theorists in the field have, therefore, argued strongly for the importance of an experimental design approach. Stice (2001b; Stice & Hoffman, 2004) has been a particularly vocal proponent of this approach. In fact, Stice has limited his reviews of prevention programs to those that were evaluated with a full experimental (pre–post; control group) design.

No one is prepared to argue that these pure experimental designs are not desirable methods. Indeed, we stipulate that they are the gold standard of methodology. Nevertheless, we also argue that it is often impossible to design such a methodology, particularly when faced with the political reality of school systems, with issues of external validity, and with funding limits. These very real concerns often reduce the likelihood that new programs undergoing their initial evaluations will be subjected to the long-term, multi-school-district experimental design that is ideal (see, e.g., Biglan et al., 2000, and Peterson, Mann, Kealey, & Marek, 2000, for such an evaluation of smoking prevention programs). Thus, we offer what we think is a realistic appraisal of common practical problems in the hopes of not overlooking a potentially useful prevention program because it was not evaluated using a pure experimental design. This does not mean that biases in evaluation can be ignored, so suggestions for how to address the challenges of practical designs are also offered.

Control Groups

Control or comparison groups are crucial in evaluation research. Failure to use such a group may actually undermine a researcher's likelihood of demonstrating the success of a prevention program (Hansen, 2002). Increases in eating and body image problems are normative developmental phenomena, at least among White girls. A successful prevention program might slow the frequency or magnitude of such increases without eliminating them (see chapter 1). If there is no control group, the researcher will be able to report only an increase in eating problems and the program will look like a failure.

However, there are two common problems in designing an evaluation using a control group. First, there is the problem of statistical power. Second, there can be contamination effects, sometimes called "spillover." This problem also raises the question of what constitutes an appropriate comparison group.

Statistical Power. The likelihood that one or two classrooms (with, presumably, 20 or so students per classroom) will provide a sufficiently large comparison group to yield a statistically significant effect is small. We must assume that real prevention program effects are no greater than moderate, and it is more likely they will be small (e.g., an η^2 value of $\leq .20$; Tobler et al., 2000; see also Stice & Shaw, 2004). Given $\eta^2 = .20$, $\alpha = .05$, and a desired power of .90 in a simple independent groups t-test comparing experimental and control groups, one needs a per group sample size of over 500 (Rosenthal & Rosnow, 1991). In a smoking prevention program enrolling more than 8,000 students from 40 different school districts, power analysis indicated that a 30% reduction in smoking prevalence could be detected (Peterson et al., 2000). Thus, the initial sample size needs to be quite large, especially in longitudinal studies where as much as one third of the sample might be lost through attrition (Hanson, 2002; Peterson et al., 2000; Smolak, 1996). If one starts with a smaller sample size, attrition must be limited by careful tracking of the participants, a procedure that is cost- and time-intensive.

Power always represents a trade-off between Type I and Type II error. Psychologists typically opt to minimize Type I error. This means that in prevention research we adopt a low alpha level (such as $p \leq .05$) in order to reduce our likelihood of claiming that a program has an effect when, in fact, it does not. It is possible that this conservative concern about Type I error has cost us in terms of Type II error. We have, perhaps, been willing to miss identifying a promising effect in the service of not erroneously claiming an effect. We need to ask whether this is a reasonable approach. The tables in chapter 9 show that many of the available prevention studies have been little more than pilots, at least in terms of sample size. In such studies, we might improve power by increasing alpha levels to at least .10. This might allow us to identify potentially valuable programs that are worthy of further research.

Contamination. Experimental designs are predicated on the assumption that the experimental group participates in the program while the control group does not. Should the control group receive any part of the experimental intervention—should the intervention somehow "spill over" to the control groups—the internal validity of the study would be undermined, as would the ability to detect a difference in performance between the experimental and control groups. In research in naturalistic settings such as schools or communities, there is a risk that the control group will be inadvertently exposed to the treatment. For example, children from a classroom randomly assigned to the experimental group might discuss lessons from their eating disorders prevention program with children from a control classroom during lunch or after school. Similarly, teachers from the experimental and control classrooms might casually discuss the lessons or techniques of the prevention program. And would we be all that surprised or disappointed if lessons designed to reduce weight- and shape-related teasing by children in the experimental classroom(s) had a positive effect on at least some children in other classrooms? In all of these cases, the control group is actually receiving at least a portion of the intervention. Although this is unintentional, the control groups' performance on outcome variables may be affected. This is known as "program contamination."

"Spillover" leading to "contamination" is particularly likely when the experimental and control groups are in the same schools. It is a good possibility, however, even when experimental and control groups are in different schools but within the same school district (Peterson et al., 2000). Children often transfer to schools within a district. Or children in comparison schools within the same county might be exposed to mass media components supplementing the school-based program. Furthermore, it is common for several elementary schools to feed into one middle school. In turn, various middle schools may send children to the same high school. Such contact between children who were originally from different schools increases the likelihood of contamination before the final, longitudinal outcome assessment.

In addition, contextual approaches to prevention often include an element of policy change (Pentz, 2000). For example, these programs may work toward changes in a school's sexual harassment policies. Schools cannot always make such policy changes without district approval. Consequently, there is some possibility that the superintendent and school board will prefer to institute such policy changes across the entire district. This means that control groups within the district will be exposed to at least this element of the program.

Solutions?   The preferred solution to these control group problems is to use several different school districts in the evaluation (see, e.g., Biglan et al., 2000). This is likely to be expensive, although collaborative research can be very helpful here.

Short of different districts, one could evaluate children who transfer into the district after the program is completed, as we did in our longitudinal prevention study (Smolak & Levine, 2001a; see chapter 9). This reduces, but does not eliminate, the threat of contamination. Moreover, these children will not have participated in the preprogram assessment, so it is possible that there will be important preexisting differences between them and the experimental group. To try to address the possibility of such preexisting differences, we measured noneating forms of psychopathology (e.g., depression) as well as knowledge of program information. The findings indicated differences between students from the experimental classrooms and the transfer students on program information and problematic eating attitudes and behaviors but not on depression (Smolak & Levine, 2001a). This preliminary information, gathered with less than $50,000 in funding over a 3-year period, encourages us to continue the development and evaluation of the program. Preliminary findings like this can, of course, also serve as the basis of grant proposals.

Another possible solution to the problem of contamination is to compare a sample to a known population (see, e.g., Piran, 1999a). This is certainly possible if one of the better validated eating disorders surveys, such as the EDI, EAT, or EDE-Q, is part of the assessment. Preprogram data from the sample can be compared to population standards to ascertain whether the sample is comparable to the population, and to validate that the target audience is appropriate for the type of prevention selected, such as universal versus targeted. Then the postprogram and follow-up data from the sample can be compared to the appropriate aged population to see if prevention has occurred.

Even if various school districts are available for participation, it is important to ensure that the districts are similar, if not matched, not only in terms of the preprogram outcome measures but also measures of the mediators. It is also crucial that efforts be made to serve the control school districts well. This process, which is important both ethically and in terms of research design, is so complex that it may require a special position on the research team (Hawkins et al., 2002; Peterson et al., 2000).

PROGRAM DELIVERY

Program evaluation cannot be fully separated from program delivery because a good evaluation addresses the process of program implementation as well as program outcomes. About 85% of all universal-selective programs for the prevention of eating problems have been delivered via a combination of lectures, discussions, and guided discussions within schools, particularly within classrooms (see tables in chapters 9 and 13). Clearly this approach has substantial advantages (Hansen, 1992; see chapter 10). It allows the researcher to use an educational and developmental setting to reach a diverse and large group of children fairly easily. Furthermore, if the program involves contextual changes, the targeted contexts will certainly include school, based on the amount of time children spend there.

Most of the school-based programs are curricula. Given that teachers are professional educators, and given that prevention education is likely to be more effective if it is integrated with the ongoing curriculum, teachers are the ideal group to implement curricular programs. Unfortunately, teachers are already overburdened by classroom sizes exceeding 30, by state-mandated curricula, and by preparations for proficiency and competency tests. It is difficult for teachers to find time to institute curricula for eating problems (Smolak, Harris, et al., 2001), despite their interest in such topics (Neumark-Sztainer, Story, & Harris, 1999). As it is unlikely that most communities will be able to mobilize mental health professionals or volunteers trained in prevention, we believe it is time to consider alternative delivery methods. Here we describe two possible alternatives: a resource coordinator and manuals.

Resource Coordinator

Our own prevention work leads us to suggest that schools assign someone the paid position of Resource Coordinator for body image and eating problems. The Resource Coordinator's responsibilities might include:

1. Working with "stakeholders" in the school, the mental health system, and the community at large to identify specific prevention needs in the school. This would likely entail a review of school policies and practices concerning teasing, sexual harassment, gender equity, nutrition, exercise, and other contextual features that might influence the development of eating problems. The needs assessment and ecological review would be followed by a proposal offering suggestions as to how positive changes in policies and practices could be made. The Resource Coordinator would also help to institute and enforce any policy changes.

2. Developing policies as to how to inform parents of children's eating problems and how to identify and refer affected children for evaluation and treatment.

3. Working with curriculum specialists and classroom teachers to assemble materials for classroom use. These materials would help educate children about proper nutrition, unacceptable teasing, an active lifestyle, media literacy, body esteem, life skills, and other topics commonly included, not only in eating disorders curricula, but also in health education and other mainstream curricula (see Tables 10.3 and 10.4). Educational materials would also likely include videos, novels, posters, pamphlets, textbooks, and computer software. Some of these resources would be used by the classroom teacher. Others might be used in programs that the Resource Coordinator would bring into classrooms.

4. Assembling materials and advice to help guide children who are concerned about friends who may be experiencing eating problems. The Resource Coordinator would also help establish and evaluate school policies in this area.

5. Assembling materials for and meeting with parents who (a) want to know more about promoting healthy eating and positive body image at home, and (b) are concerned about their daughters and sons based on what they believe are the warning signs of eating problems or eating disorders.

6. Planning and conducting in-service programs for school personnel, including teachers, coaches, school nurses, social workers, psychologists, and food service workers.

At first glance this position may appear implausible because it is seems too specialized or narrow. But it is not, really, because body image and eating issues are connected to a host of problems of immediate relevance to educators: adequate nutrition, obesity, academic underachievement, depression, substance abuse, and prejudice. Thus, the Resource Coordinator should also have information, and provide opportunities, for promoting health and well-being in the form of good nutrition, exercise and active lifestyle, safety in school, life skills, and gender equity.

If, as is likely, the Resource Coordinator is not initially a prevention specialist, someone who is would need to design both the information available to the Resource Coordinator as well as suggestions as to how the position might work. The Resource Coordinator could be a teacher (e.g., a health educator), a school nurse, a counselor or social worker, or coach. Regardless, it should be a paid position to give the person some authority and, perhaps, to attract someone with prevention experience. The Resource Coordinator would develop expertise in the field of eating problems and probably in related fields, thereby reducing the risk of inappropriate advice being given or of unfairly burdening teachers or other school personnel. It is important that someone in this position be well equipped to evaluate the needs of the particular school (or school system) so as to customize and oversee an integrated program. As demonstrated in chapter 10, this increases the chances of school and community involvement and hence program success (Hawkins et al., 2002).

Manuals

Cognitive-behavioral therapists have for many years used formal manuals to guide the training of therapists and to standardize interventions for research purposes. The use of therapist manuals led to the creation of self-help workbooks to treat at least some body image and eating problems (e.g., Fairburn, 1995; Garvin, Striegel-Moore, Kaplan, & Wonderlich, 2001). These have enjoyed some success, particularly when the client is "guided" by a professional. Cash (1997) developed the *Body Image Workbook*, which is designed to raise body esteem in both men and women. The workbook is not intended to replace professional help, but it can supplement therapy or serve as the foundation of targeted prevention of eating disorders (Cash & Hrabosky, 2004). It may also be helpful to those who do not have clinical-level problems but are nonetheless experiencing significant distress about their looks.

There are currently only a few manuals available to guide adults in *targeted* prevention work with children and adolescents (see, e.g., Scott & Sobczak, 2002; Shiltz, 1997). To the best of our knowledge, there are no readily available workbooks for the children or adolescents. It is not clear at this point whether workbooks can be used successfully by children or adolescents, even with guidance. Maybe workbooks can be used successfully by high school students but not younger children. Perhaps manuals or workbooks should be aimed at parents of high-risk girls (see, e.g., Costin, 1997). Or perhaps a combination of manuals and curriculum guides for teachers, linked to workbooks for students, should be primarily for use in the classrooms of teachers who request them. And maybe these types of resources would be most useful for relatively low-level problems. These are some of the issues that need to be investigated in regard to this type of prevention delivery method.

The same kind of statements could be made about computer programs, videos, and their supplements, such as discussion questions or reading materials. In particular, Internet-based programs focusing on improving body image have been somewhat successful with high school and college-age women (see chapter 9). Whether these can be adapted for use with children and adolescents, and under which circumstances they would be most effective, remains a question for future research. Research by Abascal and colleagues (reviewed in chapter 9) at Stanford suggests that the *Student Bodies* computer-assisted psychoeducational program can be effective in improving the body image and eating behaviors of high school students who are motivated to improve, regardless of their initial level of body image.

Program Fidelity

When researchers compare experimental and control groups on outcome variables, they want to be able to argue that any differences are due to the program's success, or that the lack of differences indicates that program is ineffective. However, the internal validity of such designs is threatened if the program is not faithfully implemented. Thus, a key element in outcome evaluation is the degree to which the actual delivery of the program matches the set of steps and processes designed by program developers. This is the dimension of "program fidelity." Lack of program fidelity can happen because of either "reinvention" or incomplete/incorrect implementation of program content or methods (Hansen, 2002; Prevention Research Steering Committee, 1993).

"Reinvention" refers to the tendency of implementers (e.g., a 7th-grade teacher of health) to modify the program to fit their own needs or interests (Hansen, 2002). One could envision this happening due to time constraints or because a prepackaged program was not particularly well suited to the developmental level or ethnic composition of students in a particular neighborhood or school. Work in schools and in the broader community requires that researchers evaluate the specific needs and resources of those contexts (Hawkins et al., 2002; Piran, 1995, 2001). Without this preparation, those implementing the program are left to do what they deem necessary to increase the program's relevance to the community.

Researchers tend to be more aware of incomplete applications, that is, the failure of teachers to fully implement a program. In the *Eating Smart, Eating for Me* program described in chapter 9 (Smolak & Levine, 2001a; Smolak et al., 1998a, 1998b), we found, for example, that only about half of the teachers completed all 10 of the lessons in their curriculum. Some teachers ran out of time; others were not particularly interested in a lesson—and perhaps the 2–3-hour training session did not inadequately train them to handle exigencies that we did not foresee. The lessons were interrelated, so this failure to complete all of them may have undermined the success of the intervention, although a lack of statistical power did not permit a full test of this possibility. Even in the well-established, well-known *Life Skills Training Program* (see chapter 10), only about two thirds of teachers actually complete the entire set of lessons (Botvin, Dusenbury, Baker, James-Ortiz, & Kerner, 1989).

So, what can be done to ensure program fidelity? First, one could employ and carefully train project assistants or managers to implement the programs. Some of the more successful programs have done this. There is, of course, a risk of "drift" or other experimenter effects in which the implementer makes some adjustments in the program along the way and thus increases or decreases its effectiveness. More important, eventually a successful program will be publicly disseminated for implementation by people not directly involved in the development of the program (e.g., teachers, health educators, social workers, parents volunteering in the classroom, or coaches). In other words, using, for example, well-educated and highly motivated graduate students to deliver a program may be helpful in the first level of rigorous evaluation, but it does not provide all the information that is ultimately needed to judge the program's success.

Researchers can also send observers to assess teacher and student fidelity to the lessons or program (Hansen, 2002). This clearly adds a layer of cost to the evaluation. Furthermore, the presence of the observer may well affect how the teacher implements the program. Nonetheless, such observations do provide the basis for modifying program training and curriculum guides to make them more "teacher friendly." At the very least, program developers involved in evaluation research should take time during teacher training to emphasize the importance of fidelity, and then follow up with survey and interview data regarding the degree and quality of program implementation. In our review of prevention outcome research in the field of eating problems, we found only a few studies that reported any data about fidelity.

Perhaps the best way to increase program fidelity is to design programs that meet the needs of teachers, parents, children, and schools. As we have already noted, it is not at all clear that teachers want or can use curricula, particularly curricula devoted exclusively to eating disorders prevention. Researchers need to gather much more information on the types of materials and delivery methods that teachers and other community members will find useful. This may ultimately involve tailoring programs to the individual community being served (Hawkins et al., 2002).

ASSESSING ECOLOGICALLY BASED PROGRAMS

Throughout this book, we have argued for the use of ecologically based models. To translate these into actual programs and their evaluation, the community itself will need to be assessed. This will involve addressing at least three major questions: Which community contexts will be considered? What elements of the community settings will be assessed? Who will provide the assessment?

Which Contexts?

Many researchers have evaluated peer, family, and media influences on body image and eating problems. Peer and media influences have also been addressed in many prevention programs (e.g., McVey et al., 2003a, 2003b; Smolak et al., 1998a; see also chapter 13), and a couple of programs (e.g., O'Dea & Abraham, 2000) have focused on the family as a factor in shaping body image and eating behavior. We believe such programs are an important step in the direction of moving beyond the individual's perception of environmental influences to changing those influences themselves.

There are other elements of the microenvironment that might be considered. Three are particularly likely to be of interest. One is the school. Recall from chapter 8 that Piran met with female students to identify aspects of their ballet school that, in their experience, contributed to their body image and eating problems. Their suggestions ranged from comments by boys to classroom comments by teachers to administrative policies concerning the reporting of harassing comments. Prior to beginning the project, Piran negotiated an agreement with the ballet school's administration to address the concerns raised by the girls. This is probably the best available example of an ecological approach to eating disorders prevention.

Although many schools will not have the resources to enable a clinical psychologist to do this type of assessment, a Resource Coordinator could gather and interpret such data in collaboration with school staff and students. If this is not feasible, it is still possible to envision classroom-based curricula that make ecological assessment a part of what the teacher and students do in the process of critically evaluating their "cultures" and of working to make these contexts more conducive to health and well-being.

In addition to schools, prevention programs might assess "proximal neighborhoods." A proximal neighborhood is the area within a relatively small radius of the child's home or school. This encompasses places such as the library or the supermarket that a child could easily visit regularly with little or no effort from parents. These are places where the child might see exemplars of the thin ideal and be exposed to prejudice against fat people, or, conversely, be exposed to opportunities to develop non-thinness-related competencies.

Finally, a program might aim to include a more "distal neighborhood." These would be places in the child's town or city that are visited with some operationally defined regularity, but in most cases less frequently than those in the proximal neighborhood. There would be exceptions to this trend. For example, we live in a very rural community with approximately 55,000 people in the entire 1,200-square-mile county. We have friends whose children were so interested in ballet or orchestra participation that the parents took them to a nearby (an hour away) large metropolitan area for weekly lessons as well as for occasional performances. For these children, involvement in these activities may have been more frequent and more salient than visiting the local YMCA. In addition to distance and frequency, these activities require more parental involvement than the more proximal ones do.

What Should Be Assessed?

We are only starting to understand all of elements of the school environment that might contribute to body image and eating problems (Neumark-Sztainer, 1996; O'Dea & Maloney, 2000; Piran, 2001). We have not yet assessed neighborhood factors such as the availability of safe playgrounds, or the frequency of visits to malls featuring a number of fashionable clothing stores, or the proximity to beaches. We can, at this point, only assume that anything that promotes the thin ideal, body objectification, and gender inequity might have a negative effect (Smolak & Murnen, 2004), whereas non-body-appearance opportunities (e.g., certain sports, music, or construction work for community causes) might serve a protective function (Geller, Zaitsoff, & Srikameswaran, 2002). Given this state of affairs, prevention research using an ecological approach can help us to clarify risk and protective factors in the etiology of eating problems.

Table 11.1 lists aspects of school, proximal neighborhood, and distal neighborhood contexts that might be assessed in preparation for devel-

TABLE 11.1
Possible Targets of Ecological Assessment in Several Community Contexts

School	*Proximal Neighborhood*	*Distal Neighborhood*
• Teacher beliefs and attitudes • Explicit or implicit rules for participation in sports or cheerleading • Gender equity in classrooms and staffing • Textbooks and videos • Magazines in the library • Posters in the classrooms and halls • Cafeteria menus • Food machines • In-school advertising • Physical education classes (availability and content) • Rule enforcement in re: teasing and sexual harassment • Systems for identification and referrals of eating problems	• Recreation opportunities, including sidewalks for walking or bicycle riding • Safety from gender- and body-related harm and harassment • Restaurants • Food stores • Posters and magazines in store windows, libraries, etc.	• Malls: Displays in stores and throughout the mall • Athletic opportunities • Opportunities in the arts • Community service opportunities • Other social-communal opportunities unrelated to body shape (e.g., religion) • Visibility of women whose success and/or substance is unrelated to the slender beauty ideal

oping an ecologically sensitive prevention program (see also Friedman, 2003; Neumark-Sztainer, 1996). In general, assessments would be designed to measure the content and availability of the listed components. We have not included family, peers, and media in this table because measures already exist to evaluate these contexts. Here, the focus is on issues that have not received much research attention.

Proximal and distal neighborhoods are part of what Bronfenbrenner's (1979) ecological model calls "microsystems," the contexts with which the child interacts daily (e.g., parents, siblings, peers, school). As discussed in chapter 4, this model also identified a contextual level called "mesosystems," which represents the interactions among elements of the microsystems. At the very least, it is likely that microsystemic forces emanating from family, peers, school, and so forth, have a cumulative and perhaps synergistic effect. For example, we found that White European middle school girls functioning in a "culture of thinness" comprised of family, peers, and mass media had poorer body esteem and a very high level of eating problems as measured by the EAT (Levine et al., 1994). One difference between boys' and girls' experiences regarding the body is that typically girls get messages about the thin ideal and disembodiment more consistently and from more sources than boys do (Smolak & Murnen, 2004; see chapter 8). Thus, challenging though this will be, we must also find ways to measure the interactions among the contexts that are evaluated.

Who Will Do the Assessments?

Piran (1999a, 2001) argues that it is very empowering, and therefore very important, for girls to participate in facilitated discussion groups that enable them to specify what aspects of their environment(s) affect their lived experiences of embodiment and disembodiment (see chapter 8). Piran's approach is relatively unstructured because it avoids generalizations or principles from previous research in other contexts. This contrasts with the highly structured methodology of Arthur, Hawkins, Pollard, Catalano, and Baglioni (2002). As part of their work with the *Communities That Care* (CTC) project (see chapter 10), these researchers designed a measure in which students self-report influences from a prearranged list of contexts. These data are then used to tailor substance abuse prevention programs. Piran and the CTC directors are working from radically different theoretical models, but a key feature of both programs is that children and adolescents provide their own assessment of the environments in which they are developing.

Adults are also an important source of information about ecological factors. For example, Friedman (2003) designed a set of assessments of the school environment, including whether puberty education and media activism are addressed. The Resource Coordinator could complete this evaluation, ideally in conjunction with others, but possibly alone. The Resource Coordinator—or the adult in charge of the prevention program, if it is a different person—then uses this information to design prevention strategies specific to the risk factors and sources of resilience operating in his or her school. This strategy should draw on a range of community resources (see chapters 13 and 15).

There are many good reasons to ask children and adolescents for their opinions as to what environmental factors negatively or positively impact their body esteem and eating patterns (see, e.g., chapters 7 and 8). However, there are at least two problems with this approach. First, girls and boys might not feel comfortable reporting certain types of problems. They might not wish to report questionable comments by coaches or teachers for fear of retaliation, for example. Indeed, Piran carefully and patiently built rapport with the girls at the ballet school by meeting with them several times before discussing body image issues (see chapter 8). Second, young children, as well as youth who are not adept at critical thinking, may be unaware of contextual influences or may be unable to effectively articulate them. In this regard Murnen and Smolak (2000) found that one cannot use broad questions or even checklists concerning sexual harassment with elementary school children. Even when participants are older, some influences may be so subtle, or acceptance of them so ingrained, that most students do not note them as problematic.

Even if valid interview or survey data are available, one would not simply want to use frequencies of student reports to determine which environmental factors need to be addressed. The Resource Coordinator and/or the program facilitator, working with their advisors, will need to decide which factors are most likely to be changeable given administrative and community support. The adults involved in this decision will also need to weigh context-specific data against findings from the research literature in order to determine which malleable factors are likely to be most severely affecting the largest groups (or at least identifiable groups) of children or adolescents.

In making these decisions, the Resource Coordinator or the program facilitator should not forget the distinct possibility that adults evaluating environments will overlook matters that are of concern to students. Adults may be trying to advance their own agendas or to protect their own interests. They may also be genuinely unaware of unhealthy attitudes and behaviors that they themselves are modeling or directing toward students or staff (Levine, 1987; Levine & Hill, 1991). Yet, there is certain information, for example, concerning the details and enforcement of school policies, that is more available to teachers, counselors, and administrators than to students.

This, then, brings us to the lesson most of us learned early in our research careers. Ideally, any research project will involve multi-informant methods. At this phase of the development of ecologically based prevention programs, this principle seems particularly important. Currently, we do not have a clear sense of what aspects of different contexts might be evaluated. We are still at the stage of gathering information about the various contexts. Information from multiple sources, reflecting differing experiences within the same environments, will help to achieve this goal of designing context-sensitive programs that are informed by a practical theory of ecological influences, such as Bronfenbrenner's (1979; see chapter 4).

CONCLUSIONS

There is much to be done in order to develop and institute effective methodologies for evaluation of prevention programs in the field of eating problems and eating disorders. Sometimes the methodological challenges reflect longstanding, familiar problems in establishing *internal* validity, such as constituting an appropriate control group, using an array of valid measures, and ensuring sufficient statistical power. As our field moves beyond pilot programs, it will become increasingly important that attention be given to these traditional issues. The twist here is that *external* validity is crucially important in prevention research, probably more so than in many traditional experimentally based fields. As we seek to improve internal validity by using experimental designs and ensuring fidelity of application, external validity cannot be sacrificed.

Some of the newer models of prevention, most notably the ecological approach, will require the development of new methodologies that permit involvement of the community. As described in chapter 7, those who espouse a Non-Specific Vulnerability-Stressor model can find some guidance in the work of Benson and colleagues at the Search Institute in assessing and improving the Developmental Assets program for community-based health promotion (Benson et al., 1998; www.searchinstitute.org). Similarly, Piran's feminist-empowerment-relational model (see chapter 8) incorporates discussion-based ecological assessment into the prevention process. Alas, at this point, we can only make suggestions as to what advocates of other models, including the most prominent approaches—social cognitive and cognitive-behavioral (see chapter 6)—might assess in the various ecologies of children and adolescents. Currently, in the field of body image and eating problems there are no validated measures available to perform these assessments. Given its importance, this is an exciting area of future research (Hawkins et al., 2002). Indeed, the excitement is increased by the fact that developing these methodologies may also improve our knowledge of risk and protective factors. With the challenge of ecological assessment firmly in mind, we turn now to the task of expanding prevention from the focus on individual participants to a focus on changing the ecology.

12

Changing the Ecology

Cognitive-behavioral therapy (CBT) is among the most effective treatments for eating disorders. Indeed, it is arguably the best available treatment and is increasingly the standard against which other treatments are measured. CBT has many components but one of the most central is the definition, deconstruction, and reconstruction of attitudes, beliefs, emotions, and behaviors concerning the self, the value of thinness, and attainment of an "ideal" body shape and weight (Fairburn, 1997; see chapter 6). These interrelated attitudes, beliefs, emotions, and behaviors constitute a "schema." Although the specifics of schema construction and maintenance vary from theory to theory, it is widely agreed that experiences in a variety of settings form the raw material for the cognitive processes that create, extend, and sustain the schema. As the schema is increasingly consolidated, it becomes a filter through which the person interprets new information and experiences so that schema-consistent material is highlighted (see chapter 6).

Whether the central schema contributing to eating problems and eating disorders is called overvaluation of weight and shape (Fairburn, 1997), a thinness schema (Smolak & Levine, 1996), weight concerns (Killen, 1996), or internalization of the thin ideal (Thompson & Stice, 2001), there is universal agreement that multiple sources of influence shape its development. Individually and in interaction with each other, the family, peers, and mass media are all seen as important contributors to the development and maintenance of the pathogenic schema (see

Thompson et al., 1999; see also chapters 4 and 5). In fact, as described in chapters 4 and 6 through 8, an emphasis on the interplay of multiple settings and systems is a feature of all the major theoretical models that have shaped the development of the specific prevention programs described in chapters 9 and 13.

It is not only theoretical perspectives that lead us to suggest that extraindividual factors must be considered in designing programs to prevent eating problems, eating disorders, and obesity. As outlined in chapter 5, available empirical data have clearly established that peers, parents, and siblings all influence the development of negative body image and disordered eating in childhood and adolescence (see, e.g., Ricciardelli & McCabe, 2001a; Smolak, 2002; Smolak & Levine, 2001b; and Thompson et al., 1999, for reviews). To reiterate, parental influence on eating patterns is evident as early as infancy and the preschool years (Fisher & Birch, 2001). Peer influence, in the form of teasing and sexual harassment, as well as in terms of peers' investment in thinness and dieting, has been documented among adolescents, and to a lesser extent, among elementary school age children (Eisenberg et al., 2003; Murnen & Smolak, 2000; Nichter, 2000; Paxton, Schutz, Wertheim, & Muir, 1999). The influence of print and video media has also been well documented, again, especially in adolescence and beyond (see chapter 13). Research documenting cultural and ethnic group differences in rates and types of eating problems underscores the influence of macrosystem factors (see, e.g., Anderson-Fye & Becker, 2004; Smolak & Striegel-Moore, 2001). Research concerning the role of these sociocultural influences in the development of eating problems among girls is much more extensive than that concerning body image and eating problems among boys. However, the limited data available suggest that boys, too, are influenced by peers, family, and media (e.g., Pope et al., 2000; Smolak, Levine, & Thompson, 2001; see Ricciardelli & McCabe, 2004, for a review).

Thus, theoretical models and empirical data converge in consistently pointing to the importance of context in developing and maintaining body image and eating problems. Yet most eating disorders prevention programs continue to emphasize intraindividual changes (see chapter 9). That is, they try to get participants, whether they are 8-year-olds or young college students, to change their own, individual attitudes, beliefs, and behaviors concerning body shape, eating, life skills, or sociocultural influences such as mass media. On some level, attempts at individual change are crucial. After all, it is an individual who ultimately adopts "problematic" attitudes and behaviors. However, as discussed in chapter 9, failing to change the environments that foster and maintain obesity or eating problems may doom programs focusing exclusively on the individual. It is probably too much to ask adolescents, let alone children, to overcome unhealthy messages from peers, teachers, coaches, parents, siblings, and media. Instead, prevention programs need to alter those messages. Our review of prevention research in the field of substance use and abuse (see chapter 10) indicates that, although the teaching of life skills and resistance skills to individuals may be effective, multifaceted approaches that transform the environment so that it becomes protective and health-enhancing are most likely to be effective in the long run for a large number of participants (see Biglan et al., 2000; Hawkins et al., 2002; Maton, 2000; Minke, 2000; Perry, 1999; Tobler et al., 2000). The purpose of this chapter, then, is to outline how prevention programs might aim to change the contexts in which body image and eating problems develop and are maintained. An extended, fictional example is provided in chapter 15.

CHANGES IN CONTEXTS

For most children and adolescents, the major influences on the development of body image and eating problems are family, school, and mass media. For our purposes, peers are considered part of the school environment. Insofar as there are important peer and adult influences associated with participation in church groups, Scouts, dance studios, community-based sports teams, or any other setting, those contexts should also be considered as potential targets of prevention programs (see chapter 15).

What needs to be changed in each of these contexts in order to reduce risk and increase resilience, that is, promote health? It is impossible to provide an exhaustive list of what will make such settings more "body friendly." Although schools, families, and media may typically share certain elements, they also differ from one another, sometimes very substantially. For example, one can imagine that a high school with a long history of football championships might see more concerns about muscularity among the boys than would a high school that does not even field a conference team. A particular coach, or the operator of the local fitness center where the boys lift weights, might encourage use of food supplements, and even steroids, to facilitate muscle development in boys who "really want to be winners." Girls attending school in areas that feature beaches and year-round mild weather might be more concerned about how they look in a bikini than will girls from a landlocked, northern state. If a particular weight-management technique is widely used by the most popular girls, others may follow suit. It is imperative, then, that program designers and facilitators are familiar not only with the general findings from prevention research, but also with school and family influences operating in their particular locale (Piran, 2001).

However, just as we can say that school, family, and media contexts are likely to be the most influential for most children and adolescents, we can point out common problems in each of these contexts. These include issues surrounding nutrition and exercise, direct comments to children that include teasing and sexual harassment, role models, opportunities for success that do not focus on attractiveness, and knowledge concerning signs and symptoms of eating disorders.

Nutrition and Exercise

Late in 2001 the Surgeon General of the United States issued a "call to action to prevent and decrease overweight and obesity." The rationale for this and for similar recent proclamations about the "obesity epidemic" was discussed in chapter 3. The percentage of children 6 to 11 years old and of adolescents who are obese currently stands somewhere between 12% and 15% (Centers for Disease Control, n.d.; Neumark-Sztainer, 1999; Troiano et al., 1995). The higher figure is almost triple the rate of obesity for these groups two decades ago.

AN, BN, and other eating disorders are much rarer among children and adolescents, especially elementary school and middle school children (see chapter 2). However, we do well to remind ourselves that AN, BN, and EDNOS all present substantial health risks, including growth stunting, osteopenia and later osteoporosis, esophageal and stomach bleeding, imbalanced electrolytes, severe dental damage, various endocrine dysfunctions, abnormal levels of neurotransmitters, and irregular heartbeats (Hill & Pomeroy, 2001; Kaye & Strober, 1999; Pomeroy, 2004). At least 5% of AN sufferers die from the disorder; rates of suicides are also elevated, at least among women with AN (Herzog et al., 2000; Nielsen et al., 1998).

Obesity and eating disorders differ in some very important ways, but one core problem in both is poor nutrition (Berg, 2001). Thus, any program aiming to prevent eating disorders, eating problems, or obesity must encourage healthy eating. But concerns about healthy eating extend beyond those with unhealthy weights or pathological eating problems (Berg, 2001). Only about 3% of Americans meet four of the five Food Guide Pyramid recommendations made by the federal government (U.S. Department of Health and Human Services [USDHHS], 2001). Government surveys suggest that approximately 40% of adolescents regularly skip breakfast, a decision that may negatively impact their academic performance (Centers for Disease Control [CDC], 1996). As many as 40% of elementary school girls may at least experiment with unhealthy calorie restriction (Smolak & Levine, 2001b).

Most schools offer some kind of nutrition education, although perhaps not consistently throughout Grades K–12 as recommended by the CDC (1996). Most children and adolescents attend school, and more than half of these students eat at least one meal there daily (CDC, 1996), so schools are a natural site for nutrition intervention. These programs should extend beyond classroom instruction (see discussion of the *Planet Health* obesity prevention curriculum in chapter 9; Gortmaker et al., 1999). Food services can provide more of the healthy and fewer of the unhealthy menu choices. Vending machines that sell candy bars or other nonnutritious foods can be outlawed in schools (as Arkansas did in 2003), or they can at least be replaced with machines offering fruit juices or milk or fruit. In this regard, school systems need to review carefully the nutritional implications of any financial arrangements that offer soft-drink and fast-food companies the opportunity for aggressive marketing of their products on school grounds.

Parents control family food choices, particularly for young children. It is not clear that families have all of the relevant information necessary to determine what constitutes healthy eating, particularly in terms of serving sizes. Families may need suggestions for quick and reasonably nutritious meals, including meals purchased at fast-food restaurants. Research suggests that parental involvement can enhance the effects of nutrition education, at least among elementary school students (CDC, 1996). Government-based food programs should aim to provide families with nutritious, low-fat foods (USDHHS, 2001).

Mass media, particularly television advertisements, also influence children's food choices. Food advertised during children's television is routinely high in sugar, fat, and "empty" calories. Consequently, it is not surprising that children who watch more television are more likely than other children to have unhealthy beliefs about food as well as poor eating habits (CDC, 1996). Consumers can protest these commercials (see chapter 13) or can, at least, mediate their effects on children by doing such things as presenting more accurate information, refusing to buy the unhealthy products, or really making moderate portions "part of a nutritious breakfast."

An active lifestyle, including exercise, is also important for good health. Regular, moderate exercise has been associated with decreased risks of heart disease, high blood pressure, colon cancer, diabetes, and depression among adults (CDC, 1997). Some of these benefits may also accrue to children and adolescents (USDHHS, 2001). Compared to normal weight individuals, and relative to caloric intake, people who are overweight or obese tend to exercise less and to be more sedentary. Exercise combined with healthy eating frequently results in weight loss, and the reduction of certain health risks, among obese people (Valdez, Gregg, & Williamson, 2002). Even critics of our culture's obsession with weight loss as the solution to obesity agree that healthy eating and regular, moderate levels of exercise are important steps in reducing health risks associated with overweight and obesity (see, e.g., Miller, 1999).

On the other hand, excessive exercise is associated with AN and BN (Davis et al., 1997; Epling & Pierce, 1996). Excessive exercise may be a risk factor for the development of AN, and it can serve as a purge mechanism in both AN and BN. Thus, the goal for health promotion and prevention of eating problems is to make moderate levels of physical activity and exercise a habitual part of daily life. Ideally, the motivation for this active lifestyle is fitness, fun, and friendship, not compulsive compensation for calories consumed or for a negative body image.

Schools can encourage physical activity by offering safe and respectful physical education levels at all grades, including high school (CDC, 1997; USDHHS, 2001). Physical education, dance, good use of recess, and other opportunities for exercise and physical play during school hours may be particularly important in neighborhoods where safety concerns preclude children from staying after school to participate in sports or even from playing outside after school. Efforts may also need to be made to increase physical activity in sprawling suburbs where schools, parks, and stores are too far away from homes to walk to them (Ewing, Schmid, Killingsworth, Zlot, & Raudenbusch, 2003). School curricula can provide information—integrated across various courses and supported by staff training—concerning the physical and mental health benefits of exercise and an active lifestyle (CDC, 1997; Gortmaker et al., 1999). School personnel should also monitor excessive interest in or commitment to physical conditioning (Ransley, 1999). The latter may indicate body image and eating problems among both boys and girls.

Families can also encourage physical activity. As of 1997, fewer than one third of American adults engaged in the federally recommended amounts of physical activity, with 40% engaging in no leisure time physical activity (USDHHS, 2001). Clearly, parents can improve their own health, and provide a better model for their children, if they increase their exercise and activity levels. Parents can include their children in at least some exercise such as walking, playing basketball and frisbee, or swimming. Parents can also support children's healthy interest in sports and dance by attending games or performances, practicing with the child, and providing transportation to and from games, practices, or rehearsals. Furthermore, parents can reduce their children's television viewing, a sedentary behavior associated with being overweight (USDHHS, 2001). This reminds us that "exercise" need not consist solely of calisthenics, jogging on a treadmill, and other forms of regimented training. Exercise can be built into a less sedentary, more active lifestyle through walking or bicycling instead of driving, taking the stairs instead of the elevator, and playing outside with friends instead of sitting in front of a TV screen or a computer monitor.

Direct Comments to Children and Adolescents

There are at least three forms of verbal comments directed toward children and adolescents that might negatively affect their body image and contribute to the development of eating problems. First, there are comments that the source views as factual. These may be negative, as in suggesting that an adolescent needs to lose weight in order to improve her appearance, or that a child is just not talented at sports and so she need not participate. Other comments are intended to be positive, as when a child is complimented on how much better he looks now that he has lost a little weight. Second, there is teasing. Appearance-related teasing is the most common form of teasing among peers. Such teasing has been prospectively related to negative body image and eating problems (Tantleff-Dunn & Gokee, 2002; see chapter 5). Third, as discussed in chapter 8, sexual harassment appears to be related to body image and perhaps eating problems.

The first step in reducing all of these harmful forms of verbal comments is to increase awareness of their effects. The sexual harassment literature in particular is full of examples in which the effects of harassment were minimized, the victim was blamed for the harassment, or the perpetrators were not punished (e.g., Stein, 1995, 1999). Schools can increase awareness of this very significant phenomenon through curricula and, more important, through regular and visible enforcement of antiteasing, antiharassment policies. Stein (1999, 2001) argued that such policies should reflect "zero indifference" rather than "zero tolerance." Her distinction captures the importance of educating school personnel, students, and parents about the effects of such comments. That brothers are more likely to harass girls than peers are (Stein, 1995) underscores the importance of getting this message out to parents.

Research also clearly demonstrates that parental comments about their children's weight and shape affect even elementary school children (Ricciardelli & McCabe, 2001a; Smolak & Levine, 2001b; Smolak et al., 1999). The research is not yet specific enough to ascertain whether these are "factual" negative comments, comments intended to be positive, or hostile teasing. It seems likely that all three play a role, although intentionally negative comments may eventually prove to be the most harmful. All of this means that it is very important for parents to refrain from making these comments and in so doing set a positive example for their children as to the inappropriateness of teasing each other about weight and shape. Similarly, in the school setting, teachers, administrators, and perhaps especially coaches and physical educators should explicitly teach and model the inappropriateness of making hurtful comments about body shape. In this regard, adults need to be educated that "hurtful" ranges from clear harassment to manipulative teasing about "fat" to subtle, disembodying messages that define people in general, and females in particular, solely in terms of body and beauty (see, e.g., Piran, 2002).

Role Models

We have already seen several examples of the importance of teachers and parents as role models for nutrition, exercise, and teasing. Adults can be encouraged to do self-evaluations as to their success in these areas, and to monitor their progress in making changes in problem areas. For example, Levine and Hill (1991) devised the Weight and Shape Attitudes Test to help teachers of their *5-Day Lesson Plan* to assess their status as healthy role models (see also Piran, 2004). A prevention program should encourage this type of self-evaluation and self-development by making both teacher in-service training and ongoing support for positive changes integral parts of school-based interventions (Piran, 2004; Wechsler, Devereaux, Davis, & Collins, 2000). Support could involve provision of charts for tracking one's behavior; convening discussion groups for continued critical evaluation of experiences in the realm of culture, the body, and eating; offering opportunities for teachers to share healthy exercise or nutritious meals with children and parents; and public recognition for salient positive steps that teachers have taken to serve as healthy role models (CDC, 1996; Piran, 2004; USDHHS, 2001).

Both girls and boys are subject to peer influences. Peers may engage in, and thereby encourage, "fat talk" or teasing (Nichter, 2000). Girls who diet are more likely to have friends who also diet (Paxton et al., 1999; Smolak & Levine, 2001b; Tantleff-Dunn & Gokee, 2002). Whether this reflects a modeling influence and/or an association preference is unclear. In either case, peer modeling helps to maintain the dieting behavior. Students, and perhaps siblings, should be made more aware of these influences. One way to do this is to work back from targeted to universal prevention. Many children and adolescents care deeply about their friends, so classroom and family discussions, or religious education, could begin with a consideration of the warning signs of eating problems and how to help a friend get help (Levine, 1987; Levine & Hill, 1991). This discussion, coupled with candid information about the challenges of identifying and treating entrenched eating disorders, becomes a logical springboard for asking: "What could friends do to help negative body image and eating problems from beginning in the first place?" A recent study by Rosenvinge and Westjordet (2004) found that Norwegian students ages 15 to 16 were very appreciative of the opportunity to discuss ways to reach to and support friends with an eating disorder, and that the students desired further opportunities for interactive classroom discussions about the issues involved.

Perhaps the most obvious, and certainly a pervasive and pernicious, role model is actually not a single model but rather the thin ideal for females that is found throughout the media (see chapter 13). In addition to being thin, this image is sexually objectified, thereby linking it to the effects of sexual harassment and sexual violence (Fredrickson & Roberts, 1997; Piran, 2002; Smolak & Murnen, 2001, 2004). Research consistently links this ubiquitous media image to body dissatisfaction and eating problems (see Table 13.1, chapter 13). Unfortunately, an increasingly muscular image for males is appearing in the media (Leit, Gray, & Pope, 2002; Pope et al., 2000). Research suggests that boys are aware of this muscular ideal, although it seems not to have the impact of the analogous thin ideal for women (Cusumano & Thompson, 2001; Smolak, Levine, & Thompson, 2001). There is, of course, the risk that this gender difference is only temporary and that, eventually, the media ideal will be as toxic to boys' self-images as it currently is to girls'.

It appears that elementary school and high school girls who actively reject a sexually objectified media image of women have a better body image than girls who accept or are ambivalent about the image (Murnen et al., 2003; Steiner-Adair, 1986). Chapter 13 is devoted to an analysis of prevention programs that revolve about literacy, activism, and advocacy in regard to mass media.

Opportunities

There are many indicators that appearance is more important in women's success than in men's (Smolak & Murnen, 2001, 2004; Thompson et al., 1999). This is true socially, academically, and in terms of career attainment. Women, more than men, are likely to be sexually objectified, that is, treated as objects that are valued mainly for the pleasurable viewing they provide to men (Bordo, 1993; Kilbourne, 1994; Fredrickson & Roberts, 1997; Smolak & Murnen, 2001, 2004). This is not to suggest that men's bodies are never objectified (Bordo, 1999; Pope et al., 2000), but rather that objectification of women's bodies is much more pervasive and acceptable. Men, and boys, typically have many options or routes for success that are not related to their body *shape*. Indeed, even when men's bodies are important to their success, it is often within the framework of sports, where athletic competence in terms of strength, agility, or endurance is more clearly valued than a particular, specific body shape. This is the case even when an imposing muscular physique is part of entertainment based on masculinity per se, such as in the enormously popular business of professional wrestling.

Academic and other non-appearance-related activities are associated with better body esteem (Geller et al., 2002). Sports are an example of the kind of opportunity that girls need. Girls who participate in non-elite, high school sports that are not appearance-related (e.g., soccer, basketball) have higher body esteem than do other adolescent girls

(Smolak et al., 2000). At least in mixed-gender schools, an emphasis on intelligence and professional success may be associated with a less severe adherence to the thin ideal (Tiggemann, 2001). Research should also investigate whether part-time employment or community service opportunities might also reduce the centrality of body shape to self-definition. Schools and families might, then, be encouraged to provide a variety of opportunities for girls to explore success that is not linked to attractiveness in general and thinness in particular. This effort will be most successful when it unfolds in schools or communities where there are numerous actual and symbolic models of female competence and "substance."

It is worth noting that this same general statement about opportunities for competence might apply to obesity. In one of the many ironies of public health endeavors, lack of exercise is associated with obesity, but obese people often feel discouraged about exercising and participating in athletic activities because of a sense of incompetence and the high probability that they will be stared at and teased (Burgard & Lyons, 1994; CDC, 1997). Obese children and adolescents may also feel incompetent socially. Efforts should be made to insure the inclusion of overweight children—and very thin, frail-looking children—in activities that are structured to enhance the sense of competency and self-esteem in all children (see, e.g., Neumark-Sztainer, Story, Hannan, & Rex, 2003).

Signs and Symptoms

Many parents and educators are uncertain as to how to determine whether a child is overweight, or is suffering from an eating disorder, or is showing behaviors or attitudes that place the child at risk for developing an eating disorder. Parents may turn to health care providers for information, but many primary care physicians are not well informed. This, then, means that another setting, health care, may need to be addressed in prevention efforts (Weiner, 1999). This is especially important in terms of identifying eating disorders, because primary care physicians are likely to be the first professionals consulted about such problems.

As children develop, they are likely to go through periods, such as at the beginning of puberty, when they seem heavier or thinner than they have been in the past. Fat deposition is a normal part of pubertal development, especially for girls. Indeed, after puberty girls normally have relatively more body fat than boys do. Many children also go through periods of marked food preferences. Adolescents, especially boys, often eat what seems to parents to be enormous amounts of food. Pediatricians, family practice physicians, and parents need to know what changes in body weight and shape, eating preferences, and food intake are normative and what signals a health or behavioral problem. This may seem obvious with respect to physicians. However, dietitians and physicians who specialize in the treatment of eating problems and eating disorders assure us that medical education about nutrition and physical development is typically brief and inadequate.

Teachers, too, need to be aware of indicators of eating problems (Levine, 1987; Ransley, 1999). As noted previously, it is not at all unusual for students to come to teachers with concerns and questions about a friend, sibling, or peer whom they suspect has an eating problem. Some students have questions about themselves. Teachers also monitor lunch or recess, where patterns of food avoidance, eating, and exercise may be easily observed. In fact, abnormal exercise patterns, as indicated by a desire to exercise as often as possible, may be more evident at school than at home. Similarly, an unusual interest in food preparation, purging techniques, or appetite-suppressing substances, or in paper topics dealing with eating disorders may indicate risk for eating problems.

Veteran clinicians are unanimous in maintaining that eating disorders are challenging to assess and to treat. Therefore, it is very important that, in addition to clear information about warnings signs and risk factors for eating problems and obesity, the network of adults involved have access to professional assistance. This network includes, not only teachers and parents, but also guidance counselors, school nurses, coaches, trainers, and administrators. Mental health professionals, and ideally eating disorders professionals, can assist schools in the development of a specific process by which parents and students can receive professional help. This process is advantageous for both the legal protection of school personnel and the well-being of troubled students and their families (Ransley, 1999). Community service agencies, including mental health clinics, might be invited to collaborate with school personnel and parent organizations to help make it easy for parents to consult with professionals in the area of eating disorders. When an adolescent is returning to school following hospitalization for an eating disorder, school personnel, parents, the student, and mental health professionals should work together to develop a plan, and a safety net of support, to enable the student to successfully reintegrate into school life. As is the case for universal-selective prevention, it is important to involve a variety of people and settings in the targeted prevention of eating disorders.

A Closing Comment

This section addressed some of the changes in family, school, and healthcare settings that might be targeted by prevention programs. We organized this section by themes rather than by settings to emphasize the need to intervene on multiple levels and to coordinate efforts so they support and reinforce each other (see chapter 15). Just as hearing a negative body image or eating message from multiple sources may increase the likelihood of a problem developing (Levine et al., 1994; Smolak & Levine, 2001b), prevention efforts that work with multiple settings are more likely to be successful (CDC, 1996; Perry, 1999; Tobler et al., 2000; USDHHS, 2001). We now turn our attention to a pioneering effort in developing a more ecological approach to the prevention of eating problems.

McVEY'S COMPREHENSIVE SCHOOL-BASED PROGRAM

In chapter 9 we reviewed a series of studies in which McVey and colleagues in Toronto, Canada, evaluated the *Every Body Is a Somebody* (EBIS) program for middle school students (Seaver et al., 1997; see Table 9.2). Encouraged by the short-term success of that curriculum- and support-group-based prevention program, McVey, Tweed, and Blackmore (2004) recently developed a school-based project to investigate the effectiveness of a more comprehensive and more ecological approach.

Goals and Structure of the Program

The goals of the *Healthy Schools–Healthy Kids* program are to reduce negative attitudes and behaviors in regard to eating, weight, and shape, while increasing positive self-esteem, body satisfaction, healthy eating, active living, and acceptance of diversity in size and shape. The principal target audience was both male and female middle school students ages

11 to 14 ($M = \sim 12$). The intervention, which lasted 8 months (i.e., almost an entire school year), had the following components.

Teacher and Staff Training. All teachers, administrators, and staff in the experimental schools were given the opportunity to participate in a 2-hour session that addressed the problem of eating disorders and allowed participants to examine their own thoughts and feelings in regard to body image and eating. The rationale offered was very similar to the arguments given earlier for ways in which adults can promote good nutrition and an active lifestyle, can reduce hurtful teasing, and can serve as healthy role models. Teachers using the prevention curriculum in their classrooms were also provided with training and monthly feedback sessions in regard to its delivery.

Parent Education. Twice per month parents were offered, at noon or in the evening, the opportunity to learn about the prevention program and learn more about topics relevant to early and middle adolescence, such as body image and self-esteem. Parents also received, as part of the monthly newsletter that the school sends home, tips for health promotion. Similar to the parent newsletters developed by Smolak et al. (1998a, 1998b) for the ESEM program (see chapter 9), the tips provided in the monthly school newsletter matched the topics covered in the in-class curriculum.

Students and the Curriculum. As part of physical education, health education, or homeroom, all girls and boys attending Grades 6, 7, and 8 were given daily lessons from the EBIS curriculum. The lessons, which were supplemented by videos made available to the teachers, covered topics such as ways to promote positive self-esteem and body image, stress management techniques, genetic influences on weight and shape, and media literacy (see chapter 13). All students also saw and discussed a 50-minute play about dealing with media and peer pressures to change the shape of one's body.

Student Groups. All girls had a chance to participate in 12 weekly 50-minute sessions of the *Girl Talk* peer support program, which is based on LeCroy and Daley's (2001) manualized program entitled *Empowering Adolescent Girls* (see McVey, Lieberman, et al., 2003a, 2003b, as reviewed in chapter 9). These groups, which are facilitated by school nurses, focus on life skills (e.g., dealing with anger, coping with stress) and a nondieting approach to both good nutrition and an active lifestyle. All boys participated in 50-minute focus groups, segregated by grade level, that discussed peer teasing and bullying.

School Environment. Posters were placed around the school to convey images and text related to empowerment, size acceptance, healthy eating, an active lifestyle, and so on. These messages were reinforced and extended by "public service" announcements (PSAs) read aloud over the PA system each morning. The PSAs were developed by the research team and, later, by the *Girl Talk* support groups.

Methods and Results

Four middle schools (matched for size, geographic location, and cultural composition) were randomly assigned to the experimental or no-intervention control. At baseline there were 784 girls and 665 boys. Of the entire sample of students, approximately 40% were White and two thirds were Canadian-born with English as their first language. Self-report assessments were completed prior to the intervention, 8 months later (postintervention), and, for students originally in the sixth and seventh grades, 6 months after that (follow-up).

The 13 dependent measures addressed self-worth, body satisfaction, awareness and internalization of slenderness as the cultural norm for ideal beauty, body size acceptance, teasing, patterns of eating and physical activity, and weight loss and muscle gaining efforts. The *Healthy Schools–Healthy Kids* project had several positive effects on the girls (irrespective of grade), whereas it had no significant positive effects on the boys when their data were analyzed separately. At 6-month follow-up, girls in the intervention schools reported greater reductions in internalization of the slender beauty ideal than did girls in the control schools. In addition, at 6-month follow-up, girls receiving the intervention reported a reduction in awareness of slenderness as the cultural beauty norm, whereas awareness scores for girls in the control condition increased significantly. At 6-month follow-up, girls who had participated in the intervention also reported skipping fewer meals than did girls in the control condition. Finally, there was a program participation effect for the number of girls currently trying to lose weight, that is, the expected difference was present at posttest but it was not maintained at follow-up. The intervention did not significantly improve body satisfaction for girls. However, when the data for girls and boys were combined, there was a significant pre-to-post-to-follow-up increase in body satisfaction for the seventh graders only.

Conclusions

This initial evaluation of the *Healthy Schools–Healthy Kids* ecological intervention (McVey, Tweed, & Blackmore, 2004) involved a relatively short follow-up period of 6 months, and the symptoms of eating disorders or serious eating problems were not assessed. Therefore, no conclusions can be drawn about whether this approach "prevents eating disorders." Nevertheless, the preliminary evidence indicates that the program is effective in reducing one major risk factor for girls: internalization of the slender beauty ideal, accompanied by beliefs that help make glorification of slenderness the sociocultural norm (see chapter 5). In addition, the program might be effective for girls in decreasing dieting behavior and skipping meals, both of which have been linked to various eating and health problems, including unhealthy weight gain. These data, as well as the positive effect on body satisfaction for seventh-grade girls and boys, support continued application and evaluation of an ecological model.

The program was not effective for boys as a category, nor were there significant intervention effects on girls for several important variables such as body size acceptance, teasing, and appearance esteem. In discussing obstacles to implementation of their program, McVey, Tweed, and Blackmore (2004) note that parent participation in the information sessions was low (see also Varnado-Sullivan et al., 2001), and that the opportunity to work with teachers was limited compared to the high level among this group of beliefs and attitudes supporting the slender beauty ideal. Both obstacles may represent limited engagement of two key elements within the ecological model. In this respect, McVey et al. (2004) also acknowledge that the research team may have erred in not using a "partnership" approach to set up the program in the intervention schools. We agree that this is a potentially significant oversight, so we turn now to a consideration of ways to build and make use of connections while working in multiple settings.

WORKING WITH MULTIPLE SETTINGS

Although working with multiple settings across various ecological levels is a widely held ideal for prevention programs, achieving a successful collaboration is very difficult. It is even more challenging to form strong collaborative relationships that will continue to function once the principal investigator of the research project or the external funding is gone (Minke, 2000). Permanent environmental transformations must be sufficiently "owned" by the host community so that the community is motivated to maintain the program on their own (Hawkins et al., 2002; Maton, 2000). Here we reiterate a critically important lesson from chapters 10 and 11: The starting point of successful, long-lasting collaborations is a thorough—and collaborative—evaluation of the needs and strengths of the target settings.

Evaluation of Needs and Strengths

Most eating disorders prevention programs are born from the vision of a single expert or from a meeting of experts. These tend to be people who are familiar with the risk factor research and who try to design a program that addresses some of those risk factors. And, typically, these professionals are trying to develop a program that can be used as a curriculum by a variety of schools. Indeed, at workshops or via e-mail, teachers or administrators often ask us for our specific recommendations about such programs.

Yet, these types of programs, like McVey's and ours, have been only moderately successful (see chapter 9). In part, this may be because, with only a few exceptions, the prepackaged curricular programs ignore the actual concerns and orientations of the people (usually educators and their students) who are supposed to use them (Piran, 1995). This "we know what is wrong and we'll tell you how to fix it" approach may lead to resentment, or at best a lack of interest, among those who are being asked to use the program. For example, in preparation for its *BodyWise* campaign the USDHHS's Office on Women's Health (1999) conducted focus groups with educators concerning what they wanted in terms of an eating disorders program. Some focus groups were indeed interested in programs to counteract dieting and the adoption of an unrealistically thin ideal. However, at other locations, the focus groups unequivocally indicated that being too thin was not the problem at their schools. Rather, they were worried about obesity. This was particularly true among groups dominated by educators from inner-city, ethnic minority schools.

In another example, we surveyed teachers in our rural, overwhelmingly European American community as to what eating disorders prevention materials they were most interested in using (Smolak, Harris, et

TABLE 12.1
Frequencies of Teacher Interest in Prevention Formats

Format	Very Likely to Use	Somewhat Likely to Use	Not at All Likely to Use
Video	14 (34%)	14 (34%)	13 (32%)
6–10 Lesson set	6 (15%)	12 (29%)	**23 (56%)**
Pamphlets re: Risk Factors	**28 (70%)**	5 (12.5%)	7 (17.5%)
Pamphlets re: How to Help	**24 (63%)**	9 (24%)	5 (13%)
Video	20 (49%)	11 (27%)	10 (24%)
School resource person	**22 (56%)**	15 (38%)	2 (5%)
Professional books	7 (17%)	18 (43%)	17 (40%)
Guest speaker	17 (42.5%)	17 (42.5%)	6 (15%)
1–3 hr. workshop	6 (15%)	22 (54%)	13 (32%)
Help change school policies	9 (22.5%)	21 (52.5%)	10 (25%)

Note. $N = 41$. Research described in Smolak, Harris, Levine, and Shisslak (2001).

al. 2001). Most of the teachers did not want a curriculum, particularly one that involved several lessons (see Table 12.1). Although we believe, based on a great deal of research (see chapter 9), that several lessons are necessary to change children's attitudes and behaviors, the teachers we surveyed saw the lessons are taking time that they did not have available. The teachers felt as if they were already overburdened with curricular requirements, especially given the recent emphasis on preparing children for proficiency testing. After all, school systems and teachers are being judged on the results of these tests. This concern is likely to intensify with President Bush's Education Act that mandates yearly testing in Grades 3 through 8.

And yet, many of the teachers we interviewed were concerned about disordered eating and related problems (e.g., depression, cigarette smoking, teasing) among their students. Surveys of small samples of teachers in Minneapolis and Toronto have produced similar findings (Neumark-Sztainer, Story, & Harris, 1999; Piran, 2004). Furthermore, the central Ohio teachers we surveyed and talked to in focus groups were unsure how they could help prevent internalization of a thin ideal or unhealthy dieting; they felt that sociocultural pressures are too multifaceted, perhaps even ubiquitous, for them to have much effect. Interestingly, then, these teachers, too, were arguing for a multifaceted, multilevel approach to prevention.

Like teachers, parents often have little spare time for attending meetings at school or evening workshops on child health (Minke, 2000). The few curricular programs that have tried to arrange educational sessions for parents have been plagued by poor attendance (see, e.g., McVey, Davis, et al., 2004; McVey, Tweed, & Blackmore, 2004; Varnado-Sullivan et al., 2001). This does not mean parents are disinterested in their children's health and development. Instead, it means that program designers need to find ways that parents can help, given their work and family demands. For example, as described in chapter 10, Dishion and Kavanagh (2000) developed a Family Resource Room that can be used to address a variety of adolescent problems when and if parents are interested.

These examples show why careful evaluation is needed prior to instituting a multifaceted, ecological prevention program. Program objectives must be applicable to the target audiences. More than this, the objectives must be meaningful to the target audiences (Perry, 1999). The "shareholders" in the program must feel that their experience, expertise, and interests are respected (Hawkins et al., 2002; Minke, 2000; Piran, 1998, 2001; see chapter 10). This means getting input from the various environmental levels included in the programs. Table 12.2

TABLE 12.2
Information-Gathering Methods From the Targeted Groups ("Shareholders")

Method	Advantages	Disadvantages
1. Existing survey data	Savings in time and money Potentially longitudinal data Potentially reliable and valid tools	May not be the targeted group Questions may not be as relevant as possible
2. New survey data	Representative sample Large sample possible Potentially reliable and valid tools	Requires time and money Questions may be limited in scope
3. In-depth interviews	Selected sample Can be open-ended Can be more personal	Usually limited to smaller sample
4. Direct observation	Selected sample Can be unobtrusive Limits reporting bias	Assesses environment and behavior only Perceptions limited
5. Focus groups	Not expensive Open-ended discussion Quick results Community involvement	Difficult to recruit sample Special training needed Difficult to schedule

Note. Reprinted with permission from Perry, C. L. (1999, p. 53). *Creating health behavior change: How to develop community-wide programs for youth.* Thousand Oaks, CA: Sage.

(Perry, 1999, p. 53) outlines several methodological approaches to gathering such information.

There are at least three broad questions that should be addressed in this evaluation. The first is, "What are the problems that exist among the youth in this community?" Specifically, are a substantial number of girls engaging in dangerous dieting? Are the girls exercising in risky ways in order to lose weight? How invested are they in the thin ideal? At a large enough school, such as a comprehensive high school with perhaps 1,500 to 2,000 students, enough girls (e.g., ~5% or 75–100; see chapter 2) may develop full-blown or subthreshold eating disorders to create significant problems (Ransley, 1999). Are the boys using food supplements, or even steroids, to "muscle up"? Is obesity more of a problem than eating disorders? Are the teachers and parents concerned about depression and suicide? If so, it would be easy to include body image concerns in a prevention program for depression and suicide, especially as poor body image contributes to depression among adolescent girls (Stice, Hayward, et al., 2000; Wichstrøm, 1999). Exercise programs may help to alleviate body image problems, obesity, and depression. By combining the methodological approaches listed in Table 12.2, program designers can respond to community concerns while still using empirical data from risk factor research.

The second question to be addressed in the preprogram evaluation is, "What contributes to the development and maintenance of these problems?" It is important to keep in mind that no one system (school, family, etc.), much less one individual, is responsible for the problem. Eating problems are multidetermined. Again, empirical data should be combined with the experiences of community members, including students, teachers, coaches, and parents, in order to create a model of the problems that makes sense in terms of the local contexts, as well as previous research.

The final question is, "How can we use our assessment data and our resources to develop ways of preventing the target problems?" Consideration of this challenge must recognize other demands on the time and resources of community members. Once priorities and constraints have been determined, the strengths of the community, including identification of influential adults and helpful organizations, need to be considered. Sources of funding should be discussed. One of the prevention programs we developed was funded by a state grant, whereas another was funded by a private individual. Private foundations as well as federal agencies have provided funding to some programs. Sometimes a local group, such as the Junior League or the Retired Teachers Association, is interested in sponsoring a program. Consideration of community strengths implicitly fosters a sense of respect and empowerment for "shareholders" in the prevention effort. Such respect and empowerment is crucial for successful collaborations and hence for successful community-based prevention programs (Hawkins et al., 2002; Maton, 2000; Minke, 2000).

Collaboration

Minke (2000) distinguishes between cooperation, coordination, and collaboration. Unlike cooperation and coordination, collaborative efforts actually result in a "fundamental restructuring of *how* individuals or agencies work together" (p. 378). Effective collaboration allows all shareholders to contribute to defining and addressing the problems of children or adolescents. This, then, enables information from other communities to work in the service of local problems rather than simply imposing on a new setting either what has worked somewhere else or what "in theory" should work on communities "in general."

Table 12.3 outlines Minke's (2000, p. 386) CORE model of collaboration. This is one example of models intended to facilitate ecologically based programs (see also, e.g., Dishion & Kavanagh, 2000; Hawkins et al., 2002; Maton, 2000; Perry, 1999; USDHHS, 2001). Three themes recur throughout these models: connection, communication, and empowerment. Connection through relationships was discussed at length in chapter 8, as it is one of the central ingredients of prevention in Piran's version of the FER model.

The second theme is communication. Beginning with the preprogram evaluation and continuing through the institution, evaluation, and revision of the program, it is crucial that all involved parties communicate. Varying perspectives need to be listened to respectfully. Disagreements should be viewed as opportunities for growth via the development of unique solutions, rather than as barriers to formulating a program (Minke, 2000). Prevention professionals need to believe genuinely in the competence of communities (Maton, 2000). This sets the stage for finding ways to develop the community's inherent capacities, while reducing the probability that time, energy, money, and other precious resources will be wasted trying to impose "programs" on a set of "toxic" environments.

TABLE 12.3
The CORE Model of Collaboration

CORE Elements	Associated Beliefs	Activities/Processes	CORE Outcomes
Connected	Others are trustworthy.	Identification of shared goals Independence Effective use of conflict	The development, implementation, and ongoing evaluation of activities and programs that create improved academic, social, and behavioral outcomes for a greater proportion of students.
Optimistic	Problems are system problems. No individual is to blame. Others are doing the best they can.	Sustained effort Commitment to individual action	
Respected	Others have different, but valid, expertise. Differences are accepted and valued. Others have something to teach me.	Inclusion of all stakeholders, including students Creative problem solving Incorporation of external ideas	
Empowered	All participants are partners. Everyone can develop new skills when given the opportunity.	Shared power and decision making Identification and development of shared resources Incorporation of internal ideas	

Note. From Minke (2000). Copyright 2000 by the National Association of School Psychologists, Bethesda, MD. Reprinted with permission of the publisher.

The final central theme is empowerment. Clearly, this is related to the concept of respectful communication. Empowerment is also the feature that most distinguishes collaboration from coordination and cooperation. In keeping with the emphasis on authentic relationships, all of the systems involved in the program must be treated as equals. Prevention experts are a resource in collaborative work, but there is no "Dr. Expert" who brings the true, correct approach to the community. Every participant is capable of—and ready to—learn new things as part of the collaborative effort (Minke, 2000). If community systems feel empowered to solve the problems, they are more likely to be motivated to fight for and continue the program after the "expert" has left (Maton, 2000). This, in turn, suggests that changes made as part of the program are more likely to be maintained over the long term. Such sustained efforts are important if substantial change in child and adolescent behaviors is to occur.

CONCLUSIONS

All of the prevention models, and a great deal of empirical data, indicate that various ecological systems are involved in fostering and maintaining eating problems in children and adolescents. However, most prevention programs focus on changing attitudes and behaviors of individual children and adolescents rather than these social systems. The central thesis of this chapter is that programs that involve multiple settings, attempting to transform the community in which the problems occur, are more likely to be successful than programs that target individual change.

Research on an ecological approach to the prevention of eating problems is very limited. The recent pioneering work of McVey and colleagues in schools in the province of Ontario, Canada, suggests that ecological approaches will likely need to extend their reach beyond the schools and into the community (Flay, 2000; see chapter 10). To that end, we have identified several themes—good nutrition, physical activity, appearance teasing, and development of multiple role models—that can be addressed in multiple settings within the school *and* within the larger community. The list was not intended to be exhaustive. Rather, we hope that these themes serve to open conversations among shareholders in the prevention effort.

The goal of working with multiple settings is to develop a program that is sensitive to the specific problems, needs, and resources of the local community. This does not mean that the extant theoretical and empirical literature concerning body image and eating problems is irrelevant. Rather, meaningful local input is necessary in order to complete an accurate assessment of risk and resilience, and in order to increase the investment of educators, parents, and other community members in the program. When local community members feel that their concerns are being addressed and that they have the power to help reduce eating problems, they are more likely to participate in, adhere to, and sustain the program. True collaboration of this sort makes permanent changes in the environment more likely. This means, for example, that children who enter the community and the schools several years after the prevention project is "completed" might still benefit from the ongoing program(s).

True collaborative programs are rare, and specific methods for facilitating collaborations and multisetting, multilevel approaches are still evolving (Maton, 2000; Minke, 2000). It is imperative, then, that research and evaluation of these and related methods continue (USDHHS, 2001). We turn next to one area of prevention that has some success in using a critical social perspective to link programs in the schools with changes in peer groups and in the community: media literacy.

13

Media Literacy as Prevention

Even though the mechanisms are poorly understood, there is substantial evidence that mass media contribute to the emergence and maintenance of negative body image, calorie-restrictive dieting, and eating disorders (Groesz et al., 2002; Levine & Harrison, 2004; Levine & Smolak, 1996, 1998; Stice, 1994; Thompson & Heinberg, 1999; Thompson et al., 1999). On the face of it, the tasks of changing the mass media or inoculating individuals against the onslaught of multinational corporations with multimillion-dollar advertising budgets strike most people as absurd and hopeless. In contrast, this chapter argues that, beginning around ages 6 to 8, audiences are active consumers who can build on their complex relationships with mass media so as to participate in two types of media literacy. The narrow type involves critical thinking about mass media in order to deepen appreciation of its many positive factors, while sharpening skills for resisting media's negative effects on health and well-being. The broad type of media literacy expands *a*wareness and *a*nalysis of media to connect them to both *a*ctivism in response to media, and *a*ccess to media for the purpose of *a*dvocating healthier messages. After we review the research on the narrow type of media literacy program, we review findings from the broad type. The latter suggest that the 5 As of media literacy (Awareness—Analysis—Activism—Access—Advocacy) are very promising for prevention because they overlap with the effective ingredients of prevention discussed in chapters 7 through 12: consciousness-raising; development of competencies and collaborative relationships; and action to change the ecology, including mass media.

MASS MEDIA AND SOCIAL INFLUENCE

Adolescents and eating disorder experts alike often dismiss the potential influence of mass media. They counter with some version of "OK, unhealthy images are all over the place, but so what? They're just images and fantasies." Because many media literacy programs include didactic and discovery-based information to dispute that proposition, Table 13.1 summarizes the current state of research on the relationship of mass media to body image and eating problems (see Levine & Harrison, 2004; Levine et al., 1999; Levine & Smolak, 1996, 1998; Thompson et al., 1999, for more detailed consideration).

MEDIA ACTIVISM

Some people do indeed "know already" that certain advertising and story-telling practices within corporate America are unhealthy for people. However, their feelings of outrage are swamped by a sense of individual helplessness. One plaintive question almost always follows a presentation about mass media, body image, and eating problems: "I mean, really, what can any of us do—really—against multibillion-dollar businesses?"

In late September of 1988, Dr. Vivian Meehan, cofounder of ANAD (see Appendix A), spearheaded a petitions and letter-writing campaign to protest Hershey Foods Corporation's advertising campaign (for a thin chocolate bar) proclaiming that "You can never be too rich or too thin." The company withdrew the ad on October 17, 1988. Similarly, in the summer of 1996, Dr. Cynthia Whitehead-Laboo of the Emory University Counseling Center and Dr. Michael Levine of Kenyon College mobilized a group of eating disorder professionals to protest a Hormel Meat Company commercial in which a 5-year-old girl refuses a piece of birthday cake because "it will go straight to my hips." The company later suspended this advertising campaign. It is inspiring to learn that an ostensibly monolithic "sociocultural factor" such as mass media can be influenced to a small degree (for now) by organized citizen action (Irving, 1999; Kelly, 2002b; Maine, 2000; Wallack, Dorfman, Jernigan, & Themba, 1993). Dr. Lori Irving was fond of closing her e-mails and her talks with a quotation from Margaret Mead: "Never doubt that a small group

TABLE 13.1
Summary of Findings From Research on Mass Media Effects on Body Image and Eating Problems

Finding	Representative Sources
Females	
In diverse cultures around the world, establishment (incursion?) of a market-driven mass media has been followed by internalization of the slender beauty ideal and resultant increases in body dissatisfaction among girls and women.	Becker (1995); Bilukha & Utermohlen (2002); Joja (2001)
White females ages 8 through 25 notice how pretty models and actresses are, and compare themselves to those standards, often despite seeing the "models" as unrealistic. African American females are more likely to reject this process.	Martin & Kennedy (1993, 1994); Milkie (1999); Then (1992); Botta (2000); Nichter (2000)
Discrepancy between a representation of the slender beauty ideal and one's body image is associated with body dissatisfaction, depression, and bulimic behavior.	Thompson et al. (1999); Thompson & Stice (2001)
Exposure to pictures of slender models or actresses causes a modest immediate increase in negative feelings about the body, an effect that is large for those who have internalized the slender beauty standard and/or already have body dissatisfaction.	Meta-analysis by Groesz, Levine, & Murnen (2002)
Trying to look like females on TV, in movies, or in magazines predicts onset of weight concerns and purging behavior in girls ages 9 through 14.	Field, Camargo, Taylor, Berkey, & Colditz (1999); Field et al. (2001)
Research on correlation between media use and negative body image/eating problems is inconclusive.	Murray, Touyz, & Beumont (1996); Stice, Schupak-Neuberg, Shaw, & Stein (1994); Thomsen et al. (2002) vs. Cusumano & Thompson (1997); Harrison (1997); Harrison & Cantor (1997); Stice (1998a)
Girls who feel subjected to pressure by media, family, and peers are particularly likely to report negative body image and disordered eating.	Levine et al. (1994)
Males	
For boys, variables such as exposure to appearance-related magazines and internalization of the muscular ideal appear to have a weak, inconsistent relationship to body dissatisfaction and weight control techniques.	Jones et al. (2004); Ricciardelli & McCabe (2001b); Smolak, Levine, & Thompson (2001)
Experimental exposure to the muscular ideal has an immediate negative impact on body-build satisfaction in young men.	Grogan, Williams, & Conner (1996); Leit et al. (2002)

of thoughtful committed citizens can change the world. Indeed it's the only thing that ever has" (Irving & Levine, 2000).

Many "thoughtful committed citizens" find purpose and strength in nonprofit organizations (see Appendix A) such as the National Eating Disorders Association (NEDA; formerly Eating Disorders Awareness & Prevention, Inc., or EDAP), About-Face (1996; formerly the Stop Starvation Imagery Campaign), and Dads and Daughters, Inc. During the late 1990s, NEDA wrote successful letters of protest to Jarlsberg Cheese, Avia, and Nicole Shoes. Activism does not consist solely of protest, so NEDA members also wrote letters praising positive images of women to Nike, Kellogg, and Champion Sportswear. Some of these companies have a history of questionable advertising campaigns, but NEDA wanted to acknowledge and reinforce specific advertisements featuring a diversity of weights and shapes, and bodies in motion for effective action, rather than objectified bodies on display. Dads and Daughters, Inc. (see Appendix D), guided by media-savvy director Joe Kelly (2002a, 2002b), has harnessed the World Wide Web to mount many effective protests through its "Take Action" campaign (see http://www.dadsanddaughters.org/actions_and_outcomes.htm). In one of the most successful protests, Swedish appliance manufacturer ASKO dropped an advertisement for energy-saving kitchen appliances. The slogan was "Like most Swedish supermodels, they consume next to nothing."

MEDIA LITERACY

Definitions

Media literacy is a general term for "the process of critically analyzing *and* learning to create one's own messages in print, audio, video, and multimedia" (Hobbs, 1998, p. 16; italics added for emphasis). "Critical viewing skills" are an important component of media literacy as a form of resistance to unhealthy cultural messages about weight and shape. Yet, most experts in media education have a much broader perspective about the meanings of media literacy than do experts in eating disorders prevention (Brown, 2001; Hobbs, 1998). In general, experts in media education/literacy assume: (a) all mass media, including documentary reportage of the "truth as it happens," are constructed representations; (b) the meaning and implications of mass media emerge from a transaction between perceiver, the "text(s)," and the cultural contexts; (c) contexts are defined on many levels, including the historical, the economic, and the political; (d) students are active, decisive, individual "information processors and consumers," rather than totally naive, gullible, and passive victims of an insidious mass media; and (e) media literacy is neither media cynicism nor blanket condemnation of "other people's pleasures."

This set of attitudes, coupled with critical viewing skills, is thought to be crucial for full participation of citizens in a democracy suffused with, if not dominated by, mass media (Center for Media Literacy, n.d.; Hobbs, 1998). Consequently, proponents of media literacy tend to favor the type of interactive, dialogue- and discovery-based learning methods featured in the prevention work of Piran and of O'Dea and Abraham (see chapters 7 and 8; see also Brown, 2001).

Goals and Processes

The essential features of media literacy programs are listed in Table 13.2. In general, the broad type of media literacy program is more likely

TABLE 13.2
Goals of Intensive Media Literacy Programs

- Develop critical thinking skills, including an enhanced ability to "read" and "decode" media messages about gender, appearance, weight, and shape
- Promote healthier body image and eating behaviors by
  —challenging the thinness schema for girls and the idealization of muscularity for boys
  —careful consideration of the benefits and costs of social comparison
  —promoting positive alternatives to restrictive dieting and to use of drugs and food supplements to build muscle and manage weight
- Foster self-confidence and a stronger sense of both personal autonomy and the power available in collaboration with peers; redefine the body as site of effective action, not shame
- Improve communication skills, including media skills, but also oral and written methods for effectively expressing outrage and the desire for change directly to businesses
- Learn advocacy skills, specifically how to "use" the mass media for the social marketing and promotion of healthy messages
- Provide participants with adult role "models" who discuss and demonstrate the availability and the benefits of a diversity of roles and identities for females as a group
- Reinforce the 4 Cs of prevention: Consciousness-raising, Competence, Connection, and Change (personal and social)

Note. Based on information from Levine et al. (1999), Irving and Levine (2000), and Piran et al. (2000).

than the prevention programs reviewed in chapter 9 to engage participants in actions (behaviors) that take them out of the classroom and into various experiences that have the potential to influence peers, their community, and mass media themselves. These activities include education, consciousness raising, activism, advocacy, and social marketing (Irving, 1999; Levine et al., 1999; Levine & Smolak, 2002; Steiner-Adair & Vorenberg, 1999).

RESEARCH ON PREVENTION OF NEGATIVE BODY IMAGE AND EATING PROBLEMS

About 10 years ago calls for media literacy programs began to appear in prevention journals (Jasper, 1993; Shaw & Waller, 1995; see also Berel & Irving, 1998). This movement was fueled in part by the promising results of theory-based media literacy programming in the prevention of positive feelings and expectations about drinking alcohol (Austin & Johnson, 1997). As noted in chapter 9, our canvassing of databases, review articles, and personal contacts with researchers yielded 12 studies that revolve around media literacy, plus a 13th (Wade et al., 2003) that was included in chapter 9's prevention statistics. The principal features and outcomes of these studies, grouped according to intensity of the program, are summarized in Tables 13.3 and 13.4.

BRIEF PROGRAMS

Young Girls

Three doctoral dissertations from the United States evaluated brief media literacy programs for girls ages 9 through 14. Strong (2000) had Southern California girls ages 10 to 14 participate in a 40-minute experiment that demonstrated the negative impact of images of ideal slender beauty (see Groesz et al., 2002). This was followed by a video about eating disorders and by a psychoeducational "lecture" focusing on media effects, the dangers of dieting, and self-acceptance. Although the methodology of this uncontrolled study is confusing, the results suggested that the program had an immediate positive effect on body image, while reducing glorification of thinness and endorsement of anorexic attitudes at the 5-week follow-up.

In a study with sounder methodology, Wolf-Bloom (1998) arranged a 2.25-hour media literacy workshop within a four-part "Sensitive Issues

TABLE 13.3
Brief Media Literacy Programs

Study	N/Gender/Age	Days/Time	Design	DID	APP	ACT	Measures	PPE	FUE	Comments
Wolf-Bloom (1998)	70 girls, 10–15 (M = 12.3)	1/135 min.	QE/RM (2)	Y	Y	N	ChEAT, FRS IBSS, SIQYA	A	BI	Sustained effect on BI
Kusel (1999)	172 girls, M = 10.8	"2-day" program	Solomon-4G (3); RA	Y	?	N	ChEAT, EDI SATAQ, MIP	A	A	Sustained effect on media skepticism & BI distortion
Strong (2000)	83 girls, 10–14	4 sessions 45 min. ea.	RM (1)	Y	N	N	ED Ideation Measure (created for study	N/A	A	At 5-wk FU, reduced both glorification of thinness & endorsement of anorexic attitude
Irving et al. (1998)	41 girls, 15–16	1/50 min.	QE/PP	Y	Y	N	EDI-BD(S) SATAQ, MAQ PASTA(S)	A	N/A	Program reduced SATAQ internalization & MAQ realism
Stormer & Thompson (1995)	112 women, M = 18.5	1/30 min.	QE/PP	Y	N	N	EDI, SATAQ, FRS, PASTA	A	N/A	Only dispositional effect was SATAQ; appearance- and weight-related state anxiety decrease
Stormer & Thompson (1998)	100 men, 144 women, students at a university	1/30 min.	QE/RM (1)	Y	N	N	EDI, SATAQ FRS, PASTA	A	A	Sustained effect on SATAQ internalization for women only
Posavac et al. (2001)	125 women, 18–25 moderate–high levels of BD	1/7 min. video	RA/PP	Y	N	N	BES-WC Free Response	A	N/A	2 control + 3 types of video interventions
Irving & Berel (2001)	110 women, 18–38 (M = 19)	1/45 min.	RA/PP No-treat C External Internal Video only	N Y Y Y	N Y Y N	N N N N	EDI-BD; MAQ PASTA(S) SATAQ	A NO NO A	N/A N/A N/A N/A	Compared video-only to media literacy (Irving et al., 1998) and media analysis + CBT group; no group diff on EDI, SATAQ, intent to diet

Note. All studies were conducted in the United States. QE = Quasiexperimental; PP = Pre–Post or Post-only; RA = random assignment; RM = repeated measures with follow-up; numbers in parentheses are approximate length of follow-up in months; DID = presence of didactic, component; APP = application of critical analysis skills; ACT = activism or advocacy experience; PPE = variables for which there was a program participation effect; FUE = variables for which there was a sustained prevention effect. For a list of variables abbreviated in the measures column, see Appendix E. In the PPE and FUE columns, A = attitudes, B = behavior.

Program" for Girl Scouts in northeast Ohio. Senior Scouts served as peer educators for *Media Magic or Madness?* The girls were shown a portion of *Slim Hopes: Advertising and the Obsession with Slimness* (see www.mediaed.org/videos/MediaGenderCulture/SlimHopes; Kilbourne, 1995; see also Irving, DuPen, & Berel, 1998). The girls also saw an episode of Joan Lunden's *Behind Closed Doors* (original airing, January 27, 1997), which shows a fashion shoot for *Cosmopolitan*, as well as a computer refashioning (to correct the "many flaws") of supermodel Cindy Crawford's image for another fashion layout (Levine et al., 1999). After the video, the girls practiced critical analysis of several forms of media popular with adolescent girls. Finally, there was a discussion of the implications of the typical discrepancy between real girls' bodies and the "perfect" images in magazines and on TV.

Media Magic or Madness? did not affect scores on measures of disordered eating or internalization of the slender beauty ideal. Nevertheless, several other results are intriguing. For example, at posttest there were no immediate positive effects on body image; if anything, intense scrutiny of media images increased the perceived–ideal discrepancy. But at follow-up this trend reversed for program participants, but not for control participants. This positive longer term effect was also seen in another, more general measure of body image. There was also some evidence, based on within-group trends, that the program reduced participants' ratings of the importance of TV images and their tendency to compare themselves to media images.

As her doctoral dissertation Kusel (1999; A. Kusel, personal communication, August 31, 1999) evaluated a media literacy program for New York girls ages 9 to 12. The theoretical foundation for the program was Erica Austin's Message Interpretation Process model (see Irving et al., 1998, in the next paragraph). During the 2-day program, videos and discussion were used to (a) dissect deceptive media techniques; (b) critically evaluate appearance-related messages (e.g., glorification of thinness and the stereotyping of overweight people); and (c) understand *and* challenge media's contributions to negative body image and poor health. Girls in the control group watched videos and then discussed stress management, as well as the pros and cons of celebrity. There were no effects for ChEAT scores, but the program did produce significant pre-to-posttest improvements in media skepticism, body image, self-esteem, and internalization of the slender ideal. Although post-to-follow-up analyses indicated a program participation effect (see chapter

9) for most of these variables, girls who received Kusel's media literacy program continued to question the media and to be aware of body stereotypes, and to have lower body image distortion (A. Kusel, personal communication, August 31, 1999).

High School Students

Irving et al. (1998) evaluated a peer-led, "one-shot" media literacy program for 24 sophomore girls (ages 15–16) in southwestern Washington State. The opening discussion of the media's glorification of slenderness began with a 15-minute segment of *Slim Hopes* (total time = 30 minutes). The segment chosen focused on the tricks (e.g., airbrushing) used to make the fashion models look "perfect." Next, a high school junior (DuPen) helped the girls to "critically evaluate and 'de-construct' media messages" (p. 125). Based on Austin's (1993) Message Interpretation Process (MIP) model, the class addressed the following questions: Do *real* women look like the models in advertising? Will buying the product being advertised make me look like this model? Does this model look like this because of this product? Does thinness really guarantee happiness and success? Finally, the peer leader encouraged her classmates to challenge and change unrealistic standards, in part through developing self-esteem in realms other than physical appearance (see chapter 12).

As was the case for the three programs for younger girls, the pretest–posttest design revealed that Irving et al.'s (1998) brief media literacy program had some limited positive effects. Compared to the control group, participating girls reported less internalization of the slender beauty ideal, and they perceived the media images as less realistic. Interestingly, there were no significant differences in body dissatisfaction, anxiety about weight and shape, the desirability of looking like slender models, or positive expectations associated with being slender.

College Women and Men

It appears that similar "psychoeducational" programs can produce this type of limited but potentially significant change in young women attending college. At the University of South Florida (USA), Stormer and Thompson (1995) assigned young women to one of three conditions: a half-hour media literacy program, a half-hour presentation about health, or no program at all. Using current and historical perspectives, the media literacy presentation considered ways in which society in general and mass media in particular promote unhealthy beauty ideals for women. Next, the young women learned how fashion models and the production staffs of magazines and movies use "cosmetic" surgery, airbrushing, computer graphics, and other technologies to *construct* the idealized *images*. This set up a consideration of the negative effects of the discrepancy between such unreal, "perfect" images and the average American woman. The program ended with a 6-minute presentation of ways to use the information in challenging internalization of the slender beauty ideal. Consistent with the previous studies of younger girls, this very brief lesson in "media literacy" had no significant between-groups effect on dispositional measures of body image or disordered eating. However, it did produce significant pre-to-postprogram reductions in appearance- and weight-related anxiety, and in internalization of the slender beauty ideal embodied by fashion models and actresses.

The next version of this program featured two additional components pertaining to gender (Stormer & Thompson, 1998; S. M. Stormer, personal communication, August 16, 1999; Thompson et al., 1999, pp. 116ff). The first helped women to correct their tendency to overestimate the degree of slenderness that males consider an attractive, ideal body size. The second was a section about males and attractiveness, paralleling the information and guidance for women. This part of the program included information about ideals of male attractiveness as conveyed in magazines such as *GQ* and *Men's Health*, and in movies featuring stars such as Antonio Banderas and Brad Pitt. This segment also emphasized the very unhealthy ways in which some men try to attain the lean, muscular ideal, for example, fanatical workouts at the gym, steroid use, obsessive attention to diet, and cosmetic surgery (see Pope et al., 2000). The principal pre-to-posttest results for both males and females were very similar to the findings of the first study. However, at 3-week follow-up attrition was high, and only the women maintained their improvement toward less internalization of the slender beauty ideal (S. M. Stormer, personal communications, August 13 & August 16, 1999).

The research reviewed thus far strongly supports the proposition that brief but very practical media-focused psychoeducational interventions produce significant improvements in state measures of appearance anxiety and media skepticism—and, for women, sustained improvement in the tendency to internalize several forms of the culture's glorification of slenderness. Yet, even a 30-minute program contains many potentially influential elements, making it impossible to know which components are most promising for further developments. One potentially important component of media literacy can be derived from a study conducted at the University of Utah (USA) by Posavac, Posavac, and Weigel (2001). These investigators presented college women who already had a negative body image with one of several versions of a "psychoeducational" intervention involving media analysis. This intervention was very brief: only 7 minutes. As predicted, after each of the interventions these at-risk women were less likely to engage in social comparison and less likely to experience body image disturbances following experimental exposure to images of slender beauty than were students who saw the same images without the prior intervention (see also Posavac, Posavac, & Posavac, 1998). The most effective "inoculation" emphasized the clash between the artificial, constructed nature of the slender, flawless, "model look" versus biogenetic realities pertaining to both the diversity of women's actual weights and shapes and to the negative effects of calorie-restrictive dieting (see Table 13.2; see also Table 10.4). This finding is consistent with the results of the brief media literacy interventions for younger audiences, and with the prevention theory and research reviewed in chapters 9 and 10.

Irving and Berel (2001) conducted a comparative evaluation of three models of media literacy as prevention. The participants were young women attending Washington State University (USA). The first intervention was the 45-minute media analysis program developed for high school students (Irving et al., 1998). The other interventions being evaluated drew on cognitive-behavioral principles (see chapter 6) to help women challenge the negative body-related cognitions activated by mass media. Women in these two conditions viewed the 15-minute segment of *Slim Hopes* described earlier and then discussed its themes and the personal impact of media messages. In the media analysis condition ("externally oriented"), the structured discussion focused on the veracity and morality of media messages (Austin & Johnson, 1997), and tactics for resisting the unhealthy sociocultural messages (Irving, 1999). The cognitive-behavioral condition ("internally oriented") provided psychoeducation to identify and correct cognitive errors activated by mass media and other sources. There were two control conditions. Women assigned to the video-only control condition saw *Slim Hopes*, followed by just an informal discussion, whereas women in the other control condition did not receive any intervention.

Irving and Berel's (2001) study yielded two important findings. First, across all these brief interventions, there were no significant group differences in EDI body dissatisfaction, SATAQ-internalization, and intention to diet. Second, the video-only "control" was, on the whole, the most effective in producing media skepticism and in stimulating a simple form of media activism. These findings are preliminary and thus in need of replication. Nevertheless, these results are pretty consistent with those of the other studies. It appears that a brief media literacy intervention, such as viewing *Slim Hopes*, can affect the logical processes involved in perceived realism of the images and in the perceived similarity between the audience and the models of beauty. For college students at least, this effect may not require further discussion. The reduction in perceived realism and perceived similarity, in turn, may temporarily improve body satisfaction while reducing internalization of the slender beauty ideal, but these outcomes are neither consistent nor robust, particularly for older audiences. Not surprisingly, one-shot programs are usually inadequate to affect deeper, more emotional processing and long-standing attitudes. Irving and Berel's (2001) study also raises the troubling possibility that the structured guidance provided in the two formal cognitive-behavioral interventions somehow stifled the desire to take personal initiative toward a simple form of media activism such as mailing in postcards developed by the activism/advocacy organization About-Face (see Appendix D). Both of these criticisms are quite consistent with the propositions underlying the FER (see chapter 8) and Stice's cognitive dissonance approach to selective-targeted prevention (see chapter 9).

LONGER, MORE INTENSIVE PROGRAMS

Young Girls

The most sophisticated media literacy study to date was conducted by Neumark-Sztainer and colleagues (2000). They randomly assigned half of 24 Minnesota Girl Scout troops (M_{age} = 10.6) to a control condition, while the remainder received the program *Free to be Me*. The themes of the six 90-minute lessons were similar to those that Kusel (1999) derived from Austin's MIP model. However, *Free to be Me* is a more ecological (and perhaps more relational-empowerment) program than Neumark-Sztainer et al.'s (1995) earlier prevention work (see chapter 6) because it

TABLE 13.4
Intensive Media Literacy Programs

Study	N/Gender/Age	Days/Time	Design	DID	APP	ACT	Measures	PPE	FUE	Comments
Neumark-Sztainer et al. (2000)	70 girls, 10–15 (M = 12.3)	6 days 90 min. ea.	RA/RM (3)	Y	Y	Y	Adaptat. of SATAQ, BSS	K, A	A	Sustained effect on SATAQ-I and on empowerment efficacy
Levine et al. (1999)	50 girls, 14–18 GO GIRLS! program	3 mos. 50 min. ea.	QE/PP	Y	Y	Y	WCS, SATAQ PASTAS, OBCS, PWBI, Empowerment	NO	N/A	2 more engaged GG groups only ones to show reduced internalization of slender ideal and reduced weight/shape concerns
Piran et al. (2000)	162 girls, 13–18 GO GIRLS! program	3 mos. 50 min. ea.	QE/PP	Y	Y	Y	WCS, SATAQ PWBI, and Empowerment	A	N/A	GG reduced internalization of slender ideal, reduced drive for thinness, greater sense of self-acceptance and empowerment
Wade et al. (2003)	53 boys, 33 girls (M = 13.4)	5 "class sessions"	RA/RM (3) Control EveryBody GO GIRLS	Y Y	N Y	N N	EDE-Q, drive-muscularity, Harter SPPA	NO A/B	NO A?	No significant effects for eating attitudes and dieting; GG had less weight concern at posttest and more perceived social competence at FU
Rabak-Wagener et al. (1998)	31 men, 75 women, students at a university	4 days 95 min. ea.	QE/PP	Y	Y	N	11-item survey created for this study	A	A	Significant postprogram effects on media skepticism, slender ideal, and body image—for women only

Note. All studies were conducted in the United States. QE = Quasiexperimental; PP = Pre–Post or Post-only; RA = random assignment; RM = repeated measures with follow-up; numbers in parentheses are approximate length of follow-up in months; DID = presence of didactic component; APP = application of critical analysis skills; ACT = activism or advocacy experience; PPE = variables for which there was a program participation effect; FUE = variables for which there was a sustained prevention effect. In the PPE and FUE columns, K = knowledge, A = attitudes, and B = behavior. For a list of variables abbreviated in the measures column, see Appendix E.

applies Bandura's concept of reciprocal determinism in three ways (see Neumark-Sztainer, 1996). First, the program was administered primarily by the Girl Scout troop leaders, who received a leader's handbook, all necessary materials, and 3 hours of training. Second, the girls were encouraged to be activists in helping peers and mass media to generate healthier norms. For example, the girls critically evaluated advertisements and then wrote letters to businesses to point out problems with advertisements and to advocate for healthier images. These letters were then posted on the NEDA Web site (see Appendix A) to promote awareness, activism, and advocacy by other girls. Finally, parents were involved through newsletters explaining the program and through take-home activities for the girls.

Free to be Me had several positive effects that were sustained at 3-month follow-up (Neumark-Sztainer et al., 2000). Participants were less likely to read *Seventeen* magazine, which promotes the slender beauty ideal and a feminine identity based primarily on appearance and fashion (Peirce, 1990). In addition, internalization of the slender ideal was reduced, while the girls' belief in their ability to be activists and thus affect weight-related social norms was increased. There was a clear program participation effect for the modest pre-to-posttest improvements in body-related knowledge and body size acceptance, although there was no effect on dieting. This study indicates that media literacy holds a great deal of promise as one component of an ecological approach to prevention.

High School Girls

Similar results emerged from two applications of NEDA's media literacy curriculum called *GO GIRLS!*™ (Levine et al., 1999; Piran, Levine, Irving, & EDAP/NEDA Staff, 2000). *GO GIRLS!*™ (further abbreviated *GG*) is an acronym for *G*iving *O*ur *G*irls *I*nspiration and *R*esources for *L*asting *S*elf-esteem. This program was developed in 1998 by the nonprofit organization Eating Disorders Awareness & Prevention, Inc. (EDAP; now NEDA: see Appendix A). The 12 weekly lessons are contained in the commercially available *GG Curriculum Guide* (EDAP, 1998; see Levine et al., 1999, for a description of the steps in the development of the program).

GG was designed to be an organized but flexible set of media-related activities that help adolescent girls understand—through experience, observational learning, *and* action—that they have a "voice" as consumers and citizens, and that together they can use that voice and their skills to effect social, corporate, and personal changes (Irving, 1999; Levine et al., 1999; Piran, 1999b, 2001). In other words, *GG* applies elements of Piran's Critical Social Perspectives model (see chapter 8) to engage girls in the cycle of activities previously referred to as the 5 As of media literacy: Awareness, Analysis, Activism, Advocacy, and Access.

The pilot application of *GG* was conducted in 1997 by Ms. Charlie Stoddard. She was assisted by Ms. Nancy Lee, MBA, a marketing expert with extensive experience in health promotion (see Kotler, Roberto, & Lee, 2002). Students in business-marketing classes at four different Seattle (USA) area high schools voluntarily participated in the program, while students in two other high schools served as the no-program comparison group. The program began with didactic presentations, but by the third lesson the students were gathering and analyzing advertisements, conducting survey research about media and other determinants of body image at their school, and discussing previous types of activism and advocacy. According to the girls, a key experience was learning about the tactics used by the fashion industry and the mass media to generate various forms of "perfect beauty," including thinness. The girls saw and discussed the *Behind Closed Doors* video, and students at two schools also discussed Cosy Sheridan's (1996) song "The Losing Game," which offers a lyrical and critical perspective on media, the drive for thinness, dieting, and self-disparagement.

About halfway through the program, Lee made a presentation about social marketing. Stoddard then used this as a platform to help students create their own advocacy projects. For example, one student led her *GG* group in mounting a campaign to persuade the Bon Marche department store to provide mannequins of varying sizes and shapes. Ultimately, this effort was unsuccessful in changing the mannequins, but the girls' work did capture the attention of the Seattle newspaper, several Seattle TV news programs, and, eventually, Channel One (which is seen each school day by more than 1 million high school students). Even if the outcome of an advocacy campaign is unsuccessful, activism and advocacy can promote a critical social perspective that may well contribute to ecological, small-group, and individual changes.

Stoddard and Lee's implementation of the first *GG* program demonstrated its potential for empowering adolescent girls to *learn-through-action* about conducting research, analyzing and producing media, and confronting businesses and advertisers. The results of the quantitative surveys were also encouraging, especially given the large within-group variances and the relatively small sample sizes (Levine et al., 1999). *GG* participants reported a small mean increase in self-acceptance and a small decrease in weight and shape concerns, whereas girls in the control group changed in the opposite direction to a modest degree (between-group ps < .10, one-tailed; see chapter 11). Furthermore, the two *GG* classes who were obviously more committed to, and engaged in, the cycle of 5 As displayed the most positive changes on 7 of the 10 dependent variables. Unlike the other two classes and the two control classes, the deeply engaged girls were the only ones to show (nonsignificant) reductions in two known risk factors for eating problems: internalization of the thin standard of beauty, and weight and shape concerns (Stice, 2001b).

In the second pilot application (Piran et al., 2000), the data from 72 participants in eight *GG* groups (most of whom were juniors or seniors) in five states were compared to a convenience sample of 90 girls from the same schools. Following an average program length of around 3 months, *GG* participants had, as predicted, a statistically significant reduction in the internalization of the slender beauty ideal and in drive for thinness, and a greater sense of self-acceptance and empowerment as citizens. The girls' personal statements and their activism projects indicate that the *GG* media literacy program helped them to critically evaluate sociocultural determinants of body image, to learn life skills, and to feel empowered as citizens capable of challenging unhealthy cultural factors. One girl wrote, "A group of girls like this is great because it gives us a chance to unite and have somewhat of an impact on things that we believe should be different." Despite these positive effects, and consistent with previous research on narrow and broad versions of media literacy, there were no between-group differences in weight concerns or dieting behavior.

Broad version media literacy programs such as *Free to be Me* and *GO GIRLS!*™ need to be improved in order to achieve the desired attitudinal and behavioral outcomes. For as yet undetermined reasons, this type of program has not been successful in motivating participants to give up or refrain from dieting based on some combination of the following: concerns about dieting's immediate negative effects (see chapter 2); a belief in one's susceptibility to eating disorders (see chapter 5); or political commitment to a vision of femininity that is not defined by restriction and restraint (Wolf, 1991).

Two lines of work indicate that improvement of the more intensive media literacy approach should be a priority for prevention of eating problems. One is the literacy-based drug prevention research of Goldberg and Elliot at the Oregon Health Sciences University in Portland (USA). This is discussed later in the chapter. The other development is ongoing in Red Wing, Minnesota, where veteran eating disorders expert and activist Sarah Stinson has led several *GG* groups. The second group began by applying the commercially available *GG* curriculum, which resulted in numerous presentations to increase media literacy in schools and communities throughout Wisconsin and Minnesota. However, at the end of the standard 3 months the cohesiveness and energy in the group was so strong that the girls and Stinson decided to continue the group. With Stinson as a facilitator, mentor, and advocate like Piran (see chapter 8), the Red Wing *GG* group has proceeded to, among other things, (a) present at professional conferences; (b) appear on TV programs; (c) incorporate as a nonprofit organization called *Higherself* (www.redwinghigherself.com); and (d) testify before Congress in Washington, DC, as part of advocacy efforts to promote the Eating Disorders Awareness, Education, and Prevention Act of 2003 (H.R. 873) and the Senator Paul Wellstone Mental Health Equitable Treatment Act (S. 486; see www.eatingdisorderscoalition.org/legupdate). In Piran's words (personal communication, June 10, 2003), the Red Wing *GG* "has certainly made itself a site of embodied agency." Further research is needed to determine if this type of *GG* group can evolve without the influence of a special professional like Stinson or Piran, and can prevent eating problems by improving body esteem, reducing internalization of the slender beauty ideal, and so forth.

A final piece of evidence supporting the viability of media literacy for adolescent girls comes from a recent study of Australian girls and boys ages 13 to 14. As noted in chapter 9, Wade et al. (2003) compared the effects of a typical personal development class to abridged and modified versions of *Everybody's Different* (O'Dea & Abraham, 2000; see chapter 7) and of the *GG* media literacy program. The commercially available *GG* program was modified to make it less didactic. The results were complex but provocative. Once again, there were no significant between-group effects for dieting, and only one such effect for the measures of attitudes toward weight, shape, and eating. At posttest (but not at follow-up: a program participation effect), boys as well as girls in the media literacy program appreciated the lessons more and reported less emotional investment in and dissatisfaction with body weight. In addition, at follow-up the media literacy group reported more competence in the area of close friendships. Thus, although eating problems were not assessed in the Wade et al. (2003) study and none of the interventions had an effect on dietary restraint, the abridged version of the *GG* program did have a promising short-term effect on two significant factors related to eating problems: competence and confidence in close friendships (Paxton, 1999) and concern about weight (Stice, 2001b).

College Women and Men

Rabak-Wagener, Eickoff-Shemek, and Kelly-Vance (1998) evaluated a "media analysis" program designed to "shift the focus of body image dysphoria from a personal failing to media exploitation" (p. 30). The intervention, carried out as part of a course at Northern Illinois University (USA), consisted of four 95-minute sessions delivered to women and men by Rabak-Wagener and the regularly scheduled instructor. The program was similar to the one devised by Irving et al. (1998). For example, participants watched and discussed *Slim Hopes*, and then critiqued advertisements from male as well as female fashion magazines. A major difference was that Rabak-Wagener et al.'s (1998) program provided an extensive assignment (lasting over 3.5 hours) to foster a critical social perspective. Small groups of students created, and actually presented to the class, several forms of advertising that challenged the stereotypical content of ads by satirizing the fashion industry's fascination with thinness, image, outrageousness, etc. Another difference was that students analyzed media by applying concepts from the study of semiotics (J. Rabak-Wagener, personal communication, February 23, 2000). At posttest the women participating in this program reported (on unstandardized instruments) significant improvements in media skepticism, rejection of the slender beauty ideal, and behaviors reflecting a positive body image. Parallel to the findings of Stormer and Thompson (1995, 1998) with a brief form of psychoeducation, men receiving Rabak-Wagener's more intensive program were no different at pretest or posttest than men in the comparison classes.

MEDIA LITERACY AND PREVENTION OF STEROID USE IN MALE AND FEMALE HIGH SCHOOL ATHLETES

The process of internalizing an unhealthy and gendered ideal ("image") of "attractiveness" and then doing potentially unhealthy, even deadly things to achieve that ideal clearly applies to some forms of the abuse of anabolic steroids and muscle-building food supplements by young males (Goldberg & Elliot, 2000; Pope et al., 2000; Smolak, Levine, & Thompson, 2001; see chapter 3). In fact, Smolak has long argued that this sort of use and abuse is probably a better male parallel to AN or BN in females than are the eating disorders in males.

The ATLAS Prevention Program

The sociocultural influences underlying use and abuse of anabolic steroids and food supplements are salient in the lives of young male athletes, particularly football players. As a result, Goldberg et al. (1996, 2000) developed the *Adolescents Training and Learning to Avoid Steroids* (ATLAS) program for male high school athletes (see also Goldberg & Elliot, 1999, 2000; MacKinnon et al., 2001; www.atlas.program.com). ATLAS is not exclusively a "media literacy program," but we describe this intervention in detail because it is an excellent example of how media literacy can become part of high quality, programmatic research with clear implications for prevention of negative body image and disordered eating (Goldberg & Elliot, 2000).

Participants in the ATLAS studies were three successive cohorts (1994–1996) of high school football players, a majority of whom were ages 14 to 16. Thirty-one schools in Portland, Oregon (USA), were matched and then randomly assigned to participate in ATLAS or a no-treatment control providing written information about the dangers of AS and the benefits of good sports nutrition. In the first cohort, ATLAS consisted of seven classroom and seven weight-room sessions; for cohorts 2 and 3 this was condensed to five classroom and three weight-room sessions.

ATLAS is rooted in the social cognitive model (chapter 6) and in several prominent theories about health promotion, such as Janz and Becker's (1984) Health Belief Model. The program intentionally incorporates at least six elements shown to be effective in prevention and health promotion (see chapters 9, 10, and 12): (a) lessons are very engaging; (b) the material adopts a critical social perspective; (c) lessons are integrated with team practice sessions; (d) classroom sessions about strength and nutrition are combined with experiences that develop behavioral competence (e.g., strength training); (e) peer facilitation of small groups whose members are already connected; and (f) participation by and training of—and overall support from—coaches, parents, and school cafeteria staff (Goldberg et al., 2000). Some players were selected by their coaches to be peer leaders. After receiving 3 to 4 hours of intensive training, these boys ("squad leaders") went on to teach about 60% of the classroom material (Goldberg & Elliot, 2000). The other classroom activities are directed by coaches who have been trained to use ATLAS program materials.

American high school football players are immersed in a culture of stereotypical "manliness"; they are encouraged to be fierce, competitive, combative, and willing to do whatever it takes in the short run and in the long run to win. In contrast, the ATLAS program encourages the boys to learn, and practice, critical thinking about culture and its impact on their body image, eating, and exercising. In addition to education about physiology and nutrition, the ATLAS program emphasizes hands-on learning of safe, effective techniques for developing strength, and of skills to resist social pressures to use anabolic steroids and food supplements. *Media literacy* training is an important part of the ATLAS package. The boys are helped to locate and analyze, not only advertisements and articles about anabolic steroids and food supplements, but also advertisements for products that are designed to treat the unspecified adverse effects (e.g., hair loss, breast enlargement, and acne) of the very steroids and steroid-like products advertised in the same muscle-building magazines. In addition, the boys work together to create, through various types of simulated media (e.g., video, posters, theatrical performances), messages that promote strength and fitness in healthier ways.

Although only 69% of the athletes were available for the 1-year follow-up, this was a sample of nearly 1,300 boys. Results indicate unequivocally that the ATLAS program had a sustained preventive effect. At 1-year follow-up, program participants knew more about exercise, anabolic steroids, and the effects of alcohol and marijuana. They were also more likely to be skeptical about the value of anabolic steroids for bulking up and about the "positive" images of supplements and steroids found in magazines. Not only did they see their coaches as less tolerant of use, program participants also reported a lower intent to use. Perhaps most important, compared to the control participants, at follow-up the ATLAS participants reported less initiation of use of the following: anabolic steroids, "athletic" supplements and other performance-enhancing drugs, and alcohol and other drugs (Goldberg et al., 2000; L. Goldberg, personal communication, August 14, 2002). Mediational analyses via multiple regression demonstrated that skepticism about media advertisements was one of the paths through which the program influenced reduced intentions to use anabolic steroids, as well as increased self-efficacy in strength training (MacKinnon et al., 2001).

The ATHENA Prevention Program

Elliot and Goldberg have also been developing a parallel prevention program for female high school sports teams, including the rally and dance teams (Elliot et al., 2002, 2004). ATHENA is an acronym for *Athletes Targeting Healthy Exercise and Nutrition Alternatives*. ATHENA is designed to prevent eating problems and unhealthy weight and shape management practices, including use of various drugs such as diet pills, nicotine, cocaine, muscle-building food supplements, and anabolic steroids. Its eight 45-minute classroom sessions and three 30-minute weight room sessions follow the structure of the ATLAS program: The material is gender-specific, the interactive activities are peer-led with some oversight from coaches, and the sessions are integrated with team practices during the season. Two other potentially relevant features are (a) neither eating disorders nor calorie-counting are explicit curricular components (though these topics do arise during discussions and sometimes are the focus of public service announcements); and (b) a cognitive-behavioral intervention for prevention of depression was included.

The first full pre-to-postseason evaluation of ATHENA has just been completed (Elliot et al., in press). Eighteen high schools from Oregon and Washington State (40 teams, N at baseline = 928) volunteered to participate. The schools were matched on a number of variables, and then nine were randomly assigned to participate in ATHENA, while nine served as no-intervention controls. Program fidelity was high, as teams covered an average of 81% of the assigned content per session.

At posttest ATHENA was relatively more effective than the comparison condition in reducing *intentions* to do the following: lose weight; use tobacco and the "muscle-boosting" food supplement creatine; and use self-induced vomiting and drugs for weight control. Girls who participated in ATHENA also reported less use of diet pills in the past 3 months. Most important, at posttest there was a prevention effect. Compared to girls in the control condition, among girls in the ATHENA groups there was significantly less *new use* of diet pills, amphetamines, and muscle-building supplements. With regard to potential mediators, as predicted, the ATHENA program was relatively more successful in increasing four potentially significant mediators: media literacy, drug resistance skills, self-efficacy in controlling mood, and the perception that few peers endorse and use body-shaping drugs. However, there was no between-group difference in body image or in perception of their coaches' attitudes. Nevertheless, it appears from a very preliminary analysis of the 2-year-follow-up data (while the girls were still in high school) that the ATHENA program resulted in a sustained prevention effect for use of diet pills, purging (self-induced vomiting, laxatives, and diuretics), anabolic steroids, and tobacco (D. L. Elliot, personal communication, July 21, 2004). The ATLAS and ATHENA programs lie somewhere between selective and targeted on the continuum of prevention. Their integration of media literacy with a number of the well-established practices in the design and evaluation of drug prevention programs is a very exciting development with broad implications for construction of more universal programs for youth ages 14 to 18.

HEALTH CAMPAIGNS, SOCIAL MARKETING, AND MEDIA ADVOCACY

Definitions

According to Merriam-Webster's online dictionary (www.m-w.com), a campaign is "a connected series of operations designed to bring about a particular result." Campaigns using mass media to bring about important social changes have a long and rich history in the United States. Mass media have been an integral part of efforts to reform slavery, lack of women's suffrage, child labor, and epidemic cigarette smoking (Brown & Walsh-Childers, 2002; Rice & Atkin, 2001, 2002). Media campaigns are very relevant for addressing eating problems and eating disorders as public health issues, because such campaigns educate, advise, advocate, and reinforce change. Good media campaigns are designed to influence large groups of people (populations), government (public policy), and other sources of focused influence, including what the media are covering (public agenda). Moreover, theory and practice in media campaigns have long acknowledged the importance of integrating media input with other modes of communication (e.g., teacher to student; parent to child; pediatrician to patient), and careful attention to the evaluation of processes and outcomes (Rice & Atkin, 2002). Recall from chapter 10 that several researchers (Flynn et al., 1994; Pentz et al., 1989) improved the effectiveness of classroom drug prevention materials by coordinating school programming with a mass media campaign (see also Perry, 1999).

Media Interventions and Campaigns

There is a long history of media interventions to reduce the initiation and continuation of substance use by youth (Derzon & Lipsey, 2002). As we consider the potential impact of media campaigns for prevention of eating problems, keep in mind that this work once again raises controversial issues surrounding the impact of mass media. For example, one skeptic, Mendelson (1968, quoted in Derzon & Lipsey, 2002, p. 232) suggests we think of "mass communication as a sort of an aerosol spray. As you spray it on the surface, some of it hits the target; most of it drifts away; and very little of it penetrates."

Even acknowledging the many challenges of conducting an effective health campaign (Rice & Atkin, 2001), this simile may be too pessimistic. To illustrate, Reger, Wootan, and Booth-Butterfield (1999) found that the "1% or Less" media campaign was successful in motivating a sustained increase in consumption of low-fat milk, as compared to baseline and to a very similar comparison community. This campaign was a media-only approach using paid advertisements and public relations events. The total cost, not including campaign development, was $43,000 for implementation and evaluation. The potential audience for TV exposure was 420,000, so the estimated cost of this successful campaign was 10 cents per person.

Derzon and Lipsey (2002) conducted a meta-analysis of 110 reports (N of studies = 72) on the effectiveness of mass communication for changing knowledge, attitudes, and behavior pertaining to substance use. With some exceptions, the effects were small but not trivial: Exposure to media messages was associated with smaller increases in use, and with improvements in attitudes and knowledge. Across these three traditional measures, better outcomes were consistently associated only with use of video as a medium and with *message content that pro-*

motes positive attitudes to nonuse. In contrast to the lessons extracted from curricular prevention programs, media messages (alone) focusing on social norms, resistance skills, or negative attitudes to substance use were *not* associated with improvement in behavior or attitudes (see chapter 10). A sequence or series of messages was much more effective than a single message, although the latter was effective.

Media Advocacy

Wallack and Dorfman (2001) define *media advocacy* as "strategic use of mass media in combination with community organizing to advance healthy public policies" (p. 393). All the models and much of the research reviewed throughout this book point to a single stark fact introduced in chapter 1: Although negative body image and the spectrum of disordered eating are painful and debilitating in intensely *personal* ways, these problems are deeply embedded in multiple strands of our fundamental *social* and *cultural* fabric. And, of course, so are mass media. If you wanted to change how our society felt about body image, would you rather have access to the curriculum of every ninth grade health class in the United States, or three episodes of the TV program *Friends*?

On February 11, 2002, an episode of the TV program *Boston Public* skillfully wove the following issue into its ongoing stories about teachers, students, and administrators at a high school: What are the motives for creating "pro-anorexia" Web sites, and what are the resultant dangers for vulnerable people visiting these sites? At the conclusion of the episode, a screen came on with the National Eating Disorders Association's logo, 800 number, and Web address. The voiceover said, "For more information about eating disorders, contact the National Eating Disorders Association." During the week of that episode, the organization's Web site received nearly 275,000 hits (each click of the mouse is a "hit"), and by the end of that month the site had received slightly over 880,000 hits (Hoff, 2002a). That monthly total was close to half the total number of hits that the NEDA Web site received throughout all of 2001.

As emphasized in chapters 4, 10, and 12, a truly ecological perspective means that people and organizations committed to advocacy for prevention need to do much more than insure that children and adolescents have adequate critical viewing skills. We need to learn more about media *advocacy* as part of an organized campaign. Wallack et al. (1993)

described a series of steps in media advocacy that could, theoretically, enable organizations to develop the tactics to "communicate their own story in their own words... and to use media to better pressure decision makers to change policy" (p. xi). Briefly, the steps are (a) identifying stakeholders with the power to create important changes; (b) developing messages necessary to influence these stakeholders; and (c) gaining access to news media and other prominent forms of media in order to frame the discourse—the problems and their prevention—in terms of public health and political power. As public policies emerge, the last step is working with mass media to promote those policies and reinforce public awareness and political pressure. Recent developments in preventing, for example, HIV infection, cigarette smoking by children and adolescents, and drunken driving, all indicate that media advocacy in the arena of public health is complicated, but capable of making a small but significant difference (see chapters by Snyder, by Dearing, and by Winsten & DeJong, in Rice & Atkin, 2001). One challenge for prevention-oriented organizations in the new millennium is learning how to collaborate with and "use" mass media to (a) promote a sociocultural perspective instead of the "individual illness" model of eating disorders; (b) insist on responsibility in advertising and business; and (c) "market" a variety of messages that advocate and represent respect for girls and women (Levine & Smolak, 2002; see also chapters 8 and 12).

But the work has begun. The National Eating Disorders Association (NEDA) collaborated with advertising giant Ogilvy and Mather to develop the "Listen to Your Body" campaign (Hoff, 2002b; click on the *Listen to Your Body* print campaign link at http://www.nationaleatingdisorders.org for more information, including the ads themselves). The target audience for this anti-dieting campaign is girls ages 12 to 17, so one ad features actor Jamie Lynn (Sigler) Discala of the TV program *The Sopranos* and two other ads feature Melissa Joan Hart of *Sabrina the Teenage Witch*. Both of these ads were used on NEDA's Eating Disorders Awareness Week posters and ran in various magazines, including *Cosmopolitan, Fitness, In Style, Nickelodeon, People, Scholastic Science World,* and *YM*. The penetration and effect of these ads are as yet undetermined, but it seems likely they are partly responsible for the enormous upsurge in visits to the NEDA Web site and calls to their 800-number hotline. In 2002 the number of hits on the Web site topped 55 million, while the number of calls to the Helpline approached 25,000.

Social Marketing and Health Promotion "Campaigns"

Despite the fact that individual people tend to deny their own susceptibility to advertising, everyone knows that "marketing campaigns" for new products can be fabulously successful in changing the attitudes and behavior of millions of people. Unfortunately, a compelling example of the power of marketing is the late 1960s campaign waged by Philip Morris (Pierce, Lee, & Gilpin, 1994) to create a desire in "modern women" (referred to as "baby") to smoke a then new cigarette called "Virginia *Slims*" (italics added to emphasize Jean Kilbourne's perceptive observation that the new product for women was not called "Virginia *Fats*" or "*Wides*," as in "Camel Wides" cigarettes for men). Could the same tools be brought to bear on the marketing of socially desirable changes in attitudes and behaviors toward, for example, body image and eating? This question is the crux of the field called Social Marketing (Coreil, Bryant, Henderson, Fortholer, & Quinn, 2001; Goldberg, Fishbein, & Middlestadt, 1997; Kotler et al., 2002).

Social marketing is neither mass communication nor propaganda. Kotler et al. (2002) define it as "the use of marketing principles and techniques to influence a target audience to voluntarily accept, reject, modify, or abandon a *behavior* for the benefit of individuals, groups, or society as a whole" (p. 5; italics added). The "five Ps" involved in meeting behavioral goals are Product, Price, Promotion, Place, and Positioning. The rough outlines of a social marketing program for reducing the objectification of girls' bodies by middle school boys is shown in Table 13.5 (see Smolak & Murnen, 2001, 2004; see also chapter 8). Social marketing is typically used in conjunction with other forms of social influence. Fishbein et al. (1997) describe in detail how five different metropolitan areas worked with academic researchers and the Centers for Disease Control to use social marketing to prevent AIDS in high-risk individuals.

CYBER-PREVENTION

The World Wide Web currently serves as a source of health-related information for many citizens, as well as a potent means of exchanging treatment and prevention information among professionals in many countries (Rice & Katz, 2001). As of August 2004, there are many informative Web sites for general information, prevention, media literacy, and me-

TABLE 13.5
**Hypothetical Example of the "5 Ps" of Social Marketing:
Reducing Objectification of Girls' Bodies by Middle School Boys**

Feature	Definition	Example
Product	The desired behavior and its benefits	Boys will stop teasing, public comments, and unwanted touching in regard to girls' bodies. Benefits: improvements in body satisfaction and confidence in girls; possible reductions in harassment of boys by boys.
Price	Monetary and nonmonetary (e.g., time, effort) costs to the target audience	Some boys will lose status, as well as a sense of power and superiority. There will be discomfort in challenging traditional gender role socialization practices.
Positioning/ Competition	Other services, products, or behaviors that compete with the "product"	Objectification is facilitated by many sources, notably older boys and men, and various forms of mass media, including video games, men's magazines, and movies.
Promotion	Messages, media, and other activities (e.g., policy changes) necessary to effect behavior change	Determining—via formative research with boys, girls, teachers, administrators, and experts on body image and gender—what types of messages are likely to be effective. Determining what policy changes (e.g., disciplinary) will support the campaign.
Place	Overlaps with promotion; the physical locations and formats for promotion	Determining—via formative research—how and where boys are most likely to be receptive to the "messages" (possibly in several languages) that are a fundamental part of the campaign. Possibilities include radio spots, posters, malls, dance clubs, and Web sites frequently visited by boys 11 through 14.

Note. Sources are Kotler et al. (2002; see, e.g., pp. 260–263) and Coreil et al. (2001, p. 217).

dia activism and advocacy in regard to body image and disordered eating (see Appendixes A through D). There are also many useful Web sites pertaining to the intersection between media literacy and child and adolescent development (Trotta, 2001). These resources are listed in Appendixes B through D. Thinking about these media resources and the "accessibility" and "reach" of the World Wide Web in general should always be tempered by the awareness that there are currently hundreds of *pro*anorexic Web sites.

The Web is already an increasingly important resource for engaging students in the analysis of media. It is likely that, very soon, media activism and advocacy will include the students' creation of their own sites for preventive education. The Web also offers various forms of interactive, health-related psychoeducation (Dede & Fontana, 1995; Franko et al., 2004; Taylor et al., 2001; see chapter 9). Dede and Fontana (1995) described the Multimedia and Thinking Skills Project (MTSP) at George Mason University, which emphasizes interactive, Web-integrated learning. "Multi-user shared environments" (MUSEs) foster independent and collaborative exploration, learning by observation and discussion, experiential learning through data gathering and simulations, hypothesis development and testing, and multimedia productions (e.g., Web sites, interactive CD-ROMs) for communication of what is learned to various audiences. It is unlikely that MUSEs can replace the potentially powerful group dynamics of interpersonal learning and empowerment through face-to-face discussion with mentors, peers, and business people (Piran, 1999b, 2001; see chapter 8). Neveretheless, this type of "virtual" project could provide a powerful extension of media literacy's focus on individual expression, collaborative learning, learning by doing, usable learning products, and more sophisticated access to and use of mass media (Levine et al., 1999).

CONCLUSIONS, CHALLENGES, AND FUTURE DIRECTIONS

Nearly 20 years ago, Steiner-Adair (1986, 1994; Steiner-Adair & Vorenberg, 1999) and Piran (1995, 1999b, 2001) began intersecting lines of work that emphasize the importance of helping girls and women to adopt a critical stance toward the body-within-culture, that is, the body politic. This critical social perspective is grounded in knowledge that is generated by dialogue and study, and affirmed and extended through actions that integrate changes in one's self, one's peers, and the culture (Levine & Piran, 2001, 2004; Piran, 2001; see chapter 8).

Our review of the research indicates that media literacy is a promising area for prevention, if three conditions are met. First, the program must be extensive and intensive in its efforts to link knowledge, practice in critical thinking, and activism. *Awareness* and *Analysis* of mass media are probably not sufficient for prevention; a cycle must be forged that incorporates *Activism* and *Advocacy*, both of which may require learning how to gain Access to media. Second, as seen in the *GO GIRLS!*™ and the ATLAS–ATHENA projects, the program must be integrated with other components of an ecological approach, including development of life skills, changing peer and adult attitudes, and, perhaps, use of mass media for health promotion, advocacy, and social marketing. Finally, those committed to prevention of negative body image and eating problems need to forge links with experts in communications and public health so as to benefit from the rich tradition of theory, research, and evaluation in regard to the mass media and health (Rice & Atkin, 2001). In this regard, organizations such as NEDA, ANAD, and the Academy for Eating Disorders (see Appendix A) would do well to follow the lead of the American Academy of Pediatrics (see Appendix C) in developing a subcommittee devoted to the study and positive transformation of mass media (Strasburger & Donnerstein, 2000).

14

Deciding the Level of Prevention: Universal, Selective, or Targeted?

For all of the debates within the field of the prevention of eating problems, there is one thing on which we all agree: Prior to designing and implementing a prevention program, you must identify a clear goal. Whose behaviors or attitudes are you trying to change? What, specifically, are the behaviors, attitudes, or beliefs that you are ultimately aiming to affect? And what are the environmental (ecological) variables and mediating psychological processes that you plan to influence in order to achieve the desired prevention effects? Various issues raised in chapter 1 (What is prevention?), chapter 2 (What are we trying to prevent?), chapters 9 and 13 (What types of prevention work best?), and chapter 11 (How does one design a good prevention outcome study?) bring us back to the fact that the first step in developing a prevention program is to delineate target behaviors, key risk and resilience factors, and a target audience.

The fact that we all agree on the necessity of identifying targets at the outset of a prevention program does not mean that we easily agree on the specifics. Indeed, one of the best-defined debates in our field focuses on the matter of goals and audiences (Austin, 2001; Rosenvinge & Børreson, 1999; Stice & Shaw, 2004). Whereas some theorists and researchers (including us) continue to argue for universal-selective (or primary; see chapters 1 and 9 for definitions) prevention programs, others propose that only targeted (or secondary) prevention has been, and is likely to be, successful (e.g., Killen, 1996; Stice & Hoffman, 2004; Stice & Shaw, 2004).

This chapter explores the universal versus targeted prevention debate within the field of eating problems. Decisions concerning the level of prevention revolve around questions of philosophy, methodology, cost–benefit, and success. This chapter is built around these four issues. It concludes by considering yet another question: Do we have to choose between universal-selective and targeted prevention?

Note that there continues to be confusion about the terms *primary* versus *secondary* prevention, and *universal*, *selective*, and *targeted* prevention. For example, in their recent meta-analysis, Stice and Shaw (2004) use the term *select*ed to encompass what Mrazek and Haggerty (1994) refer to as *select*ive and *target*ed prevention (see our discussions in chapters 1 & 9). Therefore, we will choose our words carefully and reiterate some of the material in chapter 1.

A QUESTION OF PHILOSOPHY

With some notable exceptions (see, e.g., Kater, 1998; Neumark-Sztainer et al., 2000), many people currently designing programs to prevent eating problems are psychologists or psychiatrists. As such, we have been trained to focus on the individual rather than on societal institutions. This is clear in the *DSM-IV-TR* (2000). Behavioral problems, including eating disorders, are defined in terms of signs and symptoms displayed by individuals (see chapter 2). Although very few prevention evaluations have used the criteria from specific *DSM* categories as prevention outcomes, many studies assessing "behavioral" effects draw their dependent measures from those criteria. Clinical criteria for individual signs and symptoms, as well as clinical theories about individual psychopathology, are particularly prominent in commonly used measures such as the EDI, the ChEAT, and the EDE-Q (see Appendix E).

Having established these types of individual clinical measures as the "gold standards" for operationalizing our dependent variables (i.e., our distal outcome measures), we then proceed to try to identify the proximal "causes" and "mediators" of the development of eating disorders. Risk factor research focuses on elements of individual trauma, family life, personality, and development that might increase the likelihood of the onset or maintenance of an eating problem (see, e.g., Crago et al., 2001; Stice, 2001b). The risk factors listed in Table 5.1 exemplify this focus. Mediating processes, which in prevention research are often difficult to distinguish from distal outcomes, include internalization of the slender beauty ideal (Thompson & Stice, 2001) and body dissatisfaction.

Within this approach, then, we need to prevent individuals—and especially individual girls—from developing the continuum of eating problems and eating disorders (see chapter 2) by reducing or eliminating their risk factors and mediating processes, and by increasing protective factors and sources of resilience (see chapter 5). As demonstrated in chapter 9, this is typically done by trying to change the way the *individual* girl interacts with and understands her world. Catalano and Dooley (1980) refer to this approach as *reactive primary prevention* to distinguish it from the ecological focus of *proactive prevention* (see also Austin, 2000, as well as chapters 1 and 12 of this book). So, we might try to convince the girl to react differently to unhealthy sociocultural influences by accepting her body and by ignoring or deflecting comments that belittle her appearance. Simultaneously, we might try to help the girl acquire self-affirming, empowering, and assertive coping skills so that she will neither internalize the thin ideal nor binge eat in reaction to emotional distress. We might also teach the girl about the risks of calorie-restrictive dieting. This approach occasionally addresses factors outside of the girl, such as peer teasing or parental modeling, but the emphasis is on helping individual girls.

In addition to trying to help individual girls resist or avoid risk factors, people working from the individual "illness" perspective are often interested in early identification. They seek to find ways to help parents, doctors, teachers, dentists, and other adults recognize the prodromal warning signs or the early symptoms of eating problems. For example, Gurney and Halmi (2001) found that a relatively short eating disorders curriculum, consisting of four 75-minute sessions, increased medical social workers' knowledge of assessment and treatment by about one third. Perhaps more important, participation in the program produced a significant increase in the social workers' likelihood of asking about or screening for eating disorders during routine office visits. This is an encouraging result, particularly if the program can be adapted for primary care physicians, internal medicine specialists, gynecologists, nurse practitioners, dietitians, fitness trainers, and dentists (see Weiner, 1999). These professionals may see eating disorders clients early on in their illness, and several years before a psychologist or psychiatrist is involved. Indeed, people suffering from eating disorders are more likely than those with other psychiatric disorders to seek help from their primary care provider (Ogg, Millar, Pusztai, & Thom, 1997). Yet, these medical practitioners are not always well acquainted with the warning signs or symptoms of eating disorders and do not routinely assess for them. For example, DiGioacchino, Keenan, and Sargent (2000) reported that only 28% of the dentists and 37% of the dental hygienists they surveyed routinely assessed patients for eating disorders (see also Schmidt & Treasure, 1997).

The goal of such early identification is, of course, to try to get the person into the appropriate intervention or treatment programs. Some girls identified as "at risk" will actually be in the early phases of the disorder. As such, they are likely to be referred to clinical prevention programs or practices to prevent the progression of the disorder; this is the principal meaning of *targeted* prevention (Mrazek & Haggerty, 1994). Others may be demonstrating preclinical behaviors (e.g., setting dangerous weight-loss goals, or frequent "fat talk," or overinvestment in weight and shape as defining features of self). Although identification and intervention in this instance is technically a form of *selective* prevention (Mrazek & Haggerty, 1994; see chapter 1), referral to a targeted program such as the *Student Bodies* CAPP (see chapter 9) or cognitive-behavioral bibliotherapy (Cash, 1997) is probably the best choice. The distinction between proto-symptomatic (or high risk, in relation to selective prevention) versus symptomatic (in relation to targeted prevention) is not always clear. What is clear is that early identification programs are not constructed to provide healthy children with information aimed at preventing eating disorders in and of themselves.

Proponents of targeted prevention have argued that universal approaches are not efficient (Offord, Kraemer, Kazdin, Jensen, & Harrington, 1998). In aiming for a broad audience, universal prevention typically has only small to moderate effects on individuals (see meta-analytic research by Stice & Shaw, 2004, and by Tobler et al., 2000, as reviewed in chapters 9 and 10, respectively). Across a large population containing many children and adolescents who are healthy and at low or moderate risk, the motivation for a particular child or adolescent to change is likely to be smaller than in a targeted program. In targeted programs, the potential participants are suffering from the clear precursors and/or early symptoms of the disorder, parents and friends are concerned, and the individual volunteering for the program would presumably receive substantial individual attention. Indeed, a universal-selective program (such as a curriculum for all sixth-grade girls in a large school district) may be most helpful to those who least need it (Offord et al., 1998). Existing cognitive schema will influence how children process the general messages from this type of program. For example, if a girl already diets only rarely, she may be quite receptive to the message that dieting is dangerous and therefore quite willing and able to abandon her occasional dieting. A girl who diets constantly may find an antidieting message less convincing, and she may be less able to completely change her eating habits to give up all dieting.

On the other hand, there are two major arguments in favor of universal prevention. First, we all know that it is more difficult to change a behavior if those around us are engaging in the behavior (Offord et al., 1998). If someone is trying to resist or reduce dieting while others in the cafeteria are engaging in "fat talk" (Nichter, 2000) or are severely limiting their food intake, she might feel foolish, and might even be ridiculed, for trying to diet less. Targeted prevention programs that operate in a group format may try to change norms within the group, but they do not as a rule try to change the ecology of peer groups, families, and the community (Offord et al., 1998). Consequently, these programs fail to address the ways in which individual health is embedded in public health issues. As we have repeatedly emphasized, any type of prevention program—be it universal, selective, or targeted—is likely to have effects that are limited in scope and duration if it ignores the ecology of children and adolescents.

This second argument for universal prevention is found in S. B. Austin's (2001) application of a population-based model developed by British epidemiologist Geoffrey Rose. Drawing on Rose's work, Austin begins with the empirically based assumption that risk factors such as dieting and internalization of the slender beauty ideal tend to be "more or less unimodally and normally distributed in populations" (p. 273). Furthermore, there tends to be a linear relationship between the risk factor and the cases of disorder to be prevented. Together, these two basic aspects of the concept of "risk factor" yield what might be called the "Rose Paradox" (S. B. Austin, 2001). Although by definition there will be a disproportionate number of cases arising from the high-risk group, the largest proportion of cases in the total population will emerge from the low- to moderate-risk group because there are many more people in this group. In other words, "a large number of people exposed to small risk will often produce more cases in a population than will a small number of people at large risk" (p. 274).

S. B. Austin (2001) notes further that "group" or "people" can refer to an aggregate of individuals or a collection of ecological entities like schools. In this regard, Austin applied Rose's Paradox to data from the *Planet Health* obesity prevention study (Gortmaker et al., 1999; see S. B. Austin et al., 2002, 2004, as reviewed in chapter 9). Austin demonstrated that (a) 56% of the "cases" of diet pill use and purging came from schools with moderate to low levels of dieting; and (b) if the prevalence of dieting could be reduced by 10% in all 10 of the schools in the sample (range of average dieting as a function of school = 8% to 45%), more than a third of those cases could be prevented. Rose's Paradox is a strong argument for an ecological, universal, public health approach to prevention (S. B. Austin, 2001).

A QUESTION OF METHODOLOGY

There are at least two important methodological features to be considered when deciding whether a prevention program should be more targeted or more universal. First, the more individualized the program's method of delivery is, the more likely one is to want to work with a defined group. Second, in order to conduct programs in the selective-targeted range of the prevention continuum, one must have a method for identifying at-risk or symptomatic children.

Method of Delivery

The vast majority of eating disorders prevention programs are curricula (see chapters 9, 10, and 13). This is true of both universal-selective and targeted programs. Other psychoeducational techniques, such as showing a video followed by a discussion (e.g., Moreno & Thelen, 1993) or using interactive software (e.g., Franko et al., 2004; Taylor et al., 2001), may also be fairly easily adapted to fit the goals of universal-selective or targeted programs (see, e.g., Abascal et al., 2004).

At least one method of delivering a program is not particularly well suited for universal-selective prevention programs designed to be implemented in schools with multiple classrooms of 20 to 30 students (see chapter 9). This is the feminist-empowerment-relational (FER) discussion group described in chapter 8. It is certainly the case that developers of successful programs based on the social cognitive and Non-Specific Vulnerability-Stressor models have arranged for group discussions of key material and for discovery-based learning that emerges from dialogues within a group of students (see, e.g., O'Dea & Abraham, 2000; Santonastaso et al., 1999; Stice, Mazotti, et al., 2000; Taylor et al., 2001). However, the groups developed by Piran (1999b) and Friedman (1999, 2000) differ from these discussion or work groups in that the relationships, the new norms, and the renewed "voice" constructed in the FER groups are considered essential ingredients for preventive changes.

Examples of FER discussion groups were provided in chapter 8 (Piran's work and, within a school setting, Steiner-Adair et al.'s work) and chapter 13 (*GO GIRLS!*™ program). This type of group has a variety of advantages over curricula applied in either a didactic or interactive format (see Table 14.1). FER discussion groups permit students to set at least the specifics of the agenda. The adult discussion leader may select the broad topic for the day, but the examples, connections, and details of the discussion come from the participants. Such discussion groups also provide a "safe place" for participants to explore their interests, concerns, fears, and questions. To this end, there is usually a confidentiality agreement. Furthermore, the FER discussion group will be composed of people with some similar interests or concerns. For example, girls may be invited to join the group because they have been identified as high risk (e.g., Piran, 1999b). In the hands of a skilled facilitator, this combination of safety, confidentiality, and similar experiences can lead to a strong sense of social support for the girls. Thus, the group may become a truly unique context for participants, because they are unusually free to express their opinions and emotions, and to construct a personal

TABLE 14.1
Advantages of Psychoeducational Curricula Versus Discussion Groups as Delivery Methods for Eating Disorders Prevention Programs

Advantages of Curricula	*Advantages of Discussion Groups*
Provides specific materials for use by people with minimal training	Allows more intensive coverage of material
Can be used with large groups (both boys and girls)	Can focus on the most at-risk children
Can be purchased once and used in several different classrooms	Adaptable to the needs of the participants
Can create broad ecological change	Allows individual attention
Can be coordinated across grades enabling multiple exposures	Skilled facilitator can harness group dynamics to foster new, more positive group norms
	Influence of group leader as a role model or mentor may be much more powerful

and social setting in which new norms and values replace toxic sociocultural influences (Piran, 1999b, 1999c, 2001).

FER discussion groups also facilitate individual engagement in the processes that are critical for prevention, for example, consciousness raising, competence building, and activism (see chapter 10). This is evident in responses to open-ended questions about participation in the *GO GIRLS!*™ program described in chapter 13 (Levine et al., 1999; Piran et al., 2000): For example, one adolescent girl remarked, "A group of girls like this is great because it gives us a chance to unite and have somewhat of an impact on things that we believe should be different." The group facilitator can help to monitor and encourage each girl's input, to insure everyone's involvement. This, of course, would be extremely difficult to accomplish working with a classroom of 25 students or with an entire grade level at a school.

Indeed, developing and maintaining FER groups requires all of the things that are in short supply in most schools: time, space, and personnel. Friedman's (1999) *Just for Girls* program, for example, requires that each group meet for 1.5 hours once a week over a 10- to 12-week period. Between assemblies, athletics, musical performances, special days, and mandated achievement testing, it can be remarkably difficult to create this structure, at least in public schools in the United States and Canada (see McVey, Tweed, & Blackmore, 2004). In addition, each group must be facilitated by a woman. Friedman (1999) does not specify a level of education or other experiences for a group facilitator, but she does refer to these women as having "professional lives" and being trained to be sensitive to weight and body image concerns. McVey and colleagues trained public health nurses in the province of Ontario, Canada, to conduct the Girl Talk support groups that are now an essential component of McVey's multidimensional prevention program (McVey, Lieberman, et al., 2003a; McVey, Tweed, & Blackmore, 2004; see chapter 12). In parts of the world that have such professionals well established in positions with an ongoing relationship to schools in place already, identifying and training group facilitators may be much easier than in the United States.

We agree with Friedman that it is important for prevention specialists to be knowledgeable about and comfortable with children and adolescents. We also think it important that an FER group leader have strong connections to children, adolescents, and adult stakeholders in the system (see chapters 4, 8, 10, and 12). Therefore, although a few schools will have on their staff a social worker, health educator, or nurse who meets Friedman's criteria, we presume that in most schools a teacher, coach, counselor, or administrator would fill the role of group facilitator. Certain teachers could function as a facilitator for an FER discussion group if the group could be scheduled as a regular class, as has sometimes been done with the *GO GIRLS!*™ program. But if the discussion group(s) must meet after school, many teachers will be unable to participate, as will girls who rely on school bus transportation to get home or who have commitments to sports or work. Time and money for training might also decrease the likelihood of some teachers' participation. Again, training scheduled in the evening or on weekends may be difficult for teachers. From an ethical perspective and in terms of modeling professional respect for working women, teachers who give up some of their nonteaching time to be trained for a prevention program should receive remuneration. Finally, group meetings need to occur in a place with sufficient privacy that the girls feel comfortable discussing difficult issues. Based on our experience with the *GO GIRLS!*™ program, this can be surprisingly difficult to arrange in the many schools where space, as well as time and human resources, is in short supply.

Programs using an FER discussion group format are designed to enable girls to raise concerns about the environment in which they live (Friedman, 1999, 2000; Piran, 1999b, 1999c). More specifically, girls may suggest that the behaviors of certain peers, teachers, or coaches contribute to their poor body image and eating problems. As discussed in chapter 8, for her program Piran carefully and patiently negotiated an explicit agreement with the ballet school's administration that they would address the ecological-contextual issues raised by the girls' discussions of their "lived experiences." Other schools may find such an approach (based on empowerment and changing the ecology) threatening rather than enlightening. Thus, without substantial background advocacy work within the school system and local community, schools may be actively and passively resistant to addressing many issues raised in the discussion groups (Friedman, 1999). If this happens, the groups may be allowed to proceed, but they may become frustrating and discouraging rather than empowering for the participants.

Method of Identification

Selective or targeted prevention may be more efficient than universal prevention if the children (or adolescents) who are most at risk are substantially helped by focused programs for a lower total cost than would be involved in a more universal, public health effort (Offord et al., 1998). This improved level of efficiency is possible only if one can identify at-risk or proto-symptomatic children using a relatively inexpensive, valid, and practical technique. One must not identify a substantial number of children as high risk when their likelihood of developing the problems is actually low to moderate (Offord et al., 1998). Thus, the method employed to identify at-risk children (or adolescents) for a selective-targeted prevention program is of critical importance. There are fundamentally two ways to do this. One can group children according to some known risk factor such as Type I insulin-dependent diabetes mellitus (a form of selective prevention; see Olmsted et al., 2002, as reviewed in chapter 9), or one can use a measure of body dissatisfaction or eating problems to identify groups (a form of prevention that falls closer to the targeted category; Stice, Mazotti, et al., 2000).

Risk Factors. Chapter 5 outlined some of the empirically investigated risk factors associated with body image and eating problems. It is much easier to discuss such factors for girls than for boys. Research on body image problems among boys is still in its infancy (Ricciardelli & McCabe, 2004; see chapter 3). Hence, most of what we discuss here applies only to girls. We note findings about boys wherever possible.

At present, some risk factors such as internalization of the thin ideal can be ascertained only via questionnaire or interview. These sorts of measures are discussed in the next section of this chapter. Other risk factors reflect either demographic factors or group membership and so can be easily identified without pretesting.

Many programs have been aimed at adolescent girls because it is during adolescence that we see a precipitous drop in body image among girls (Smolak & Levine, 1996). This means that several prevention programs have involved exclusively middle school girls (e.g., Killen et al., 1993), high school girls (Santonastaso et al., 1999), or young women in college (e.g., Taylor et al., 2001). But, as noted in chapter 9, programs for these audiences are really a form of prevention that falls between universal prevention (designed for large groups of nonsymptomatic girls) and selective prevention (as a "group," adolescent girls are at high risk for a variety of reasons). It is not true selective prevention. At least half the participants in the program are not at substantial risk of developing eating problems. Conversely, the groups participating were not established on the basis of some valid or even reasonable criterion of being "at high risk."

In developing a selective prevention program, one could further narrow the groups of high-risk girls by focusing on those who participate in certain activities, most notably dance and cheerleading (Smolak et al., 2000; see, e.g., Elliot et al., in press). Similarly, boys who participate in bodybuilding, wrestling, and, perhaps, football might be at particular risk for muscle dysmorphia, steroid use, and food supplement abuse (Goldberg & Elliot, 2000; Pope et al., 2000).

Body weight and fat might also be a defining risk factor for selective prevention. Children who are overweight or obese are clearly at risk for a variety of health problems, particularly diabetes (see chapter 3). Research suggests that girls who are heavy are also at risk for developing eating disorders, although findings in this regard are inconsistent (Stice, 2002). Overweight adults appear to be more likely to binge eat (Striegel-Moore, 1993). Similarly, some currently unknown percentage of overweight girls in all ethnic groups is already engaging in binge eating (Douchinis et al., 2001). This means that, unavoidably, a minority of overweight or obese girls identified for selective prevention would be more appropriate for targeted prevention.

Whether they are overweight or not, children and adolescents who are teased about their bodies are at increased risk of developing body image and eating problems (Thompson et al., 1999). Teachers may be able to easily identify children who are teased. However, before teasing can be effectively used to identify potential prevention program participants, researchers must provide evidence that teacher selections are consistent with children's own self-reports.

It is also increasingly clear that girls who are victims of child sexual abuse are at increased risk for serious body image and eating problems (Connors, 2001; Smolak & Murnen, 2002, 2004). A minority of sexual abuse victims, at least, comes through the children's services or criminal justice systems. Selective prevention programs should be developed to reduce the risk that these girls will develop eating problems.

Measures for Targeted Programs. Recall that targeted (or "indicated") programs are designed to prevent the development of serious, chronic problems in people who are already showing significant warning signs or symptoms of the disorder (Mrazek & Haggerty, 1994; see chapter 1). Currently, there are a variety of measures to assess body image and eating problems in children and adolescents (see Gardner, 2001; Netemeyer & Williamson, 2001; Smolak, 2004; see Appendix E). Several widely used adult measures—including the Eating Disorders Inventory (EDI-2; Garner, 1991), the Eating Attitudes Test (EAT; Garfinkel & Garner, 1982), and the Eating Disorders Examination (EDE; Fairburn & Cooper, 1993)—have been adapted for use with elementary and middle school children. Limited psychometric data are available for the Children's Eating Attitudes Test (ChEAT; Maloney et al., 1989; Smolak & Levine, 1994b) and the Eating Disorders Inventory–Children (EDI-C; Garner, 1991). The children's version of the EDE interview has been shown to correlate with diagnoses of eating disturbance in a pattern similar to that seen in adults (Bryant-Waugh, Cooper, Taylor, & Lask, 1996). Thus, if one is seeking to identify a group of children who are showing signs of serious eating disturbance, the Children's EDE is probably the best measure to use. One could also consider using the Kid's Eating Disorder Survey (KEDS; Childress, Brewerton, Hodges, & Jarrell, 1993) to identify possibly symptomatic children. However, there are fewer psychometric data for this questionnaire than for the EDE children's interview.

Some of the analyses in Stice and Shaw's (2004) meta-analysis of prevention programs indicate that selective-targeted programs will be most effective with people age 15 and older. Thus, it is fortunate that there is a greater choice of instruments to identify a variety of problems among adolescents (see Appendix E). Adult measures, including the EDI, the EAT, and the restraint subscale of the Dutch Eating Behavior Questionnaire (DEBQ; Van Strien et al., 1986), have been used in several studies with adolescent participants. In addition to the DEBQ restraint scale, the Dietary Intent Scale (DIS; Stice, 1998b) has been developed for use with adolescent girls. These measures may help to identify girls who are problem dieters, on the assumption that chronic dieting behavior, accompanied by a "dieting mentality," is related to eating problems, particularly binge eating (Heatherton & Polivy, 1992; Polivy & Herman, 1985). In this regard, there is also evidence that dieting predicts later development of obesity among adolescent girls (Stice et al., 1999). Targeted prevention programs that recruit girls based on dieting may be able to address both eating disorders and obesity.

Most of these measures have not been thoroughly examined in prospective studies in which the outcome variable is a clinical or subthreshold eating disorder. Thus, it is difficult to identify specific scores on the scales that are associated with development of a serious eating problem. This is especially true in elementary school samples, which have never been followed long enough for an analyzable number of eating disorders (clinical or subthreshold) to develop. With adolescents, two measures have been found to predict later development of disordered eating. The first, the Weight Concerns Scale, has been shown to predict the onset of subthreshold eating disorders over a 3-year period (Killen, 1996; Killen et al., 1996). Girls scoring in the highest quartile in middle school (ages 11–14) were significantly more likely to develop eating problems before the end of high school.

Recently, The McKnight Investigators (2003) developed a four-question screen to identify girls at risk for subthreshold or clinical forms of BN or BED. The four questions and the necessary scores on each (on a 5-point scale, with 1 being *never*) are shown in Table 14.2. The most important statistics in the evaluation of a screening tool are shown in Table 14.3. The McKnight screen has a sensitivity of .72, a specificity of .80, and an efficiency of .79. As expected for a set of disorders in which the base rate is relatively low, this screen tends to overidentify cases; that is,

TABLE 14.2
The McKnight Risk Factor Screen

Question	Criterion Score*
How often have you been on a diet to lose weight?	≥ 4
How often does your weight make boys not like you?	5
Average of the following two items:	
How often do you change your eating around boys?	
How often do you change your eating around girls?	$M \geq 3.5$

Note. *All items are scored on a 5-point scale with 1 = *never*. From The McKnight Investigators (2003).

TABLE 14.3
Statistical Factors to Be Considered in Assessing Screening Measures

Factor	Definition
Sensitivity	The percentage of children developing the problem at T_2 who were correctly identified as high-risk by the screen at T_1
Specificity	The percentage of children without the problem at T_2 who screened negative at T_1
Positive Predictive Value (PPV)	The percentage of children who screened positive at T_1 who develop the problem at T_2
Negative Predictive Value (NPV)	The percentage of children who screened negative at T_1 who do *not* develop the problem at T_2
Efficiency	The percentage of children whose status (positive or negative with respect to the criterion problem) at T_2 was correctly predicted by the screen at T_1

Note. T_1 refers to the first time of testing and T_2 refers to the second time of testing.

it tends to yield a significant number of false positives. Thus, in the sample used to develop the screen ($N = 1,103$), the measure would have identified 242 girls (21.5%) as being at risk. Of this group, 23 (9.5%) actually developed at least subthreshold eating disorders; this is the "positive predictive value" (see Table 14.3). The screen would have missed 9 of the 32 girls (sensitivity = $23/32 = .72$) who later developed clinically significant levels of eating problems. The screening instrument yielded a correct prediction of no disorder in 852 of the 1,071 girls who did not develop the disorder, so the specificity is $852/1,071 = .80$. Of the 861 girls whom the screen identified as low risk, only 9 developed one of the criterion disorders, so the "negative predictive value" is $852/861 = .99$. Overall, the screen correctly predicted 875 of the actual outcomes (efficiency = $875/1,103 = .79$). Whether this screen is sufficiently sensitive, specific, and thus efficient in identifying high-risk girls depends on the costs and goals of the prevention program. Although we would ideally always know the sensitivity, specificity, and efficiency, as well as the positive and negative predictive values of a measure, these important statistics are not readily available for most eating disorders measures.

If a measure does yield a substantial number of false positives, that is, it has a low positive predictive value, it might be desirable to use a second screening device to further narrow the group of students who would be referred for participation in a targeted program (Offord et al., 1998). Perhaps, for example, one could move to an interview technique, such as the EDE or the McKnight Eating Disorders Examination (MEDE; The McKnight Investigators, 2003). Clearly, addition of an interview-based screen would be considerably more expensive to administer than would a four-question survey. This cost must be weighed against the gain of more accurately specifying the at-risk group.

A QUESTION OF COSTS AND BENEFITS

Assuming the cost–benefit ratio of doing nothing about the spectrum of eating problems is so unacceptably high that we can ignore this passive option, the criterion against which any prevention effort must be measured is the cost and success of attempting to treat people who are suffering. As discussed in chapter 1, it is unlikely that the majority of people with eating disorders are currently receiving treatment. Yet, they (and their families) are suffering from significant medical risks or problems that are part of the cost of failing to prevent the disorder. These problems cover a wide range, including dental enamel erosion caused by vomiting, organ damage due to long-term steroid abuse, osteoporosis from calcium deprivation, and death due to malnutrition, esophageal hemorrhage, or cardiac arrhythmia. Body dissatisfaction and dieting may be causal factors in the development of depression and obesity (e.g., Field et al., 2003; Stice et al., 1999; Stice, Hayward, et al., 2000; Wichstrøm, 1999), two health problems that themselves carry substantial costs for society. Thus, an emphasis on treatment has at least two types of costs. First, there is the cost to the individual, to distressed family and friends, and to society of serious conditions that are not treated at all for various psychological and socioeconomic reasons, or are treated inadequately. Second, if the individual has access to and will indeed participate in treatment, there is the cost not only of psychological therapy, psychopharmacological agents, and psychiatric hospitalizations, but also dental and medical care and time lost from work or school.

Intuitively, prevention would appear to be more efficient and more cost-effective than treatment (see chapter 1). This has certainly proven to be the case with medical prevention programs. Consider, for example, the cost of preventing polio, smallpox, or AIDS, compared to treating each or to the suffering and loss of life associated with these diseases. Eating disorders are potentially fatal; in fact, untreated they are much more likely to result in death than all but the most severe psychiatric disorders such as schizophrenia or bipolar disorder. Eating disorders are also difficult and expensive to treat. Treatment typically requires a team of specialists consisting of a dietitian, an internist (and possibly other physicians such as an endocrinologist or cardiologist), a psychiatrist, a psychologist, and various therapists. Brief hospitalization and other forms of residential care, for either medical or psychological problems (including suicide attempts), are not unusual. Nonetheless, it would be easier to gain political and therefore financial support for prevention efforts if we were able to *demonstrate* the efficacy of prevention versus treatment.

What would be required for such a cost–benefit analysis? First, we need solid epidemiological data on the rates of various eating disorder diagnoses, including Eating Disorders Not Otherwise Specified (EDNOS; see chapter 2). Some data are available for some groups, but overall there is a lack of good epidemiological data (Striegel-Moore & Smolak, 2001). This is particularly true for ethnic groups other than

Whites. There are better data available for obesity (see chapter 3). There are a number of large-scale studies of dieting and body dissatisfaction, especially for girls, and even though some use excellent sampling and measurement techniques, none is truly population based. There are a few estimates of steroid use by adolescent boys (see, e.g., Goldberg & Elliot, 2000), but the extent of food supplement abuse by children and adolescents is unknown.

Epidemiological data are important in several ways. First, they help convince funding agencies that a problem is a significant issue for public health. Second, they can be used to estimate the overall cost of treatment, by multiplying the cost of identification and treatment per person by the number of expected cases. Finally, they can be used to assess the effectiveness of both screening tools and prevention programs. The most important measure of the success of a prevention program is a reduction in the rate of the onset (i.e., the incidence) of new cases of a disorder (see chapter 1).

It is also important to have an estimate of the cost of treatment per case, as well as the costs associated with leaving the problem untreated. These values can then be compared to the cost of the prevention program per person. The cost of prevention must include screening expenses for selective and targeted programs. The cost per person of prevention would then be multiplied by the number of participants in the prevention program. The reduction in the number of new cases must also be considered. Thus, the direct costs of the prevention program must be assessed, but the real "benefit" or "savings" is in terms of the reduction in the number of people requiring treatment (Offord et al., 1998).

Presently, we do not have strong data concerning the effectiveness of most prevention programs, particularly in regard to the reduction in incidence over long periods of time. The material reviewed in chapters 9 through 11 and in chapter 13 indicates that most of the available evaluations of programs are limited or flawed when compared to the standard for good prevention research in the fields of epidemiology and public health. Furthermore, most of the prevention programs have been aimed at White girls, so it is unclear how effective they may be with other groups. This state of affairs, in conjunction with the lack of epidemiological data, makes it impossible for us to do meaningful cost–benefit analyses for prevention programs. Even though this is true of most child and adolescent psychiatric problems (Offord et al., 1998), we need to make it a priority to collect the data necessary to do these cost–benefit evaluations if we are to be effective advocates of prevention and to compete successfully for public or private funding.

We have been discussing cost–benefit analysis as if the prevention programs in question were aimed at clinically significant eating problems. Yet most prevention programs are designed to reduce or prevent body dissatisfaction, dieting, or some general amalgam of "eating disordered attitudes and behaviors." Certainly there is a much higher prevalence of body dissatisfaction or dieting than eating disorders in countries such as the United States, Great Britain, Spain, Italy, and Australia. And a focus on body image would clearly permit both genders to be involved in the prevention program. Dieting is an appealing target behavior because it is widespread, with perhaps 40% to 60% of high school girls dieting, and because it is often cited as a precursor to eating disorders (Austin, 2000, 2001; Smolak et al., 1998b). Given the difference in base rates—about 50% for dieting compared to 5% to 10% for clinically meaningful eating problems among girls (see chapter 2)—it should be easier to demonstrate a significant effect of a dieting prevention program. However, in the context of cultures that glorify slenderness and vilify fat and fat people, it may be more difficult to convince funding agencies of the importance of combating body dissatisfaction or dieting. Linking prevention of dieting and body dissatisfaction to prevention of not only eating disorders but also depression (Stice, Hayward, et al., 2000; Wichstrøm, 1999) and obesity (Field et al., 2003; Irving & Neumark-Sztainer, 2002; Stice et al., 1999) may help "sell" such programs. Again, we need to generate estimates of the cost of body dissatisfaction and dieting, as well as the cost and efficacy of prevention programs, in order to offer more cogent proposals for competitive grants, as well as more powerful advocacy for allocation of grant monies to support research in our field.

A QUESTION OF SUCCESS

Several important researchers in the field of eating problems have suggested that programs in the selective-targeted range of the prevention continuum are more effective, if not *much* more effective, than universal prevention programs such as general classroom curricula (see, e.g., Stice & Shaw, 2004; Taylor et al., 2001; see also chapter 9). In fact, the greater success of several of the targeted prevention programs reviewed in chapter 9 has led to pessimism about the likelihood of an effective and efficient universal prevention effort. Before accepting such a claim, it is important to consider at least two methodological issues.

First, prevention programs have tended to look for *reductions* in risk factors such as thin-ideal internalization, dieting, or extreme weight-loss techniques like purging. In a broad, unselected sample—particularly of elementary school children ages 6 to 11—the preintervention levels of these attitudes and behaviors may be too low to demonstrate a statistically reliable *change* over the relatively short time periods that are typical in such research (Smolak, 1996; Smolak et al., 1998b). Researchers need to take one or both of two steps to remedy this problem. They can arrange for much longer follow-up periods in order to compare the *development* of risk factors and, perhaps, disorder in the experimental group versus a comparison group. Or they can better identify dependent variables that are more likely to show significant *decreases* or *increases* following a universal program. For young audiences, such variables might include attitudes about fat and fat people, beliefs ("knowledge") about weight and shape, and healthy eating and exercise patterns.

Second, because universal programs are by definition less intensely focused on individuals (Cowen, 1973, 1983; see chapter 1), these programs are less likely to have a substantial effect on individual behavior (Offord et al., 1998). The immediate benefits might more clearly be to the ecology of the school or community than to the individual student. As in Piran's (1999a, 1999b) research, the long-term benefits would emerge in terms of, and be assessed as, a reduction in the incidence of disorders (eating problems, obesity, depression) over a long period such as 5 to 15 years. Again, we need to define and learn to assess ecological dependent variables in ways that capture both the intended changes in the environment and further changes set in motion by, for example, a "new" school setting (see chapter 12). In general, psychologists and psychiatrists are not trained to measure such ecological effects, so we may need to turn to the literature in community psychology, public health, sociology, and anthropology for valid measures.

The combination of low base rates, less impact on individual behavior, and elusive epidemiological data makes it is more difficult to demonstrate an effect in a universal prevention program (Offord et al., 1998). This is the nature of universal prevention. Nevertheless, the greater and more consistent success to date of selective-targeted over universal-selective programs (Stice & Shaw, 2004) must be acknowledged in thinking about the allocation of prevention resources.

DO WE HAVE TO CHOOSE?

In 1997 Mann and her colleagues at Stanford University published a paper that, for better or for worse, deeply affected prevention advocates and researchers. Mann et al.'s (1997) research revealed a temporary iatrogenic effect of a one-shot eating disorders prevention "program" that, by their definition, combined universal and targeted prevention (see chapter 9). The impact of this study extended to the general public because the "negative results of prevention" received extensive coverage in *The Washington Post*, *The New York Times*, and other influential newspapers. The study and resulting furor (see, e.g., Cohn & Maine, 1998, vs. Carter et al., 1998; Mann & Burgard, 1998) had an unintended polarizing effect. Mann, Burgard, and colleagues hoped their findings would demonstrate the inadvisability of combining both forms of prevention in a particular way that is often seen on college campuses (T. Mann, personal communication, August 20, 1999). Nevertheless, many people committed to eating disorders prevention felt pushed to defend prevention qua prevention, and to "choose" either the universal or targeted form.

Many experts in the broader fields of psychopathology and public health argue that the aims and audiences for the different levels of prevention require separate types of programming (e.g., Mrzaek & Haggerty, 1994; Offord, 2000; Offord et al., 1998). Similar arguments have been advanced by experts in the field of eating problems, and some limited progress has been made in integrating universal (or at least more general), selective, and targeted types of prevention within universities (Hotelling, 1999; Schwitzer, Bergholz, Dore, & Salimi, 1998) and within special settings such as an elite ballet school (Piran, 1999b) or an Israeli kibbutz (Latzer & Shatz, 1999). For example, Latzer and Shatz helped psychologists and nurses on the kibbutz to implement a combination of education for adolescents and their families, training for professionals, and provision of skilled counseling, treatment, and support services. This well-orchestrated plan integrated programs with a wider, more universal scope (e.g., raising the community's awareness of how sociocultural factors contribute to many challenges faced by adolescent girls), a moderate, more selective scope (e.g., helping families with teenage girls understand the impact of the pubertal transition on body image), and a narrow, targeted focus (e.g., the necessity of helping girls evincing the warning signs of disordered eating). A program evaluation has not been published, but there was some evidence for an increase in public awareness about the nature and causes of eating disorders, an increase in early identification of disordered eating (targeted prevention), and a possible reduction in the incidence of serious eating disorders (Latzer & Shatz, 1999).

Although it would be ideal to offer all levels of prevention—universal, selective, targeted, and clinical—in every school system or community, the realities of time, space, and money often preclude such broad-based intervention. Consequently, many program designers and researchers, working with school systems and public officials, feel the pressure of having to choose one level or the other. We acknowledge this practical matter, but we hope that prevention specialists, school administrators, and community leaders will think creatively about ways to integrate, to some degree, different types of prevention.

For example, consider the position of Resource Coordinator proposed in chapter 12. This position fits nicely with the growing trend in the United States toward social work and health promotion in the schools, including the nascent movement called "school-based health care centers." With a similar set of materials and activities, the Resource Coordinator could educate students and staff about risk factors for eating problems, obesity, depression, and substance abuse. Through an arrangement like the Family Resource Center (Dishion & Kavanagh, 2000; see chapter 10), preventive education could be extended to parents, grandparents, and siblings. As part of the education and training effort for teachers and staff, the Resource Coordinator can address warning signs, humane and ethical ways of reaching out to students who are suffering, and referral to effective treatment and support services. The resource person might be able to provide a discussion group or psychoeducational program for one or two small groups of high-risk girls. Thus, if a school and its stakeholders are willing to support a Resource Coordinator, she or he might be able to combine levels of prevention.

The recent work of Abascal and colleagues (2002, 2004; see chapter 9) has demonstrated that it may also be possible to tailor computer or Internet programs to meet the needs of different audiences (see also Taylor et al., 2001). A Web-based program could start with a sensitive and specific screening device that then links the user to a particular package; this might employ the same technology that allows you to follow a path to men's or women's clothing at the Web sites of well-known retailers. Or a school could purchase two programs for its local network and then differentially assign children to them based on risk. If the school already has computers with Internet access, the cost will not be substantial. Indeed, links could be established such that children can access the program from home. Particularly among White families, home computers are the norm. If there is a computer available, program cost may be minimal. There is also the potential for a school to buy access to a Web site, as one might do with a newspaper subscription, and then provide free use of the site to a certain number of parents and children. Certain community organizations, such as the Retired Teachers Association or the Rotary, might also be willing to contribute to programs that combine computing, education, and prevention.

It should be noted that compliance with computer-assisted psychoeducational programs (CAPPs; Taylor et al., 2001) has been mediocre. As researchers work to improve adherence (see Celio et al., 2002), two points might be kept in mind. First, the availability of CAPPs at home raises the attractive possibility of easily involving parents. It has been difficult to effectively involve parents in prevention programs (see chapter 12). Parents have time constraints and may be unwilling to admit in a public place like a school meeting that there is an eating problem, or even a concern about the possibility of one developing, in their families. Working with a CAPP in the privacy of their own home alleviates both of these problems.

Second, young women have shown poor adherence to CAPPs. It appears this is partially attributable to women's desire for connection and relationships, so recent versions of *Student Bodies* have incorporated some time in face-to-face group meetings (Celio et al., 2002; Taylor et al., 2001). This means that, despite the provision of online discussion opportunities, and despite the fact that face-to-face meetings are not necessary to improve compliance (Celio et al., 2002), the CAPP format may be too impersonal for many girls and women. Moreover, a significant number of girls and women are not very comfortable with their computer competency. Boys still seem to make greater use of computers, and video games continue to be designed primarily for boys' interests. Thus, boys may be more comfortable with computers. In addition, boys may be quite embarrassed to admit body shape concerns; discussions about weight and shape probably are not as normative among boys as girls (Jones et al., 2004). All of these factors make it likely that adherence to CAPP will be greater for boys than it is for girls. In thinking about ways to integrate levels of prevention and to engage boys as well as girls, researchers should evaluate gender differences in the effectiveness of various delivery methods.

CONCLUSIONS

The ongoing debate as to whether eating disorders prevention ought to occur primarily at the universal-selective end of the prevention spectrum or the selective-targeted end is unlikely to be resolved easily or soon. Given the limited time and financial resources available to most schools or communities, and given the long-standing tensions between the clinical–medical versus community–public health approaches, this discussion is likely to continue and perhaps even grow more heated.

In this chapter we have tried to consider in depth four issues that are involved in the evaluation of universal-selective versus selective-targeted prevention. In terms of philosophy, the more clearly committed people are to an ecological model, the more likely they are to favor universal prevention. Conversely, even if they accept the Rose Paradox (Austin, 2001), people committed to a more individual medical model may well believe that the most effective strategy is a focused, clinical intervention that targets the children and adolescents most seriously at risk.

In terms of methodology, in order for a targeted program ultimately to be more efficient that a universal one, there must be an effective, relatively low-cost screen. If such a screen exists, then another argument in favor of selective-targeted programs is that they are much better able to accommodate both the facilitator–participant relationship and the intensive, individualized style inherent in FER discussion groups.

Third, there is the important question of costs and benefits. We probably need to more clearly estimate costs and benefits if we wish to convince politicians and funding agencies of the value of prevention work. Unfortunately, we currently do not have the data to do this very well. Research on the prevention of eating problems needs to be designed so that three types of information can be analyzed: (a) good long-term outcome data for the experimental and control conditions; (b) the monetary costs of the experimental program per person in the target population or group; and (c) the costs of the experimental program in terms of negative effects on some individuals. Comparisons of effects in the experimental and control conditions over time, coupled with an estimate of the costs of treating those people in the control condition whose condition might have been prevented (1 – the preventive fraction; see chapter 9), can yield a rough estimate of a benefit in the form of money saved through prevention.

Cost–benefit analysis brings us back to the question of differential success. Although the targeted prevention programs have generally been more successful than the universal programs (Stice & Shaw, 2004), this may be due in part to biases in program content and evaluation methodology that favor targeted programs. Moreover, Rose's Paradox reminds us that even a universal prevention program with a small but consistent effect could produce a greater reduction in the absolute number of new cases than a targeted program with a moderate effect, even though the proportion affected by the program may be higher in the latter condition.

The complexities of all four questions raise a fifth, overriding question: Do we actually have to choose between the two? Several experts have described how prevention, treatment, and support services can be integrated within special systems such as private schools, universities or colleges, and kibbutzim. However, the overall effectiveness of this multidimensional approach is unknown, and it is likely to be very difficult to implement in large public schools, public school systems, and communities. Nevertheless, we believe that certain relatively low-cost options can be effectively combined to achieve our ideal picture of all levels of prevention being available in a setting. The next chapter offers, as our concluding thoughts, our recommendations for that ideal.

V

CONCLUSIONS AND FUTURE DIRECTIONS

15

Conclusions and Future Directions

Levine and Piran (1999) wrote that there is "little doubt that prevention of the continuum of eating problems is an immense task: immensely complicated and challenging, but also immensely interesting, exciting, important, and even transformative for those engaged in the collaborative process" (p. 319). Although the intervening years provide no compelling reasons to revise this conviction, the upsurge of studies (see chapters 9 and 13) and reviews (e.g., Austin, 2000; Levine & Piran, 2004; Stice & Shaw, 2004) published after 1998 has helped to clarify the challenges and provide some directions for meeting them. This final chapter revisits the questions raised in chapter 1 in order to offer direct answers that we hope will have practical implications for advancing the field. These questions are reproduced in Table 15.1.

RESPONSE TO QUESTIONS 1 AND 2: PREVENTION IS FUNDAMENTALLY DIFFERENT FROM TREATMENT

There is overlap between prevention and treatment, so several prominent experts (e.g., Mrazek & Haggerty, 1994) use a continuum of intervention, rather than distinct and contrasting categories. For example, cognitive-behavioral therapy (CBT) is recognized as effective for many clients who have eating disorders. CBT for individuals suffering from negative body image is a form of selective-targeted prevention of full-blown, serious, and potentially chronic eating disorders (see chapter 9). In turn, cognitive-behavioral techniques are a prominent feature of many school curricula designed to be universal-selective prevention (see chapters 6, 9, and 13).

TABLE 15.1
Basic Questions in the Prevention of Eating Problems

(1) What is prevention and how is it distinct from treatment?
(2) What is the rationale for an emphasis on prevention?
(3) What exactly are we trying to prevent?
(4) What is the role of models of problem etiology and preventive change in the development of prevention programs?
(5) What is the status of evidence for the effectiveness of prevention programs, especially universal and targeted prevention programs?
(6) What specifically have we learned about program development, evaluation, and refinement?
(7) What can eating disorder prevention specialists learn from current theory and research regarding the prevention of health problems, such as cigarette smoking?
(8) What are the implications for prevention of recent developments in neuroscience?
(9) Are prevention programs, however well-meaning, potentially dangerous?
(10) What is the relationship between efforts to prevent disordered eating and public health concerns about obesity in children and adolescents?
(11) (a) What is it about the experience of growing up female that contributes to the development of eating problems and disorders? (b) What is the position of males as target audiences for change, as agents of prevention, and as obstacles to prevention?

Nevertheless, prevention of problems before they occur by promoting health and resilience to illness is not the same thing as treatment (see chapter 1). We agree with those who have argued that the medical model of detect-it-and-treat-it (or head it off) will be inadequate to prevent the range of body image and eating problems. In this regard, even proponents of targeted prevention acknowledge that one of its disadvantages is the typically limited power of screening devices to predict future disorder (see chapter 14). Even if the screening devices were refined considerably, the same problems discussed in chapter 1 would still apply: Too many segments of society do not have access to professional care, and, even if they did, there are nowhere near enough capable experts, especially for work with children, adolescents, and ethnic minorities. Equally important, the attitudes and behaviors that comprise high risk for disorder, or early forms of disorder, are often too strong to change easily, not only because they have become habitual over the years, but because they are so deeply embedded in unhealthy cultural influences.

Although there is definitely a place for selective-targeted interventions, the solution to a continuum of *widespread* and *culturally supported* eating problems is a return to Cowen's (1973, 1983) definition of prevention. We need to take a more ecological approach to prevention as the promotion of public health and well-being through policies and other interventions that target, not high-risk *individuals*, but rather institutions, communities, and other large groups (see chapters 4, 10, 12, and 13). The solutions to a set of problems that are so clearly rooted in sociocultural factors must themselves be clearly rooted in sociocultural changes.

RESPONSE TO QUESTION 3: OUR GOAL SHOULD BE TO PREVENT A RANGE OF EATING PROBLEMS BY PROMOTING A RANGE OF HEALTHY CONTEXTS AND PRACTICES

The prevalence and seriousness of AN, BN, and various forms of EDNOS (e.g., binge-eating disorder) in many countries throughout the world is certainly a cause for concern (Gordon, 2000). But so is the spectrum of negative body image and eating problems (see chapter 2), which itself intersects with other significant health problems that can be arrayed on a continuum. These include obesity, inactivity, depression, abuse of anorexic stimulants such as tobacco, and malnutrition in girls with wholly adequate access to food (see chapter 3). Public health efforts should focus on the universal-selective prevention of these interrelated problems (Neumark-Sztainer, 2003). Social programs to promote positive influences on health—such as safety and respect for girls at home, in school, and in the mass media—should also reduce the likelihood that genetically vulnerable girls will encounter the trauma and other stressors that help transform genetic and psychological vulnerability into severe and chronic eating disorders.

RESPONSE TO QUESTION 4: MODELS OF PROBLEMS, PREVENTION, AND CHANGE NEED TO BECOME MORE PROMINENT IN PREVENTION RESEARCH

The Big 3 Paradigms

Chapters 6 through 8 discuss three broad theoretical perspectives that have guided most of the prevention work to date: social cognitive/cognitive-behavioral theory; the Non-Specific Vulnerability-Stressor perspective; and the feminist-empowerment-relational model. Prevention outcome research in the fields of eating problems and substance use indicates that each of these paradigms can contribute to the development of effective universal-selective and selective-targeted prevention programs (see chapters 9, 10, and 13). We urge future researchers to follow the lead of Killen (1996; social cognitive model), Taylor et al. (2001; cognitive-behavioral model; see also Stewart, 1998), O'Dea and Abraham (2000; Non-Specific Vulnerability-Stressor model), Piran (1999a, 1999b, 2001; feminist-empowerment-relational model), and Stice (dissonance-based approach; Stice et al., 2001) in offering a clear theoretical rationale for the specific prevention methods and outcome variables employed in their studies.

Future researchers also need to pay much more concrete attention to two other broad and interrelated theoretical perspectives. The implications of the ecological perspective (see chapters 4, 10, and 12) are outlined later in this chapter. The second overlooked perspective incorporates the developmental psychology of body image, eating issues, and preventive education (see chapters 4 and 10). We urge future researchers to think about specific ways the content, learning experiences, and outcome variables of a prevention program should be structured according to the developmental level of the target audience.

The Need for Explicit Models

Many studies of risk factors for eating problems offer a clear theoretical *and* pictorial model to help readers understand the hypotheses being tested and the methodology being used. In contrast, although some prevention studies offer a set of solid theoretical propositions with direct links to prevention techniques, most of the propositions are just that—broadly theoretical. We could not locate a single prevention outcome study that provided a detailed model for understanding the interplay between risk factors, preventive interventions, mediating processes (proximal outcomes), and prevention (distal) outcomes (see chapter 11). We strongly encourage prevention theorists, researchers, dissertation advisors, editors of journals and books, and so forth, to make such models a standard part of the "introduction" to program development and evaluation.

Progress Through Analysis of Specific, Basic Processes

Social cognitive theory, cognitive-behavioral approaches, the Non-Specific Vulnerability-Stressor model, and the feminist-empowerment-relational paradigm are the basis for preventive interventions that seek to instill or change beliefs, attitudes, and behaviors. Consequently, it is surprising how rarely programs have been guided by theory and research concerning attitude change. For example, Ajzen and Fishbein's theory of "Reasoned Action" explains how norms, beliefs, values, and expectations combine to shape intentions and behaviors (see Carter, 1990, for a review). This has clear implications for understanding and deterring a controllable behavior like dieting. Similarly, the "Health Belief Model" (see Janz & Becker, 1984) argues that the likelihood of preventive action by an adolescent girl is determined by a threat–benefit analysis in which she weighs her perceived susceptibility to a condition she considers serious and her beliefs about the benefits of and the barriers to prevention. These sorts of models have helped researchers understand attitudinal and norm-related determinants of various health behaviors, including contraception, physical activity, and seat-belt use (see review by Kohler et al., 1999). However, with the exception of Grodner's (1991) preliminary attempt to apply the Health Belief Model to bulimia nervosa, until recently such focused models of attitudinal and behavioral change have been notably absent in the field of eating problems prevention.

This trend may be changing. Stice's "dissonance reduction" approach to targeted prevention (see chapter 9) and Sanderson's application of "social norm theory" (see chapters 9 and 10) demonstrate how a narrower, process-oriented theory may be applied to prevention. Also encouraging is a line of research by Wertheim, Paxton, and colleagues in Australia. For example, in an extension of research reviewed in chapter 9 (e.g., Heinze et al., 2000; Withers et al., 2002), Paxton, Wertheim, Pilawski, Durkin, and Holt (2002) examined how middle school girls responded to seven different sets of 2- to 3-minute messages about strict dieting. Each set represented themes found in many prevention programs. In terms of relevance, believability, emotional effect, and impact on intention to diet, Paxton et al. (2002) found that the most persuasive message addressed media literacy: "Don't be fooled by the fad diets promoted in the media" (p. 479). The theme of the next most persuasive message was "Skipping meals makes you feel starved so you overeat and feel bad" (p. 479). Consistent with the fact that it is much more difficult to change attitudes than prevent them, Paxton et al. found that girls who reported high levels of dieting and body dissatisfaction were much more resistant to those messages. There is a clear need for more of this type of theory-driven and systematic microanalysis of the healthpromotion messages and practices that make up preventive interventions (see also Sanderson & Holloway, 2003).

RESPONSE TO QUESTIONS 5–6 AND 10–11: PREVENTION IN SCHOOLS CAN WORK BUT IMPROVEMENTS IN UNIVERSAL-SELECTIVE AND SELECTIVE-TARGETED PROGRAMS ARE NECESSARY

Effectiveness

It sounds so simple and obvious: A truly effective prevention program would reduce the number of new cases, that is, the incidence, of eating disorders or eating problems by minimizing the existence or the impact of risk factors such as negative body image. Compared to a similar group of healthy people in general (for universal prevention), or healthy but at-risk people (for universal-selective prevention), who did not receive the preventive intervention, valid assessment of program participants would reveal that they developed fewer instances of disordered eating over a meaningful period of risk (e.g., from ages 13 to 20).

To date, only 4 (4.4%) of the 90 universal-selective programs reviewed in chapters 9 and 13 have included follow-up assessments of 2 or more years in duration. Within this small subset, Killen et al.'s (1993) well-designed social cognitive program was ineffective, Neumark-Sztainer et al.'s (1995) social cognitive program had limited positive long-term effects, and Smolak and Levine's (2001a) social cognitive and developmental program had positive effects on body esteem and weight management only in relation to a potentially noncomparable control group. Piran's 8-year evaluation of three different sets of girls at the elite ballet school where she applied her FER and ecological program (see chapters 8 and 12) yielded very promising results, but there was no control so the results must be seen as preliminary.

One could argue, as indeed we have in this book, that there are a number of *promising* school-based curricular approaches to universal-selective prevention. It is possible that these programs and others in development (e.g., the ecological work of McVey and colleagues in Ontario, Canada; see chapter 12) will turn out to be effective when they are thoroughly and carefully applied (i.e., fidelity is high) and when they are subjected to more rigorous longitudinal evaluations (see chapter 11). Yet the frequency with which classroom curricula yield significant posttest effects that dissipate at follow-up (i.e., the frequency of the "program participation effect") suggests that the impact of classroom programming as it has traditionally been constructed and applied is limited (see chapters 9 and 10). Before considering an ecological approach that extends prevention within the schools and well beyond, we offer a few suggestions for improving curricular programming in the schools.

Multimodal, Integrative Education

The power of information to shape attitudes and influence behavior is enhanced when lessons are integrated across topics within a given school year and reiterated in synchrony with the development of students throughout, for example, middle school (see Gortmaker et al., 1999; Perry, 1999, for examples). With respect to Question 11 (see Table 15.1), gender equity and appreciation of diversity in weight and shape are very relevant to prevention of negative body image and disordered eating, as well as to promotion of safer, more supportive schools (see chapters 8 and 12). Following the themes discussed in chapter 10, these practices could be addressed in interesting and creative ways in a wide variety of classes for girls *and* boys, including biology, history, social studies, health, media studies, English, and the arts. People committed to prevention need to collaborate (see chapter 12) with graduate programs in public health, education, and educational psychology in order to develop broader, more creative, and more developmental approaches to integrative education.

Interestingly, the only program to date that employed an integrative approach to education and that clearly prevented eating problems over the course of its 2-year application was the obesity-prevention program *Planet Health* (Austin et al., 2002, 2005; Gortmaker et al., 1999; see chapter 9).

Integrating Obesity and Eating Problems Prevention

With regard to Question 10 (see Table 15.1), people engaged in preventing negative body image and eating problems can no longer afford either to ignore obesity, or to be content to blame those who refuse to ignore it for fanning the flames of weightist prejudice (see chapters 2 and 3). Obesity is a major health concern for our country, and, increasingly, the United Kingdom and Europe. If we are to collaborate respectfully and effectively with educators, parents, medical professionals, and community leaders, all of whom want to promote positive body image and healthy eating and exercising, we must acknowledge the clear, undeniable links between the development of obesity and of many critical elements in the spectrum of disordered eating. These include body dissatisfaction, disturbances of interoceptive awareness, unhealthy dieting, maladaptive weight management practices (e.g., diet pills and self-induced vomiting), binge eating and other forms of chaotic food consumption, inadequate nutrient intake, and personal factors such as low self-esteem and lack of skills to cope with negative affect and depression. Notice that this list of shared features and issues also links the prevention of obesity and eating problems to prevention of another very significant problem for females that emerges in early adolescence: depression (Bearman et al., 2003). Obesity and eating problems also appear to be influenced in similar ways by certain sociocultural factors. Prominent examples are media messages about indulgence and restraint, and lifestyles that have all but eliminated two important phenomena: (a) casual "family meals" as a time for sharing nutritious foods and emotional support; and (b) more casual activity and exercise, such as walking to school or to the store, playing at neighborhood parks, and school physical education programs. Integration of efforts to prevent obesity and eating problems faces real conceptual and political obstacles (Cogan & Ernsberger, 1999; Irving & Neumark-Sztainer, 2002), but it is a vitally important direction for our field. Those seeking guidance in this integration are referred to the recent work of Neumark-Sztainer and colleagues (Neumark-Sztainer, 2003; Neumark-Sztainer et al., 2003) and of Berg (2001, 2004).

FED: A Synthesis

There is great variety in current approaches to universal-selective prevention, and the results of many programs are limited or inconclusive (see chapters 9 and 13). This makes it difficult to offer guidelines for prevention based on compelling empirical evidence. Nevertheless, many of the successful programs and promising interventions for children ages 10 and older (see chapters 9, 10, and 13) construct special opportunities for students to investigate, discuss, and think critically about sociocultural factors that have a positive or negative influence on body image and eating. With proper guidance from adults, what will likely emerge from such active, student-oriented education is what Piran (personal communication, July 15, 2000) calls "cultural literacy," a type of intellectual and emotional insight into forms of injustice that foster objectification and disembodiment. Cultural literacy subsumes media literacy but is not confined to analyses of media. This relational knowledge can motivate individual and collective actions to change unhealthy influences.

We believe that school-based programming can contribute significantly to prevention if we focus on ways to mobilize the schools in promoting the 4 Cs of prevention and health promotion (Levine, Piran, & Irving, 2003): *C*onsciousness raising (education), *C*ompetency building (skill development), *C*onnections with others (meaningful relationships with peers, adults, and community), and *C*hange in community norms, practices, and systems (development of community assets within an ecological framework). Although the 4 Cs reflect some behavioral elements of the social-cognitive-behavioral model, they draw much more heavily from theory and research in the feminist-empowerment-relational model (consciousness raising, connections, and change), the Non-Specific Vulnerability-Stressor model (competency, connections, e.g., support, and change), and the developmental model (competency, connection, change). These three models expressly emphasize the ecology of development. In addition, the NSVS model is similar to the developmental model in fundamental ways, such as the focus on nonspecific risk factors and on social support. Therefore, with the 4 Cs we are arguing for school-based programming that is feminist, ecological, and developmental. This perspective is captured by the acronym *FED*. One meaning of this word, according to Merriam-Webster's online dictionary (www.m-w.org), is "to furnish something essential to the growth, sustenance, maintenance, or operation" of an organism.

RESPONSE TO QUESTION 7: IMPORTANCE OF CHANGING NORMS, LIFE SKILLS, AND ECOLOGIES—HEALTH PROMOTING SCHOOLS

The 4 Cs of prevention predict what is demonstrated in chapters 9, 10, and 13: *Curricular* programs for universal-selective prevention will have limited effects, in part because such programs tend to focus on the knowledge, attitudes, and skills of *individual* participants. It is strange that, although the *social* cognitive and vulnerability-*stressor* models are the dominant influences on prevention of eating problems, the role of *environments* has typically been limited to *individual* skills for appraising and coping with either specific sources of social pressures for thinness (see chapter 5) or general developmental stressors of adolescence (see chapters 4 and 7). Theory and research in the prevention of cigarette smoking and other substance use is consistent with major theories of prevention in our field in emphasizing the necessity of ecological changes (see chapter 10).

The Theory of Health Promoting Schools

One ecological approach to prevention that is worthy of attention is the "Health Promoting Schools" movement, developed in the 1980s by the World Health Organization (O'Dea & Maloney, 2000; Piran, 1999d). We introduce this approach here because it offers an excellent opportunity to take what the social cognitive, cognitive-behavioral, Non-Specific Vulnerability-Stressor, and feminist-empowerment-relational models contribute to the 4 Cs of prevention and embed these practices in the FED framework.

Health Promoting Schools (HPS) are founded on the assumption that the education and development of students, teachers, and staff are facilitated by good health. Good health requires environments that are safe, responsive to people's needs, and unambiguously caring. Another core belief is that environments will be more caring and more responsive when they apply democratic principles of participation and equity. Consequently, health promoting schools challenge the traditional rigid hierarchies of education (administration "over" teachers "over" students) in order to create student–staff–community partnerships committed to healthy development.

This expansion and organization of stakeholders (see chapters 8, 10, and 12) is designed to promote a number of positive factors that we have advocated in this book, including gender equity, dissociation of women's authority from physical beauty and sexuality, and values and policies that support freedom from various forms of teasing, harassment, and objectification (see chapters 8 and 12). But, perhaps as important, the principles of participation and equity are designed to empower students. Responsibility for constructing and evaluating a healthier school environment is situated directly in the "communities" formed by interactions between students, staff, parents, and the community at large. Consistent with the principles of feminism (chapter 8) and prevention-oriented community psychology (chapters 10 and 12), the real basis for clarifying problems and deciding on solutions is not top-down expertise backed by bureaucratic power. Rather, it is a combination of discussion, relationship building, and critical thinking. In fact, this feature of the HPS model was one of the inspirations for Piran's (1995) early feminist-empowerment-relational prevention work and her current Critical Social Perspectives model. According to the HPS philosophy, this participatory-action approach increases the probability that changes in individual behavior, teacher training, teaching styles, school policies, school norms, and so on, will be sustainable.

The HPS philosophy is explicitly holistic. Nevertheless, for the purpose of constructing more effective, ecological prevention and intervention programs, the realms of a health promoting school can be separated into three categories.

School Organization, Ethos, and Environment

Research from the European Network of Health Promoting Schools confirms the value of a designated Resource Coordinator (see chapter 11) or Health Education Coordinator who takes initial responsibility for overseeing the HPS project (Healy, 1998). The Resource Coordinator's first task is to facilitate discussion among stakeholders in order to clarify school-wide goals concerning health promotion. These goals are likely to include increasing tolerance of and respect for diversity in weight and shape, and promoting positive body image, good nutrition, and physical activity. The process of determining these goals helps to construct working principles (see chapter 1), such as (a) no one is to blame for negative body image and disordered eating, but everyone is responsible for prevention and health promotion; (b) stigmatization of fat people and glorification of dieting are unhealthy, so educators should never dispense weight-loss advice, regardless of the child's size; and (c) racism limits opportunities to be something other than a voiceless body, so multiethnic teams of staff are important for modeling and otherwise teaching respect for diversity in ethnicity as well as in weight and shape.

The Resource Coordinator can lead groups of stakeholders to examine many different aspects of the school environment and, if deemed necessary, to try to make them more healthy. Table 11.1 provided an example of an Ecological Review Checklist. This checklist is a good place to start, but it is very important that each particular ecological review work from the ground up by asking girls and boys, separately, several basic questions:

- What happens at school that helps or makes girls and boys feel *good*—strong, capable, positive—about their bodies or about being "in" their bodies?
- What happens at school that helps girls and boys feel *bad*—anxious, self-conscious, weak, helpless, negative—about their bodies or about being in their bodies?

School environments are complicated and fluid, so assessment of policies, practices, and the physical setting needs to be an ongoing process. In addition to leading the analysis and improvement of environments, the Resource Coordinator should also serve as an advocate and sounding board for students and staff, and as a catalyst for interactions between the school, the parents, and the community.

The health-promoting qualities of a school's ethos are heavily dependent on the knowledge, attitudes, and behavior of influential individuals, most notably administrators, teachers, and coaches. The content of classroom lessons and other structured educational experiences is, of course, very important in the process of health education (see chapter 10). But so is the presence of positive role models and strong advocates for the health and well-being of young people. We acknowledge that telling people "how to live" or "how to teach" is often a futile and even risky proposition. Nevertheless, as adults committed to young people and to education, educators can be helped to consider the nature and importance of their own behavior inside and outside the classroom. Table 15.2 offers some recommendations for ways in which teachers and those who teach them (e.g., a Resource Coordinator) can work to be good role models and solid advocates for health.

Surprisingly, relatively little has been written about the specifics of training teachers in education for preventing eating problems (see, e.g., Levine, 1987; Piran, 2004; Shisslak et al., 1990). Several preliminary studies suggest that a 60- to 90-minute training session can help high school faculty and staff learn more about eating problems and become more aware of their potential role in selective and targeted prevention (Chally, 1998; Toledo & Neumark-Sztainer, 1999). As noted in chapter 12, the USDHHS's Office of Women's Health (1999) worked with expert clinicians, prevention researchers, and nonprofit organizations to develop the *BodyWise* program (see Appendix B). It is designed to motivate, educate, and support middle school teachers, counselors, administrators, and parents who want to participate in all the levels of

TABLE 15.2
10 Sample Practices for Educators in Being a Healthy Role Model

- Eliminate jokes, stories, pictures, self-disparaging remarks, and so forth, that glorify slenderness and vilify fat and fat people.
- Promote safety and respect for females and males of all ages and all shapes. In particular, take girls and women seriously, regardless of their size, shape, weight, age, and such.
- Refuse to play the "body disparagement" game. Do not engage in calorie-restrictive dieting and in making negative remarks about your own body.
- Bring in and eat—and share—healthy and fun snacks.
- Exercise for fun, fitness, and friendship—not to compensate for calories eaten or other forms of "being bad." Take advantage of opportunities for physical activities at school: stretch, take walks, participate in (and maybe organize) teacher events at track and field days.
- Exercise your right to dance, swim, play, and dress with your own style, regardless of body shape and body weight.
- Compliment other adults—in their presence and when they are not there—about things they do well. It is fine to compliment appearance occasionally but include compliments for people who look different from the societal ideal.
- Encourage others to say and think positive things about themselves. Help them recognize their own skills and strengths.
- Show respect for the concerns people express (e.g., about prejudice, teasing, limitations due to gender roles). Try to help them find active solutions rather than just telling them to ignore or tolerate the problem.
- Study culture, cultures, history, gender, resistance, and change. Share (and create) stories of resistance to unhealthy cultural influences, and in so doing try to provide alternative images of pride, competence, care, and respect.

prevention by serving as personal agents of influence inside and outside the classroom. Other, similar resources are listed in Appendix B.

One major shortcoming in current curricular programs to prevent eating problems has been insufficient attention to teachers, coaches, and other key educational personnel. It is important to conduct educational and dialogical forums with teachers, coaches, and parents, prior to intervening with students. In addition to basic education about body image and adolescent development, these conversations help adults examine their own prejudices and experiences in the body domain, and identify unhealthy and healthy aspects of particular school systems. In a pilot study, Piran (2004) found that, after a 3-hour workshop about body image development, teachers increased their intentions to not continue promoting weightist attitudes, as well their awareness of how powerful school norms are transmitted by educators and peer groups. These interactive sessions may be a very significant first step in helping teachers and other adults to be active partners in the process of critical thinking and constructive change.

Curriculum, Teaching, and Learning

As noted previously, a multimodal, integrated, and developmentally sensitive curriculum can immerse students in the 4 Cs of prevention and help them learn life skills necessary for making and sustaining positive changes in their lives (see chapters 9 and 10). The Health Promoting Schools movement agrees that curriculum development, including teacher training, is a key feature of a school's ethos. In this respect, styles of teaching (and the training of teachers) should reinforce that classrooms are safe and respectful places for girls and boys, that cultural "literacy" training is valuable for teachers as well as students, and that, in addition to facts (e.g., genetic influences on weight and shape), students should learn life skills such as problem solving and assertive advocacy of a position. Furthermore, schools continue to champion the value of opportunities for student leadership and citizenship. Therefore, across the curriculum, girls and boys should be encouraged to get involved in activities that deemphasize appearance, obsession with weight and shape, and self-preoccupation. Community service projects are particularly desirable in this regard because they promote the simultaneous development of individual and community assets (see chapters 7, 10, and 12); that is, they promote Connection, Competencies, and positive individual and social Change.

School–Community Partnerships

Many adults in the community have a stake in creating health promoting schools. The Resource Coordinator and collaborators within the school need to engage parents, mental health professionals, leaders of service organizations, and so forth, in conversations that deepen connections between school and community. These discussions may have at least four positive outcomes for an ecological program that integrates universal, selective, and targeted prevention. First, they help stakeholders appreciate how negative body image and unhealthy eating patterns are connected to other parental concerns: academic and athletic underachievement, low self-esteem, depression, eating disorders, obesity, problems relating to peers, poor coping skills, prejudice and teasing, cigarette smoking, and lowered ambitions. Second, school–community conversations can provide student participants with an expanded set of role models, and possibly mentors, in the person of women and men who care more about community service and participatory citizenship than about the size of their thighs. Third, carefully developed connections between the school and community leaders can establish the avenues necessary for student activism and advocacy that improve the environments and services provided by the community. Finally, these conversations help the Resource Coordinator work with school staff and community mental health professionals to establish or improve a system for identification, referral, and treatment of students who have an eating disorder or its warning signs.

Parents. Parents are particularly important in school–community partnerships. It is a given that most parents are by necessity extremely busy, and thus they have precious little time for meetings and volunteer activities. However, it is also a given that most parents are committed to education and to the health and well-being of their children. This means that many parents will be motivated to participate in and thereby promote prevention. A few parents will be excited about the prospect of working with school staff and with local businesses and media to help students construct activism and education projects that make the community a better place. The energy, expertise, and connections of these parents should be used and honored.

Whether they are focused on their own families or on the school–community partnership, parents need accurate information about topics such as nutrition, pubertal development, media literacy, and physical fitness. Many parents want and need to know how to respond to questions such as "Mommy, am I fat?" or "Does this dress makes me look fat?" Many parents also want to know how to respond to the painful, anguished silence of boys who have been brutally teased for being "small" and "wimpy." Professionals designing curricular prevention programs should include student homework assignments that encourage dialogues with parents. The Resource Coordinator should try whenever possible to connect parents (and staff) to organizations such as the National Eating Disorders Association (see Appendix A) and Dads and Daughters (see Appendix D). In addition, parents can be included in the process of psychoeducation by being invited to evening seminars and by newsletters sent home that are synchronized with in-class lessons for students.

We are well aware that previous attempts to include parents in psychoeducational programs at school have generated low levels of enthusiasm and participation by parents. However, we also know that prevention specialists in other areas have had some success in this regard (see, e.g., Perry, 1999; Weissberg et al., 1997; see chapter 7). This suggests that the role of parents in collaborative health promotion is an important area for researchers and graduate students who want to make a significant contribution to the prevention of eating problems.

RESPONSE TO QUESTION 7 (CONTINUED): CHANGING NORMS, LIFE SKILLS, AND ECOLOGIES— AN ECOLOGICAL MODEL OF COMMUNITY-BASED, INTEGRATED PREVENTION

Consistent with the tenets of the Health Promoting Schools model, the theory and research discussed in chapters 7, 10, and 12 indicate that universal and selective prevention of eating problems will be facilitated when various forms of health promotion in the school are coordinated with efforts to improve the environments that make up a community. Bronfenbrenner's (1979) ecological model of developmental influences remains a useful tool for conceptualizing environments and how they may be improved for the purpose of preventing a range of problems pertaining to body image and eating (see chapters 4 and 12). In this section, following a brief review of previous community-based prevention efforts, we offer our vision of a comprehensive community-based program for preventing eating problems.

Formative Efforts in Integrated, Community-Based Prevention

In the field of eating disorders there is not much to draw on in formulating a truly ecological prevention program. Outside of the work of Lazter and Shatz (1999; see chapter 14) on an Israeli kibbutz, we are aware of only two major efforts to construct a large-scale, integrated program. In Norway, the National Board of Health and the Ministry of Education created an educational package called "Adolescence and Eating Disorders." In the early 1990s it was distributed free to all secondary schools, colleges, and school health services, as well as to all advanced schools of education and nursing in Norwegian universities (Gresko & Rosenvinge, 1998). This campaign was supplemented by training courses that reached 10,000 school and health care personnel, and by advocacy work to establish regional treatment and prevention centers.

Around the same time, Susan Paxton and seven other clinicians, educators, and activists in Melbourne, Australia, created a nonprofit organization eventually known as Body Image and Health, Inc. From 1990 to 2000 this organization used various sources of funding and alliances with higher education, hospitals, and public health agencies to create a set of interlocking programs. Their focus was mass media, the fashion industry, health and education professionals, fitness centers, schools (using the HPS framework), and public health organizations (Body Image and Health, Inc., 2000). The objective was to promote size acceptance, positive body image as part of self-acceptance, and healthy eating and exercising. As but one example, Paxton and colleagues used data from their own research projects in collaborating with a community health center, various women's groups, and local retailers to develop the *Fashion for Every Woman Project*.

Our Ecological Model of Community-Based, Integrated Prevention

Figure 15.1 presents our working model of one possible ecological approach to prevention. In addition to Bronfenbrenner's nested levels of ecological influence, this model also draws on Blum, McNeely, and Nonnemaker's (2002) application of the principles of developmental psychopathology (see chapter 4) and of the Non-Specific Vulnerability-Stressor paradigm to promotion of resilience and healthy development in adolescents. Blum et al.'s broad construal of Bronfenbrenner's model helps establish preventive interventions that could have positive effects on multiple aspects of adolescent health, not just eating or weight management.

Table 15.3 demonstrates how our ecological model might be specifically applied. To make our application more manageable, we focused on preventing negative body image and eating problems in middle school students living in a single community of 100,000 people. Aspects of the Health Promoting Schools (HPS) approach, as discussed in the previous section, will be applied in the schools (see Fig. 15.1), but they are not reiterated in Table 15.3. Thus, for example, individual teachers and perhaps a coach and a school administrator are part of the microsystem for a middle school student, but programs for them are omitted from that table. Similarly, efforts by adults participating in parent–teacher–administrator associations to promote healthy food choices and exercise options in school would fall under the first entry in Table

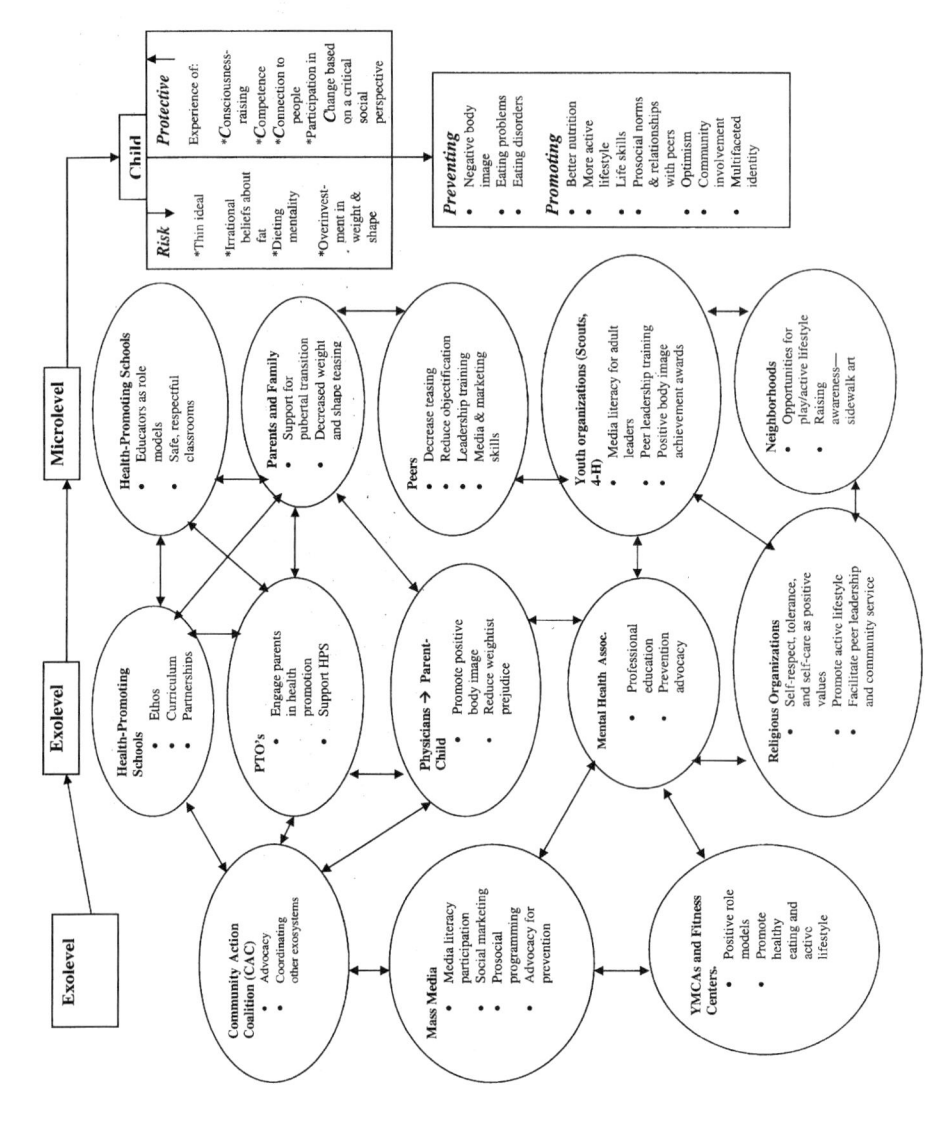

FIG. 15.1. An ecological approach to the prevention of eating problems in middle school students.

TABLE 15.3
Application of a Bronfenbrenner-Type Ecological Model
to Preventing Eating Problems in Middle School Students

Target	Desired Outcomes	Proposed Activity/Program
Microsystem		
Parents	Increase knowledge about pubertal changes and body image.	Mass media + direct mailing = information and motivation.
	Increase ability of mothers and fathers to communicate with children about pubertal changes and body image.	Interactive, experiential "Family Fun Nights" at school or church. Homework assignments requiring collaboration of student and parents and/or grandparents.
		Active recruitment of parents to be part of community coalition overseeing entire ecological program.
	Decrease weight- and shape-related teasing within the family.	Community Action Coalition (CAC) works with Dads and Daughters, Inc. (see chapter 13 and Appendix D) to develop campaign to educate, motivate, and train fathers.
Peers	Reduce weight- and shape-related teasing.	Training of and collaboration with youth group leaders, including older adolescents.
	Reduce objectification.	Poster and public service announcement campaign in theaters, malls, markets, and libraries.
		Peer-led social marketing via t-shirts, posters, etc., created with peer art work.
		Peer leadership programs in middle and high school provide peers for participation in CAC and in prevention in the classroom and neighborhood.

(*Continued*)

379

TABLE 15.3
(Continued)

Target	Desired Outcomes	Proposed Activity/Program
Microsystem *(cont.)*		
Neighborhoods	Increase/reinforce opportunities for play and exercise. Increase neighborhood involvement in supporting prevention.	Peer-designed projects (from school and/or youth groups) to raise awareness, funds, and commitment in neighborhoods. CAC works with banks, local government, and developers to place parks, playgrounds, walking and bike paths, etc., in new neighborhoods, to restore lapsed areas, and to offer indoor activities (e.g., basketball, dance) where outdoors is unsafe.
Scouts & 4-H & Boys and Girls Clubs (and schools)	Increase media literacy skills. Increase awareness of value of positive body image. Decrease teasing.	Education of adult and peer leaders. Development/application of media literacy program, along with projects, badges, and awards to be covered by media (see Exosystem, next). Peer leadership training by adults, with emphasis on (a) what can be done in schools and neighborhoods (note adult–peer–neighborhood–school = mesosystem for child), (b) skill development unrelated to weight and shape, and (c) healthy exercise opportunities.
Exosystem *(Note:* Health Promoting School is assumed)		
Parent–Teacher–Administrator Organizations	Increase commitment of PTOs to Health Promoting Schools. Increase actions of PTOs in supporting healthy food choices and exercise options at school.	PTO involvement in Community Action Coalition. Educational programs for PTOs, supported by prevention-oriented benefits to participating schools.
Mental health professionals in community	Increase awareness of MHA members of spectrum of eating problems, and Bolder Model of prevention.	Involve Mental Health Association (MHA) in community organizing, direct action, and exosystem-level planning. MHA coordinates community-wide ED Awareness Week, including campaign to help mental health professionals and business people reduce objectification of women's bodies (see NEDA in Appendix A).

	Increase awareness of mental health professionals as to what they can do in their daily practice to facilitate prevention. Integrate universal, selective, and targeted prevention.	Coordinate development of a plan whereby mental health professionals work with schools to set up services for selective-targeted prevention, as well as universal-selective prevention. Expert-led workshops, supported by continuing education credit, to provide training in the ways that a prevention philosophy can be synergistic with good "clinical services" in, for example, medicine, public health, social work, psychology.
Physicians (and especially those working with parents and children)	Increase awareness of weightist prejudice in medical personnel.	MHA works with medical association and community funding sources to develop programs that train physicians about ways to promote positive body image, healthy eating, and (when necessary) weight loss, without glorifying thinness and stigmatizing fat people.
	Increase awareness of citizens in general. Increase commitment of key citizens to involvement in prevention.	Construct the CAC: Involve prevention specialists and other public health professionals, parents, medical personnel, MHA, adolescents, religious leaders, and so on, to coordinate entire ecological prevention effort. Mass media campaign.
Citizens in the community		
MHA–Business–Community Connection	Increase involvement of business community in prevention. Increase social marketing of prevention messages (health promotion) to adolescents and parents. Increase awareness of and commitment to acceptance of diversity in size and shape.	Community Action Coalition works with business service groups (e.g., Rotary) to plan and fund outreach to parents. Community Action Coalition works with business professionals and business service groups to plan and fund social marketing in high-traffic areas such as supermarkets, post offices, and libraries. Educational presentations to local civic groups. Develop or restore (a) parks, bike and walking paths, and safe playgrounds, including school playgrounds; and (b) safe, available spaces for indoor activities. Develop *Fashion for Every Woman* size-acceptance project.

(Continued)

TABLE 15.3
(Continued)

Target	Desired Outcomes	Proposed Activity/Program
Exosystem *(cont.)* YMCA, Gyms, Fitness Centers, and Churches (with youth groups & camps)	Increase awareness of personnel to what they can do to help prevent eating problems.	Community Action Coalition works with YMCA leaders to make local YMCA(s) a point of promotion for social marketing consistent with goals of both organizations. Train YMCA coaches, camp counselors, and fitness center instructors, promoting positive body image, respect for diversity, and an active lifestyle.
Mass Media	Increasing awareness of mass media professionals in the community about the *positive* and *negative* effects of mass media on body image, gender roles, eating habits, and so forth. Increase media messages that promote respect for diversity in size and shape, positive body image, rejection of restrictive dieting, and so on.	Involve media professionals in all steps of development of mass media and social marketing campaigns. Involve media professionals in process of developing media literacy programs in local schools. Media literacy programs in school and youth groups will direct activism and advocacy toward local media. Same as above.
School Board(s) and local, state, and federal governments	Increase funding and other support for prevention, for community athletic and recreation centers, and for parks. Increase legal and political support for antiharassment policies in schools.	Lobbying efforts coordinated by the CAC.

15.3 for the "exosystem," but they are assumed to be part of the school–community partnerships in a health promoting school.

As you think critically about this ambitious proposal, keep two other things in mind. First, in accordance with principles discussed in chapter 8 and in chapters 10 through 12, in all phases of prevention we would seek to facilitate prevention through genuinely collaborative, respectful relationships with stakeholders in the community. Second, we would try very hard to involve a wide variety of clinical professions (e.g., psychology, medicine, public health, social work, dietetics, dentistry) in this project. Consequently, the leadership team would focus education, training, and advocacy on integrating improved treatments with all forms of prevention.

Four-Step Model of Program Evaluation

We approached the methodological challenge of community-based, integrated prevention in this hypothetical community by using the Four-Step Model of Program Evaluation developed by Linney and Wandersman (see Dalton et al., 2001, pp. 408–416). Step 1 of this approach is to specify the prevention (distal) goals as established by a needs assessment. As described in Table 15.4, in our hypothetical example the prevention goals are to decrease the prevalence, the incidence, and the severity of negative body image, pathogenic weight management (e.g., skipping meals, using diet pills), subclinical eating disorders (EDNOS), and full-blown eating disorders. In order to achieve the distal prevention goal, we want certain groups to change in particular ways. Those changes constitute the mediating, proximal outcomes of our prevention program. In this example the target groups include teachers and other school staff, parents, peers, neighborhoods, Scouts, 4-H clubs, parent–teacher organizations, and so on (see the far left column in Table 15.3). In order to create the desired changes in the critical groups, we design certain prevention activities or programs. Thus, Step 2 in our evaluation documents the development and implementation of the prevention activities designed to achieve the proximal outcomes for each of the target groups. Step 3 is an evaluation of those proximal outcomes. Table 15.5 provides an example of Steps 2 and 3 for the parents-as-microsystem component of our hypothetical ecological program.

Step 4 is the "impact evaluation." Here we assess whether or not the distal outcome goals, that is, the desired prevention goals, have been achieved. Table 15.4 presents some of the design and measurement de-

TABLE 15.4
Steps 1 and 4: Impact Evaluation—Did Prevention Take Place?

Desired Impact: Prevention Goals for Middle School Girls and Boys	*Basic Design*
Decrease the incidence, prevalence, and severity of: 　Negative body image 　Pathogenic weight management 　Subclinical eating problems 　Full-blown eating disorders	Quasiexperimental: with matched control community in different media market Five-year longitudinal-sequential design of 6th–8th grade boys and girls Begin with baseline measures

Measures From Youth
Stage 1: Self-report measures of beliefs, attitudes, and behaviors related to these constructs
Stage 2: Follow-up structured interviews of samples with high scores on these measures
Stage 3: Focus group data concerning "eating problems at your school"

Other Measures
Surveys of and interviews with parents of middle school children as to what they have observed
Surveys of and interviews with middle school teachers, counselors, and nurses as to what they have observed
Archival data from and interviews with samples of physicians and mental health professionals as to cases treated

---

tails of Step 4 in our hypothetical program. The quasiexperimental design of our impact evaluation is adapted from the methodology of Biglan et al. (2000; see chapter 10). There would be a control (comparison) community of similar size and socioeconomic composition, but from a completely distinct media market. In each community there would be a longitudinal-sequential collection of data. This would allow a comparative determination of the number of new cases emerging over time (i.e., the incidence) in the experimental versus comparison communities, as well as a determination of incidence based on independent successive samples from the same grade(s) in the experimental community. Similarly, this design would allow cross-community comparisons of prevalence (new cases plus continuing cases), as well as longitudinal assessment of within-cohort changes in prevalence and severity of the target problems. The extended time frame is necessary to detect the impact of community-based changes that probably require several years to

TABLE 15.5
Steps 2 and 3: Process and Outcome Evaluation Worksheet for Parents and Family (in the Microsystem) Component

Activity	Process Evaluation	Outcome Evaluation
Mass media and direct mailing re: puberty and body image	How many TV and radio "spots"? How many direct mailings? What percentage of parents read the mailings and were exposed to the TV and radio "spots"? Which ones were valuable?	Parents' scores on surveys of knowledge, attitudes, and behaviors (e.g., successful communication experiences); include knowledge of the specific content contained in mailings and media messages.
"Family Fun Nights" (FFNs) at school or church	How many FFNs, and where? Attendance in raw numbers and as percentage of attendance goals.	(1) Interviews with, and surveys of parents and middle school children about family communication. (2) Interviews with pediatricians and adolescent medicine specialists about adolescents' knowledge and reports of communication with parents. (3) Teacher ratings of parent interest in and involvement in relevant topics.
Collaborative homework assignments involving parents and grandparents	Assignments returned as a percentage of those given out. Number of parents and grandparents participating; and information on who participated: mom, dad, gender of child, GPA of child?	
Recruiting parents for involvement in Community Action Coalition	Types of recruiting activities and number of parents involved.	Interviews with parents who participated to determine what the experience was like and whether those parents have become more "culture-wise."
Coalition works with Dads and Daughters, Inc., to educate, motivate, and organize fathers	Description of interactions with this organization and of resulting events and programs. Number of fathers participating.	Interviews with and surveys of fathers of middle school girls to assess attitudes and behaviors in regard to promoting positive body image.

Note. Process evaluation would also address time spent, problems encountered, and other useful feedback for improving the program.

385

become well established (see chapter 12). Although, admittedly, this design is complicated, it would enable one to apply advanced multivariate techniques to determine how well program participation predicts prevention outcomes (adjusted for covariates such as age, and nested within units such as schools), and to evaluate at least some of the major mediating processes. The application of these statistics (e.g., multilevel analysis of coefficient modeling, or latent growth curve modeling in structural equation modeling analyses) is discussed in MacKinnon and Lockwood (2003).

The plan articulated in Fig. 15.1 and Table 15.3 may strike some readers as naive and grandiose, or, more charitably, as impractical. But this impression is just that: an impression, or at best a null hypothesis. The program we are proposing is based on the specific practices in several successful prevention programs in other fields (see chapter 10). Significant increases in the 4Cs have been achieved by a number of programs that constitute the vanguard of the "Youth Development" movement in adolescent health (Roth & Brooks-Gunn, 2003). Moreover, our ecological proposal embodies the empirically based principles of coordinated programming set forth by representatives of the American Psychological Association's Task Force on Prevention: Promoting Strength, Resilience, and Health in Young People (Weissberg, Kumpfer, & Seligman, 2003; see, e.g., Wandersman & Florin, 2003). In this regard Biglan, Mrazek, Carnine, and Flay (2003) offer a review of several large-scale resources for community-based programming to prevent interrelated problems such as violence, conduct disorder and delinquency, substance abuse, and depression. Examples include the University of Kansas' *Community Tool Box* (http://ctb.lsi.ukans.edu), the University of Illinois' *Collaborative for Academic, Social, and Emotional Learning* (http://www.casel.org) and the Substance Abuse and Mental Health Services Administration's (SAMHSA, under the United States Department of Health & Human Services) *Center for Substance Abuse Prevention* (http://prevention.samhsa.gov/About/contact.asp).

We are well aware that ecological, community-based interventions are not easy to conceptualize, to fund, or to carry out—and that controversy about outcomes cannot be ignored (see, e.g., Stevenson & Mitchell, 2003). Moreover, significant resources, including time, are going to be required in developing, evaluating, and integrating the individual components of coordinated ecological programming in the community. Nevertheless, we believe that the development of components (e.g., as described in Table 13.5, a peer-led social marketing campaign to reduce teasing and objectification) and their integration into ecological, community-based interventions is a critically important part of the future of prevention in our field. The multilevel, ecological focus is dictated by the status of current research in eating disorders prevention, by many developments in the more advanced fields of prevention and health promotion (see Weissberg et al., 2003), and by the environmental focus of all prevention models emphasized in this book.

RESPONSE TO QUESTIONS 8 AND 9: CRITICISM IS HEALTHY, NOT FATAL, AND DIALOGUE IS IMPORTANT

The Challenge of Neuroscience

The spectrum of eating problems, like the continua of mood and anxiety disorders, comprises a set of serious disturbances that can be conceptualized at multiple levels, ranging from the genetic and biochemical to the interpersonal and sociocultural. Consequently, when proponents of the powerful biopsychiatry movement challenge the ability of a sociocultural perspective to explain individual differences in disordered eating, their methodological and empirical concerns must be taken seriously.

However, the biopsychiatric critique of prevention lacks the logic and the evidence to support the oft-heard contention that sociocultural factors are irrelevant and, therefore, universal-selective prevention is futile and ill-advised. There is a great deal of solid evidence for the contention that (a) there has been a substantial rise in the incidence of anorexia nervosa over the past 50 years (Hoek & van Hoeken, 2003); (b) bulimia nervosa and related, subclinical conditions are new psychiatric problems in the last 40 years (Russell, 2004); and (c) sociocultural and interpersonal factors play very important roles in the development, maintenance, and treatment of negative body image and disordered eating (see chapter 5). Furthermore, genetic vulnerability to a spectrum of eating and weight-management problems is still poorly defined (see chapter 3), and so far it has yet to explain the preeminent fact in the field: the extraordinarily gendered nature of eating problems (see chapters 2 and 8). Moreover, the same twin research and liability modeling that supports genetic vulnerability also establishes the importance of nonshared *environments* as sources of vulnerability. It has long been recognized in the study of schizophrenia, mood disorders, and substance abuse that genetic liability operates in some families, but disorders also emerge in people for whom there is no clear-cut genetic vulnerability; and that genetic vulnerability interacts or transacts with psychosocial experiences in order to produce a spectrum of disorder (Merikangas & Avenevoli, 2000; Rende, 1996).

That said, proponents of universal prevention based on a sociocultural perspective cannot ignore either advances in neuroscience (see chapter 3) nor the modest success of selective-targeted (indicated) prevention in reducing negative body image and eating problems (see chapters 9 and 14). Both sets of findings point to a need for improvements in identifying and helping individuals who are at high risk. In this regard it must be acknowledged that one source of risk is genetic vulnerability to eating disorders per se, whatever the nature of that vulnerability may be. In the language of genetic epidemiology (Merikangas & Avenevoli, 2000), prevention specialists need to address the range of preventive interventions dictated by a triangulation of "environmental" factors (e.g., objectification, weightist prejudice) with the "agents" of the problem (e.g., dieting) and with factors pertaining to the "host" (e.g., genetic vulnerability). More universal forms of prevention are needed to address the environmental factors, agents, and certain host factors. The Rose Model of prevention demonstrates that this approach could have a powerful cumulative effect on low-risk individuals, such that the population incidence could be significantly reduced (see chapter 14). But an emphasis on the "host" and individual differences in vulnerability also points to importance of selective-targeted prevention. One such selective-targeted approach to prevention that needs to be developed and evaluated is family-based programming for high-risk daughters of mothers (or, in rare cases, fathers) who are receiving treatment for an eating disorder. This emphasis on individual differences in vulnerability may be particularly important for the goal of preventing full-blown, potentially chronic eating disorders.

Is Prevention Dangerous?

Critics, and even some supporters (e.g., O'Dea, 2000, 2002b), of universal-selective prevention often contend that prevention is potentially dangerous, that is, iatrogenic. That is a serious charge, so this statement needs to be dissected carefully. Analogous to showing children how marijuana is used and then telling them not to use it, certain forms of prevention, such as informing children about purging for weight loss in order to frighten them into avoiding this technique, are indeed probably very unwise (see chapter 10). More subtly, it is possible that raising children's awareness about the glorification of slenderness in the mass media and about the unfair disparity between the range of ordinary bodies and the ideal may result in that disparity becoming more salient—and, thus, in body esteem worsening (see O'Dea, 2000; Smolak et al., 1998b). Conversely, efforts to combat "fear of fat" and to educate about the body's wisdom in weight management may be misinterpreted as "eat anything you like."

There is certainly the potential for negative effects, not just null effects. However, the recent meta-analysis by Stice and Shaw (2004) found little evidence for iatrogenesis in the prevention of eating problems, especially at follow-up. It has long been known that various forms of psychotherapy have a negative effect on a minority of clients and patients. And pharmacotherapy, a cornerstone of the biopsychiatric approach to eating disorders, mood disorders, anxiety disorders, and so on, has a number of well-established negative effects operating under the misnomer of "side" effects. The response to such negative treatment outcomes has been to improve the efficacy and ethics of both these major types of therapies because they have the potential to make a big difference. The same should be true of prevention.

A CONCLUDING STATEMENT: MORE THAN EVER, PREVENTION REQUIRES "THE BOLDER MODEL"

The model of graduate training for clinical psychology in the United States was ratified by the American Psychological Association in 1949 at a conference in Boulder, Colorado. The "Boulder Model" mandates that clinical psychologists be educated as "scientist-practitioners." Based on the feminist principle that "the personal is the political," our late friend and colleague Lori Irving (1999) argued that prevention requires a *Bolder* model of training and practice. This means that professionals committed to prevention of eating problems need to integrate their professional activities as "scientist" and "practitioner" with both political advocacy for multidimensional ecological change and personal commitment to serving as a model of healthy beliefs, attitudes, and practices (see Table 15.2; see also, e.g., Maine, 2000; Kelly, 2002a). This is true not only for clinical and counseling psychologists, but also for psychiatrists, social workers, dietitians, public health educators, and so forth.

We agree. To reiterate: Sociocultural factors are the foundation for the spectrum of eating problems; therefore, sociocultural changes must be the proximal and, ultimately, the distal goal of prevention. This reminds us yet again that, in order to promote the 4 Cs, the field of eating problems prevention needs further advances in theory, programming, and research methodology that address the intersection between developmental–ecological psychology and the psychology of gender. But the Feminist-Ecological-Developmental (FED) perspective also means that those committed to prevention—and to engagement of daughters and sons, students and colleagues, spouses and parents, and, indeed, everyone we encounter in the process—must embrace the desired changes in attitudes about gender, weight, body shape, eating, and health by embodying these changes in their own lives. This lifestyle will at times be ambiguous, anxiety provoking, and alienating, but also invigorating, exciting, and enriching. But, then, true activism, which has resulted in many significant improvements in the health and well-being of women and men over the past 200 years, always is.

Introduction to Appendixes

Whether one is a professional or not, people committed to prevention often have to be very versatile. In addition to requiring a variety of skills, prevention work typically involves contact with, and knowledge about, a wide variety of topics, people, and settings. Consequently, we offer the following appendixes as resources.

If you and your colleagues know of other practical and relatively inexpensive resources, we would appreciate your sharing that information with us. To do so, e-mail either of us at levine@kenyon.edu or smolak@kenyon.edu, or write to either of us at Department of Psychology, Kenyon College, Gambier, OH 43022-9623 USA.

Disclosure

The following lists of organizations, books, curriculum guides, and measures are intended to provide the reader with some guidance, in the form of choices, for prevention programming and for research. Whenever it is relevant, we indicate whether a program has been empirically evaluated. All the measures in Appendix E have some level of the standard forms of reliability and validity.

Of course, we have our own opinions and biases about the different resources. Michael has a long-standing relationship as a volunteer (and former president of the Board of Trustees) for what is now the National Eating Disorders Association. Since 1990, Michael and Linda have contributed a number of educational documents to that organization and its predecessor (EDAP, Inc.). Several times we mention Gürze Books (see www.gurze.com) as a very convenient source for purchasing various books, curriculum guides, and treatment manuals in the field of eating disorders. It is important to note that the current proprietors of that company are friends of Michael's, and that both Linda and Michael benefit from the sale of our books by that company. Furthermore, having worked in this field since the mid-1980s, we know and respect a great many of the women and men whose works and organizations are noted. Some of those people (e.g., Sandra Friedman, Gail McVey, JoAnne Ikeda, Joe Kelly, Margo Maine, Dianne Neumark-Sztainer, Jennifer O'Dea, Susan Paxton, and Elizabeth Scott) kindly provided various forms of support for this book.

With these disclosures in mind, please be informed that the inclusion of any particular resource is not an endorsement of that resource for your particular needs. It is crucial, as we have noted in this book, that you work closely with various stakeholders to clarify your particular prevention needs and goals, and to assess firsthand which of several possible resources might best meet those particular needs and goals.

Appendix A: Eating Disorder Organizations and Web Sites

These organizations and Web sites offer a wealth of information about the nature and treatment of eating disorders, choosing a therapist, meeting the challenges for recovery, getting involved in activism and advocacy, opportunities for prevention, and so on. Some of the organizations sponsor specific programs such as Eating Disorders Awareness Week (e.g., NEDA); some offer guidelines for developing support groups (e.g., ANAD); some have advice and extensive resources concerning children and weight (see, e.g., BodyPositive); and some are engaged in lobbying and other political action at the national level (e.g., Eating Disorders Coalition). Most have well-organized lists of resources and links to other sites.

It is recommended that you consult at least two when seeking specific types of information concerning prevention or any other important topic (e.g., choosing a therapist).

Organizations (in alphabetical order)

Body Image Coalition of Peel
c/o Peel Health,
9445 Airport Road
3rd Floor, West Tower
Brampton, Ontario
L6S 4J3
CANADA

www.bodyimagecoalition.org
info@bodyimagecoalition.org

APPENDIX A

**Eating Disorders Coalition
for Research, Policy, & Action**
611 Pennsylvania Avenue
Washington, DC 20003-4303
USA

www.eatingdisorderscoalition.org
Phone/Fax: 202-543-9570

**Eating Disorders Foundation of
New South Wales, Inc.**
P.O. Box 532
Willoughby NSW 2068
Australia

www.edf.org.au
Phone: (61) 9412 4499
e-mail: edf@edf.org.au

**National Association of
Anorexia Nervosa and
Associated Disorders (ANAD)**
Box 7
Highland Park, IL 60035
USA

www.anad.org
Phone: 847-831-3438
Fax: 847-433-4632

**National Eating Disorders
Association (NEDA)**
603 Stewart Street, Suite 803
Seattle, WA 98101
USA

www.nationaleatingdisorders.org
Phone: 206-382-3587
Treatment Referral:
              1-800-931-2237

**National Eating Disorder
Information Centre (NEDIC)**
CW 1-211, 200 Elizabeth Street
Toronto, Ontario M5G 2C4
CANADA

www.nedic.ca
Phone: 416-340-4156 (in Toronto)
              866-633-4220
Fax: 416-340-4376

**The National Centre for Eating
Disorders**
54 New Road
Esher, Surrey KT10 9NU
United Kingdom

http://www.eating-disorders.org.uk
Phone: 01372 469493

**Victorian Centre of Excellence in
Eating Disorders (CEED)**
8th Floor, CCB
Royal Melbourne Hospital
Grattan St.
Parkville
Melbourne, Victoria 3052
Australia

http://www.rch.org.au/ceed/
Phone: (03) 9342 7507
Fax: (03) 9342 8216
e-mail: ceed@mh.org.au

Other Web Sites

Eating Disorder Referral www.edreferral.com
and Information Center www.edreferral@aol.com

BodyPositive.com Great source of information and resources (e.g., links to other Web sites) concerning ways to promote positive body image in people of all ages.

Mirror-mirror.org/eatdis.htm *Eating Disorders* and *Getting Help* sections contain a wealth of solid, introductory information.

Something-fishy.org Extensive Web site providing information and support in regard to many aspects of eating disorders.

Appendix B: Resources for Educators and Clinicians Committed to Prevention

A number of the resources for educators, such as the books for elementary school children, or the Web sites, would also be fine resources for parents.

BOOKS ON BODY IMAGE, WEIGHT AND SHAPE ISSUES, TEASING, AND EATING DISORDERS
[see www.hedc.org and click on "children's reading list"]

Elementary School Fiction

Mills, A., Osborn, B., & Neitz, E. (Illustrator). (2003). *Shapesville.* Carlsbad, CA: Gürze.
Newman, L. (1991). *Belinda's bouquet.* New York: Putnam & Sons.
Zeckhausen, D., & Boyd, B. (Illustrator). (2003). *Full mouse, empty mouse.* Atlanta, GA: Eating Disorders Information Network (EDIN; see www.edin-ga.org for information about this children's book and 5-day companion lesson plan).

Late Elementary/Middle School Fiction

Blume, J. (1974). *Blubber.* New York: Bantam Doubleday.
Jasper, K. (1988). *Are You Too Fat, Ginny?* Toronto: Is Five Press. [out of print]

PREVENTION CURRICULUM AND PROGRAM GUIDES

General Guide for School Staff

Victorian Centre for Excellence in Eating Disorders and the Eating Disorder Foundation of Victoria. (2004). *Eating disorders resource for schools. A manual to promote early intervention and prevention of eating disorders in schools.* Victoria, Australia: Author(s). A PDF version of this 93-page resource may be downloaded from the CEED Web site: http://www.rch.org.au/ceed/.

Elementary School

Ikeda, J., & Naworski, P. (1992). *Am I fat? Helping young children accept differences in body size.* Santa Cruz, CA: ETR Associates. [Outstanding, but out of print]

EDAP, Inc. (NEDA). (1996). *Prevention Puppet Project.* Puppets, scripts, follow-up activities, and facilitators' guide by Linda Smolak is available from NEDA at www.nationaleatingdisorders.org. See Irving (2000) for evaluation.

Kater, K. (1998). *Healthy body image: Teaching kids to eat, and love their bodies, too!* Curriculum for Grades 4–6 is available from the NEDA at www.nationaleatingdisorders.org or Gürze Books. See Kater et al. (2000, 2002) for evaluation. Revised version available in late 2005.

Menassa, B. N. (2004). *Preventing eating disorders among pre-teen girls: A step-by-step guide.* Westport, CT: Greenwood Publishing/Praeger [www.greenwood.com]—not evaluated.

Zeckhausen, D., & Boyd, B. (Illustrator). (2003). *Full mouse, empty mouse.* Atlanta, GA: Eating Disorders Information Network (see www.edin-ga.org for information about this book and 5-day companion lesson plan)—not evaluated.

Middle School

U.S. Department of Health & Human Services, Office of Women's Health. (2003). *BodyWise* program (updated 2003). Created with consultation from a variety of educators and eating disorders experts, this packet provides school personnel and policymakers with specific ideas for preventing and responding effectively to eating disorders. If you have access to the Internet and if you have Adobe Acrobat or some other reader, go to: www.4woman.gov/BodyImage/bodywise/bodywise.htm or call National Women's Health Information Center: 1-800-994-WOMAN.

Dalle Grave, R., & De Luca, L. (1999). *Prevenzione dei disturbi dell 'alimentazione* [Prevention of eating disorders]. Verona: Positive Press [www.positivepress.net/aidap]. See Dalle Grave et al. (2001) for evaluation. [In Italian]

Friedman, S. S. (2003). *Just for girls: Facilitator's manual* [updated]. Vancouver: Salal Books. Available from Salal Communications, Ltd. [see www.salal.com]—not evaluated.

Friedman, S. S. (2003). *Nurturing GirlPower: Integrating eating disorder prevention/intervention skills into your practice* [updated]. Salal Books. Available from Salal Communications, Ltd. [www.salal.com].

Gortmaker, S. L., et al. (1995). *Planet Health* [curriculum that aims to increase activity, improve dietary quality, and decrease inactivity]. Cambridge, MA: Harvard University Prevention Research Center on Nutrition and Physical Activity. See http://www.hsph.harvard.edu/prc/proj_planet.html, or call (617) 432-1358. See Gortmaker et al. (1999), Austin et al. (2002, 2005), and chapter 9 for evaluation.

Manley, R. (1996). *Teaching body confidence: A comprehensive curriculum for girls.* See www.gurze.com; not evaluated.

O'Dea, J. (1995). *Everybodys different* [handbook of activities]. Available from the University of Sydney, Faculty of Education, Building A35, NSW, 2006, Australia. See O'Dea and Abraham (2000) and chapter 7 for evaluation.

Partnership for Women's Health. (2003). *Helping girls become strong women.* Columbia University. For more information, call 212-326-8860; no published evaluation.

Pryor, T., & Konek, J. (2002). *RSVP: Respect Self Value People: Middle school student lesson and activity guide.* See www.gurzc.com. Not evaluated.

Scott, E., & Sobczak, C. (2002). *Body aloud! Helping children and teens find their own solutions to eating and body image problems.* Berkeley, CA: The Body Positive [2550 9th Street, 204B, Berkeley, CA 94710; 510-548-0101]. Not evaluated.

Seaver, A., McVey, G., Fullerton, Y., & Stratton, L. (1997). *Every BODY is a Somebody: An active learning program to promote healthy body image, positive self-esteem, healthy eating and an active lifestyle for adolescent females: Teachers Guide.* Brampton, ON: Body Image Coalition of Peel. For more information: www.bodyimagecoalition.org (see McVey et al., 2003a, and McVey, Davis, et al., 2004, for evaluation); also available in French.

High School: Body Image and Eating Disorders

Levine, M. P., & Hill, L. (1991). *A five-day lesson plan on eating disorders: Grades 7–12.* Seattle, WA: National Eating Disorders Association. Not evaluated.

NEDA. (1998). *GO GIRLS!* Seattle, WA: Author. [Media Literacy program]—see program and evaluation details in chapter 13.

Neumark-Sztainer, D. (1992). *The weigh to eat! A program for the prevention of eating disturbances among adolescents.* Contact Dr. Neumark-Sztainer, Division of Epidemiology, School of Public Health, University of Minnesota, Minneapolis, MN 55455. See Neumark et al. (1995) & chapter 6 for evaluation. [note: Contact Neumark@epi.umn.edu for information about her other programs, such as *Free to be Me* (see chapter 13) and *New Moves* (see Neumark-Sztainer et al., 2003)]

High School Girls: Weight, Shape, and Drugs

Elliot, D., Goldberg, L., et al. (1996). *Athletes targeting healthy exercise and nutrition alternatives* (ATHENA). Portland, OR: Oregon Health & Science University (Division of Health Promotion & Sports Medicine CR110, 3181 SW Sam Jackson Park Road, Portland, OR 97201). See http://www.ohsu.edu/hpsm/athena.html. See also chapter 13 for evaluation.

High School Boys: Shape and Steroids

Goldberg, L., & Elliot, D. (1999). *Athletes training and learning to avoid steroids* [ATLAS]. Portland, OR: Oregon Health & Science University (Division of Health Promotion & Sports Medicine CR110, 3181 SW Sam Jackson Park Road, Portland, OR 97201). See http://www.ohsu.edu/hpsm/atlas.html. See also Goldberg et al. (2000) and chapter 13 for evaluation.

TARGETED PREVENTION

Middle School and High School

Shiltz, T. J. (1997). *Eating concerns support group curriculum grades 7–12.* Greenfield, WI: Community Recovery Press (P.O. Box 20979, Greenfield, WI 53220).

College

Inflexxion, Inc. (2003). *Food, mood, and attitude*® [computer software]. Newton, MA: Author. Go to www.inflexxion.com or write to Inflexxion® , Inc., 320 Needham Street, Suite 100, Newton, MA 02464 (toll free: 800.848.3895).

RESOURCES COMPILED FOR OR WITH ATTENTION TO ETHNIC MINORITY OR NON-ENGLISH-SPEAKING GROUPS

Spanish

Calvo Sagardoy, R. (2002). *Anorexia y bulimia: Guía para padres, educadores y terapeutas* [Anorexia and bulimia: Guide for parents, educators, and therapists]. Barcelona, Spain: Planeta Practicos/Editorial Planeta.

Centers for Disease Control. Entire Web site available in Spanish. For example, on July 25, 2004, clicking on http://www.cdc.gov/spanish/prevencion.htm resulted in *Prevención: Lucha contra la obesidad epidémica* [Prevention: Combating the obesity epidemic].

Grupo Zarima-Prevención. (n.d.). *Guía practica: Prevención de los trastornos de la conducta alimentaria* (Segunda edicion) [Practical guide: Prevention of disordered eating behaviors]. Contact Dr. Pedro Manuel Ruiz Lázaro at pmruiz@aragob.es.

Ruiz Lázaro, P. M. (2002). *Bulimia y anorexia: Guía para familias* [Bulimia and anorexia: Guide for families]. Zaragoza, Spain: Libros Certeza (certeza@certeza.com).

New Mexico Media Literacy Project. (n.d.). *Medios y remedios: La alfabetización de los medios de communicación para la salud* [Media and remedies: Media literacy for health]. Free media literacy CD-ROM—available in Windows/Mac. See NMMLP Web site: www.nmmlp.org.

U.S. Department of Health & Human Services, Office of Women's Health. (2003). *BodyWise* program. Described earlier under Middle School Prevention Curricula and Program Guides. See, for example, the reproducible handout *Jóvenes Latinas: Hoja de información sobre los desórdenes de la alimentación* [Latina youth: Information sheet about eating disorders].

African American and Other Non-White Groups

Nichter, M., Vukovic, N., & Parker, S. (1999). The Looking Good, Feeling Good Program: A multiethnic intervention for healthy body image, nutrition, and physical activity. In N. Piran, M. Levine, & C. Steiner-Adair (Eds.), *Preventing eating disorders: A handbook of interventions and special challenges* (pp. 175–193). Philadelphia, PA: Brunner/Mazel.

Thompson, B. W. (1994). *A hunger so wide and so deep: American women speak out on eating problems*. Minneapolis: University of Minnesota Press.

MEDIA LITERACY AND ACTIVISM: SAMPLE RESOURCES

Action Coalition for Media Education (ACME) 6400 Wyoming Blvd, NE Albuquerque, NM 87109	www.acmecoalition.org Phone: 505-828-3377 Fax: 505-828-3142	Media literacy skills, advocacy for democratic media systems

APPENDIX B

Center for Media Literacy 3101 Ocean Park Blvd, #200 Santa Monica, CA 90405	www.medialit.org cml@medialit.org Phone: 310-581-0260 Fax: 310-581-0270	Resources, best practices, and professional development
Just Think Foundation 39 Mesa St. Suite 106 San Francisco, CA 94129	www.justthink.org think@justthink.org Phone: 415-561-2900 Fax: 415-561-2901	*MyBody Image* Curriculum + Teacher's guide
Media Education Foundation 26 Center Street Northampton, MA 01060	www.mediaed.org Phone: 800-897-0089 Fax: 800-659-6882	Offers videos of the work of J. Kilbourne & others addressing gender, media, athletics, etc.
Media Literacy Online Project Center for Advanced Tecnology University of Oregon Eugene, OR 97403	http://interact.uoregon.edu/MediaLit/mlr/home [click on resource links]	Wonderful source for many different types of information and links in regard to media literacy
Mind on the Media P.O. Box 1816 Burnsville, MN 55337	www.mindonthemedia.org tbio@mindonthemedia.org Phone: 952-210-1625	"Promote healthy body image & expand the definition of what makes people beautiful"
New Mexico Media Literacy 6400 Wyoming Blvd. NE Albuquerque, NM 87109	www.nmmlp.org e-mail: nmmlp@nmmlp.org Phone: 505-828-3129 Fax: 505-828-3142	Leader in media education, activism, and advocacy
Ontario Media Literacy Project	http://angelfire.com/ms/MediaLiteracy	Great introduction to media literacy for K–12 teachers

OBESITY, HEALTHY EATING, AND ACTIVE LIFESTYLE
(www.bodypositive.com/childwt.htm [Resources on Children & Weight Programming] was the source of some of these Web sites)

Center for Weight & Health J. P. Ikeda, Co-Director College of Natural Resources University of California 101 Giannini Hall #3100 Berkeley, CA 94720-3100	www.cnr.berkeley.edu/cwh/	Outstanding source on obesity, children, and spectrum of eating problems

Action for Healthy Kids 4711 West Golf Road Suite 806 Skokie, IL 60076	actionforhealthykids.org	Collaborate with local & state resources to create health promoting schools
National Center for Chronic Disease Prevention and Health Promotion Centers for Disease Control & Prevention 4770 Buford Highway, NE, MS/K-24 Atlanta, GA 30341-3717	www.cdc.gov/nccdphp/dnpa/index.htm Phone: 770-488-5820 Fax : 770-488-5473	CDC site for information about overweight, obesity, physical activity, and nutrition
Society for Nutrition Education 7150 Winton Drive, Suite 300 Indianapolis, IN 46268	www.sne.org [click on "positions and resolutions"] Phone: 800-235-6690	*Guidelines for Childhood Obesity Prevention Programs* (2003)

UNDERSTANDING, RESPECTING, AND CELEBRATING DIVERSITY IN GENDER, SIZE, AND SHAPE

American Association of University Women. (undated). *Harassment-free hallways.* Guide, along with report, can be downloaded free from the following: http://www.aauw.org/k-12/

Council on Size & Weight Discrimination, Inc. Contact this organization at P.O. Box 305, Mount Marion, NY 12456, or 845-679-1209, or www.cswd.org. They have a Size Discrimination Packet and a Kids Project Packet available for only a couple of dollars each.

National Women's History's Project, 7738 Bell Road, Windsor, CA 95492-8518. [www.nwhp.org]. The Spring 2000 catalogue offers a variety of resources, including a classroom activity kit, bookmarks, Women Who Dare calendars, and illustrated books such as *Remarkable Women of the 20th Century, The Thinking Girl's Guide to the Hippest Women in History*, and the resource guide entitled *Once Upon a Heroine: 450 Books for Girls to Love*.

New Moon Magazine is a professionally produced, advertisement-free magazine created by and for girls ages 8–14. New Moon Publishing has attracted considerable attention for its award-winning "Turn Beauty Inside Out" campaign. Contact the publication at P.O. Box 3587, Duluth, MN 55803-3587; 800-381-4743; or at www.newmoon.org.

Tolerance.org describes itself as "is a principal online destination for people interested in dismantling bigotry and creating, in hate's stead, communities that value diversity." Contact this organization at www.tolerance.org or Tolerance.org c/o The Southern Poverty Law Center, 400 Washington Ave., Montgomery, AL 36104; Phone: (334) 956-8200; Fax: (334) 956-8488.

Appendix C:
Resources for Parents

BOOKS AND ARTICLES ON BODY IMAGE, WEIGHT/ SHAPE PROBLEMS, AND EATING DISORDERS

Eating, Weight, and Body Image

Berg, F. M. (2001). *Children and teens afraid to eat: Helping youth in today's weight-obsessed world.* Hettinger, ND: Healthy Weight Network. [www.healthyweight.net/]

Berg, F. M. (2004). *Underage & overweight: America's childhood obesity crisis—What every family needs to know.* Long Island City, NY: Hatherleigh Press.

Cordes, H. (2000). *Girl power in the mirror: A book about girls, their bodies, and themselves.* Minneapolis, MN: Lerner Publishing. [See also www.gurze.com]

Friedman, S. S. (2000). *When girls feel fat: Helping girls through adolescence.* Toronto: HarperCollins.

Friedman, S. S. (2002). *Body thieves—Help girls reclaim their natural bodies and become physically active.* Vancouver, BC (Canada): Salal Books. [see www.salal.com]

Kater, K. (2004). *Real kids come in all sizes: 10 essential lessons to build your child's body esteem.* New York: Broadway Books.

Kelly, J. (2002a). *Dads and daughters: How to inspire, understand, and support your daughter when she is growing up so fast.* New York: Broadway Books.

Maine, M. (2004). *Father hunger* (2nd ed.). Carlsbad, CA: Gürze.

Waterhouse, D. (1997). *Like mother, like daughter: How women are influenced by their mothers' relationship with food—and how to break the pattern.* New York: Hyperion.

Obesity

Ikeda, J. P. (2004). *If my child is overweight, what should I do about it?* [pamphlet]. Available by calling 800-994-8849 or through UC Agricultural and Natural Resources online catalog: http://anrcatalog.ucdavis.edu [prod. Code 21455]

Kosharek, S. M. (2003). *If you child is overweight: A guide for parents* (2nd ed.). Order from American Dietetic Association, 216 West Jackson Blvd., Chicago, IL 60606-6995, (800) 877-1600 ext. 5000 [www.eatright.org].

Moran, R. (1999). *Evaluation and treatment of childhood obesity*. Article retrieved July 25, 2004, from Web site of the American Academy of Family Physicians, http://www.aafp.org/afp/990215ap/861.html.

Eating Disorders

Bryant-Waugh, R., & Lask, B. (2004). *Eating disorders: A parents' guide* (rev.). London & New York: Brunner-Routledge.

Costin, C. (1997). *Your dieting daughter. Is she dying for attention?* New York: Brunner/Mazel.

Herrin, M., & Matsumoto, N. (2002). *The parent's guide to childhood eating disorders.* New York: Henry Holt (Owl Books).

Natenshon, A. (1999). *When your child has an eating disorder: A step-by-step workbook for parents and other caregivers*. San Francisco: Jossey-Bass.

Sherman, R., & Thompson, R. A. (1997). *Bulimia: A guide for family & friends* (rev.). Lexington, MA: Lexington Books.

Siegel, M., Brisman, J., & Weinshel, M. (1997). *Surviving an eating disorder: Strategies for family and friends* (Revised & updated). New York: HarperPerennial.

ORGANIZATIONS AND WEB SITES

American Academy of Pediatricians
141 Northwest Point Boulevard
Elk Grove Village, IL 60007-1098

http://www.aap.org/family/mediaimpact.htm
Phone: 847-434-4000
Fax: 847-434-8000

Understanding the Impact of Media on Children & Teens—section of Web site for parents

Harvard Eating Disorders
WACC 725
15 Parkman St.
Boston, MA 02114

www.hedc.org
Phone: 617-236-7766

List of children's books promoting (a) respect for diversity in weight, shape, gender, etc.; (b) healthy lifestyles

Healthy Weight Network
402 South 14th Street
Hettinger, ND 58639

www.healthyWeight.net
Phone: 701-567-2646

Health at Every Size approach to eating, activity, weight, and weight management in children and adults

National Institute on Media and the Family
606 24th Avenue South
Suite 606
Minneapolis, MN 55454

www.mediafamily.org
Voice: 612-672-5437
Phone: 1-888-672-5437
Fax: 612-672-4113

National nonprofit, nonpartisan, and nonsectarian organization to maximize benefits and minimize harm of media use

APPENDIX C

Changing the Channels
Cornelius Foundation
P.O. Box 10307
Winston-Salem, NC 27023

www.changingchannels.org
Phone: 336-945-5016
Fax: 336-945-2780

Nonprofit, faith-based organization offers research-based articles and tips for making healthy use of media

Appendix D: Resources for Advocacy and Activism

Note that many of these resources have information or features that are designed for educators and/or parents.

GUIDE FOR COMMUNITY ORGANIZING AND PLANNING: BODY IMAGE

State Government of Victoria Australia, Department of Human Services. (2002). *Shapes: Body image program planning guide*. This 32-page document is available on the Web at: http://www.health.vic.gov.au/healthpromotion/quality/body_image.htm

BOOKS ON BODY IMAGE, EATING DISORDERS, AND CULTURE

Kilbourne, J. (1999). *Deadly persuasion: Why women and girls must fight the addictive power of advertising.* New York: Free Press.

Maine, M. (2000). *BodyWars: Making peace with women's bodies. An activist's guide*. Carlsbad, CA: Gürze.

WEB SITES

About-Face
P.O. Box 77665
San Francisco, CA 94107

www.about-face.org
Phone: 415-436-0212

Combats negative & distorted images of women in media.

Dads and Daughters
34 East Superior St., Suite 200
Duluth, MN 55802

www.dadsanddaughters.org
Info@dadsanddaughters.org
Phone: 888-824-3237

Leader in activism and advocacy, and in importance of fathers.

APPENDIX D

Girls International Forum P.O. Box 16007 St. Paul, MN 55616	www.girlsforum.org forum@girlsforum.org Phone: 651-270-7798	Works to empower girls to take action on sports, media, employment, and other issues affecting them.
Henry J. Kaiser Family Foundation: Entertainment, Media Partnerships 2400 Sand Hill Road Menlo Park, CA 94025	www.kff.org Phone: 650-854-9400 Fax: 650-854-4800	Works with entertainment industry to help convey health messages to the public.
Mind on the Media 710 St. Olaf, Suite 200 Northfield, MN 55057	www.mindonthemedia.org Phone: 952-210-1625	Girls, politics, empowerment & voice
New Moon Publishing 34 E. Superior St., Suite 200 Duluth, MN 55802	www.newmoon.org newmoon@newmoon.org Phone: 1-800-381-4743 Fax: 218-728-0314	*New Moon* magazine (by and for young adolescent girls); *Turn Beauty Inside Out* campaign
Reel Grrls Project 911 Media Arts Center 117 Yale Ave., N Seattle, WA 98109	www.reelgrrls.org Phone: 206-682-6552 Fax: 206-682-7422	Curriculum combines consciousness-raising & art and activism.
Red Wing, MN *GO GIRLS!*™ Attn: Sarah Stinson 1407 W. 4th Street Red Wing, MN 55066 Office Tel: (651) 267-3506	www.redwinggogirls.com sarah@redwinggogirls.com see also redwinghigherself.com	Example of what a mentor can do with adolescent girls committed to cultural literacy.

Appendix E: Abbreviations for Validated Measures Used in Prevention Studies

(In Alphabetical Order)

Abbrev.	Measure	Reference
BES-C	Body Esteem Scale—Children	Mendelson & White (1993)
BES-WC	Body Esteem Scale (Weight Concern Subscale)	Franzoi & Shields (1984)
BSQ	Body Satisfaction Questionnaire	Cooper, Taylor, Cooper, & Fairburn (1987)
ChEAT	Children's Eating Attitudes Test	Maloney et al. (1989)
DEBQ	Dutch Eating Behavior Questionnaire	Van Strien et al. (1986)
DIS	Dietary Intent Scale	Stice (1998b)
EAT	Eating Attitudes Test	Garfinkel & Garner (1982)
EDE	Eating Disorder Examination—Structured Interview	Fairburn & Cooper (1993)
EDE-Q	Eating Disorder Examination—Questionnaire form	Fairburn & Beglin (1994)
EDE-Ch	Eating Disorder Examination—Children's version	Bryant-Waugh et al. (1996)
EDI-2	Eating Disorders Inventory—2nd edition	Garner (1991)
IBSS	Ideal Body Stereotype Scale	Stice et al. (1994)
KEDS	Kid's Eating Disorder Survey	Childress et al. (1993)
MAQ	Media Attitude Questionnaire	Irving et al. (1998)

APPENDIX E

MEDE	McKnight Eating Disorders Examination	The McKnight Investigators (2003); see chapter 14.
MRFScr	McKnight Risk Factor Screen	The McKnight Investigators (2003)
MRFSur	McKnight Risk Factor Survey	Shisslak et al. (1999)
OBC(S)	Objectified Body Consciousness Scale	McKinley & Hyde (1996)
PASTAS	Physical Appearance State and Trait Anxiety Scale	Reed, Thompson, Brannick, & Sacco (1991)
PWBI	Personal Well-Being Inventory	Ryff (1989)
FRS	Figure Rating Scale	Fallon & Rozin (1985)
SATAQ	Sociocultural Attitudes Towards Appearance Questionnaire	Heinberg, Thompson, & Stormer (1995); Smolak, Levine, & Thompson (2001)—boys
SIQYA	Self-Image Questionnaire for Young Adolescents	Petersen, Shulenberg, Abramowitz, Offer, & Jarcho (1984)
SOQ	Self-Objectification Questionnaire	Noll & Fredrickson (1998)
SPPA	Self-Perception Profile for Adolescents	Harter (1986)
WCS	Weight Concerns Scale	Killen et al. (1994); Killen (1996)

References

Abascal, L., Brown J. B., Winzelberg, A. J., Dev, P., & Taylor, C. B. (2004). Combining universal and targeted prevention for school-based eating disorder programs. *International Journal of Eating Disorders, 35,* 1–9.

Abascal, L., Bruning, J., Winzelberg, A. J., Dev, P., & Taylor, C. B. (2002). An Internet delivered intervention to enhance body image in high school students [Abstract]. *Annals of Behavioral Medicine, 24* (Suppl.), S117.

Abood, D. A., & Black, D. R. (2000). Health education prevention of eating disorders among female college athletes. *American Journal of Health Behavior, 24,* 209–219.

About-Face. (1996). *About-face: About time.* Pamphlet and other prevention materials available from About-Face, P. O. Box 77665, San Francisco, CA 94107 (415-436-0212).

Ackard, D., Neumark-Sztainer, D., Hannan, P., French, S., & Story, M. (2001). Binge and purge behavior among adolescents: Associations with sexual and physical abuse in a nationally representative sample: The Commonwealth Fund survey. *Child Abuse & Neglect, 6,* 771–785.

Albee, G. W. (1983). Psychopathology, prevention, and the just society. *Journal of Primary Prevention, 4,* 5–40.

Albee, G. W. (1996). Revolutions and counterrevolutions in prevention. *American Psychologist, 51,* 1130–1133.

Albee, G. W., & Gullotta, T. P. (1997). Primary prevention's evolution. In G. W. Albee & T. P. Gullotta (Eds.), *Primary prevention works* (Issues in children and families' lives, Vol. 6, pp. 3–22). Thousand Oaks, CA: Sage.

Allen, J., Philliber, S., Herrling, S., & Kuperminc, G. (1997). Preventing teen pregnancy and academic failure: Experimental evaluation of a developmentally based approach. *Child Development, 64,* 729–742.

Allison, D. B., & Saunders, S. E. (2000). Obesity in North America. *Psychiatric Clinics of North America, 84,* 305–332.

Altabe, M., & Thompson, J. K. (1996). Body image: A cognitive self-schema construct? *Cognitive Therapy and Research, 20,* 171–193.

Altman, T., Killen, J., Bryson, S., Shisslak, C., Estes, L., McKnight, K., Gray, N., Crago, M., & Taylor, C. B. (1997). Attachment style and weight concerns in preadolescent and adolescent girls. *International Journal of Eating Disorders, 23,* 39–44.

American Association of University Women Educational Foundation (2001). *Hostile hallways: Bullying, teasing, and sexual harassment in school.* Washington, DC: American Association of University Women.

REFERENCES

American Psychiatric Association (2000). *Diagnostic and statistical manual of mental disorders* (4th ed., Text Revision; DSM-IV-TR). Washington, DC: Author.

Andersen, A. E. (1985). *Practical comprehensive treatment of anorexia nervosa and bulimia.* Baltimore: Johns Hopkins University.

Andersen, A. E., Cohn, L., & Holbrook, T. (2000). *Making weight: Men's conflicts with food, weight, shape & appearance.* Carlsbad, CA: Gürze.

Anderson, I. M., Parry-Billings, M., Newsholme, E. A., Fairburn, C. G., & Cowen, P. J. (1990). Dieting reduces plasma tryptophan and alters brain 5-HT function in women. *Psychological Medicine, 20,* 785–791.

Anderson-Fye, E. P., & Becker, A. E. (2004). Sociocultural aspects of eating disorders. In J. K. Thompson (Ed.), *Handbook of eating disorders and obesity* (pp. 565–589). New York: John Wiley.

Anesbury, T., & Tiggemann, M. (2000). An attempt to reduce negative stereotyping of obesity in children by changing controllability beliefs. *Health Education Research: Theory & Practice, 15,* 145–152.

Antoniadis, A., & Lubker, B. B. (1997). Epidemiology as an essential tool for establishing prevention programs and evaluating their impact and outcomes. *Journal of Communication Disorders, 30,* 269–284.

Arthur, M., Hawkins, J. D., Pollard, J., Catalano, R., & Baglioni, A. (2002). Measuring risk and protective factors for substance use, delinquency, and other adolescent problem behaviors. *Evaluation Review, 26,* 575–601.

Atkins, D., & Silber, T. (1993). Clinical spectrum of anorexia nervosa in children. *Journal of Developmental and Behavioral Pediatrics, 14,* 211–216.

Attie, I., & Brooks-Gunn, J. (1989). Development of eating problems in adolescent girls: A longitudinal study. *Developmental Psychology, 25,* 70–79.

Austin, E. W. (1993). Exploring the effects of active parental mediation of television content. *Journal of Broadcasting & Electronic Media, 37,* 147–158.

Austin, E. W., & Johnson, K. (1997). Immediate and delayed effects of media literacy training on third graders' decision making for alcohol. *Health Communication, 9*(4), 323–349.

Austin, S. B. (1999). Fat, loathing and public health: The complicity of science in a culture of disordered eating. *Culture, Medicine, & Psychiatry, 23,* 245–268.

Austin, S. B. (2000). Prevention research in eating disorders: Theory and new directions. *Psychological Medicine, 30,* 1249–1262.

Austin, S. B. (2001). Population-based prevention of eating disorders: An application of the Rose prevention model. *Preventive Medicine, 32,* 268–283.

Austin, S. B., Field, A. E., & Gortmaker, S. L. (2002, April). *The impact of a school-based nutrition and physical activity intervention on onset of disordered eating behaviors in early adolescent girls over two years.* Paper presented at the Academy for Eating Disorders' International Conference, Boston, MA.

Austin, S. B., Field, A. E., Wiecha, J., Peterson, K. E., & Gortmaker, S. L. (2005). The impact of a school-based obesity prevention trial on disordered weight control behaviors in early adolescent girls. *Archives of Pediatrics and Adolescent Medicine, 159,* 225–230.

Bahrke, M., Yesalis, C., Kopstein, A., & Stephens, J. (2000). Risk factors associated with anabolic-androgenic steroid use among adolescents. *Sports Medicine, 29,* 397–405.

Baker, D., Sivyer, R., & Towell, T. (1998). Body image dissatisfaction and eating attitudes in visually impaired women. *International Journal of Eating Disorders, 24,* 319–322.

Bandura, A. (1986). *Social foundations of thought and action: A social cognitive theory.* Englewood Cliffs, NJ: Prentice Hall.

Bandura, A. (1997). *Self-efficacy: The exercise of control.* New York: W. H. Freeman.

Baranowski, M. J., & Hetherington, M. M. (2001). Testing the efficacy of an eating disorder prevention program. *International Journal of Eating Disorders, 29,* 119–124.

Baranowski, T., Perry, C. L., & Parcel, G. (2002). How individuals, environments, and health behavior interact: Social Cognitive Theory. In K. Glanz, F. M. Lewis, & B. K. Rimer (Eds.), *Health behavior and health education: Theory, research, and practice* (3rd ed., pp. 153–178). San Francisco: Jossey-Bass.

Barlow, S. E., & Dietz, W. H. (1998). Obesity evaluation and treatment: Expert committee recommendations. *Pediatrics, 102,* 11 pages. Available at www.pediatrics.org/cgi/content/full/102/3/e29.

REFERENCES 411

Bates, J. (1987). Temperament in infancy. In J. Osofsky (Ed.), *Handbook of infant development* (2nd ed., pp. 1101–1149). New York: Wiley.

Battle, E. K., & Brownell, K. D. (1996). Confronting a rising tide of eating disorders and obesity: Treatment vs. prevention and policy. *Addictive Behaviors, 21,* 755–765.

Bearman, S. K., Stice, E., & Chase, A. (2003). Evaluation of an intervention targeting both depressive and bulimic pathology: A randomized prevention trial. *Behavior Therapy, 34,* 277–293.

Beck, A. T., Rush, A. J., Shaw, B. F., & Emery, G. (1979). *Cognitive therapy of depression.* New York: Guilford Press.

Becker, A. E. (1995). *Body, self, and society: The view from Fiji.* Philadelphia: University of Pennsylvania Press.

Belensky, M. F., Clinchy, B. M., Goldberger, N. R., & Tarule, J. M. (1986). *Women's ways of knowing: The development of self, voice, and mind.* New York: Basic Books.

Benedikt, R., Wertheim, E. H., & Love, A. (1998). Eating attitudes and weight-loss attempts in female adolescents and their mothers. *Journal of Youth and Adolescence, 27,* 43–57.

Bennett, W. B., & Gurin, J. (1982). *The dieter's dilemma: Eating less and weighing more.* New York: Basic Books.

Benson, P. L., Leffert, N., Scales, P. C., & Blyth, D. A. (1998). Beyond the "village" rhetoric: Creating healthy communities for children and adolescents. *Applied Developmental Science, 2,* 138–159.

Berel, S., & Irving, L. (1998). Media and disturbed eating: An analysis of media influence and implications for prevention. *Journal of Primary Prevention, 18,* 415–430.

Berg, F. M. (2001). *Children and teens afraid to eat: Helping youth in today's weight-obsessed world* (3rd ed.). Hettinger, ND: Healthy Weight Network.

Berg, F. M. (2004). *Underage & overweight: America's childhood obesity crisis—What every family needs to know.* Long Island City, NY: Hatherleigh Press.

Berg, M. L., Crosby, R. D., Wonderlich, S. A., & Hawley, D. (2000). Relationship of temperament and perceptions of nonshared environment in bulimia nervosa. *International Journal of Eating Disorders, 28,* 148–154.

Bergen, A., & The Price Foundation Research Collaborative (2003). Candidate genes for anorexia nervosa in the 1p33–36 linkage region: Serotonin 1D and delta opioid receptors display significant association to anorexia nervosa. *Molecular Psychiatry, 8,* 397–406.

Bergin, A. E., & Lambert, M. J. (1978). The evaluation of therapeutic outcomes. In S. L. Garfield & A. E. Bergin (Eds.), *Handbook of psychotherapy and behavior change: An empirical analysis* (2nd ed., pp. 139–189). New York: Wiley.

Biglan, A., Ary, D. V., Smolkowski, K., Duncan, T., & Black, C. (2000). A randomized controlled trial of a community intervention to prevent adolescent tobacco use. *Tobacco Control, 9,* 24–32.

Biglan, A., Mrazek, P. J., Carnine, D., & Flay, B. R. (2003). The integration of research and practice in prevention of youth problem behaviors. *American Psychologist, 58,* 433–440.

Bilukha, O. O., & Utermohlen, V. (2002). Internalization of Western standards of appearance, body dissatisfaction and dieting in urban educated Ukrainian females. *European Eating Disorders Review, 10,* 120–137.

Bloom, M. (1996). *Primary prevention practices* (Issues in children and families' lives, Vol. 5). Thousand Oaks, CA: Sage.

Blum, R. W. (1998). Healthy youth development as a model for youth health promotion. *Journal of Adolescent Health, 22,* 368–375.

Blum, R. W., McNeeley, C., & Nonnemaker, J. (2002). Vulnerability, risk, and protection. *Journal of Adolescent Health, 31S,* 28–39.

Body Image and Health (BIH) Inc. (2000). *Body Image and Health Inc. final report.* Melbourne, Australia: Author. For information, contact Dr. Susan Paxton at Susan.Paxton@latrobe.edu.au.

Bordo, S. (1993). *Unbearable weight: Feminism, Western culture, and the body.* Berkeley: University of California Press.

Bordo, S. (1999). *The male body: A new look at men in public and in private.* New York: Farrar, Straus & Giroux.

Botta, R. A. (2000). The mirror of television: A comparison of Black and White adolescents' body image. *Journal of Communication, 50,* 144–159.

Botvin, G. J. (1996). Substance abuse prevention through life skills training. In R. D. Peters & R. J. McMahon (Eds.), *Preventing childhood disorders, substance abuse, and delinquency* (pp. 215–240). Thousand Oaks, CA: Sage.

Botvin, G. J. (2000). Preventing drug abuse in schools: Social and competence enhancement approaches targeting individual-level etiologic factors. *Addictive Behaviors, 25,* 887–897.

Botvin, G., Dusenbury, L., Baker, E., James-Ortiz, S., & Kerner, J. (1989). A skills training approach to smoking prevention among Hispanic youth. *Journal of Behavioral Medicine, 13,* 279–296.

Botvin, G. J., & Griffin, K. W. (2002). Preventing substance use and abuse. In K. M. Minke & G. G. Bear (Eds.), *Preventing school problems—Promoting school success: Strategies and programs that work* (pp. 259–298). Bethesda, MD: National Association of School Psychologists.

Boutelle, K. N., Neumark-Sztainer, D., Story, M., & Resnick, M. (2002). Weight control behaviors among obese, overweight, and nonoverweight adolescents. *Journal of Pediatric Psychology, 27,* 531–540.

Braet, C., & Van Strien, T. (1997). Assessment of emotional, externally induced, and restrained eating behaviour in nine to twelve-year-old obese and non-obese children. *Behaviour Research and Therapy, 9,* 863–873.

Brewerton, T. D. (1995). Toward a unified theory of serotonin dysregulation in eating and related disorders. *Psychoneuroendocrinology, 20,* 561–590.

Bronfenbrenner, U. (1979). Toward an experimental ecology of human development. *American Psychologist, 32,* 513–531.

Brooks-Gunn, J., Newman, D., Holderness, C., & Warren, M. (1994). The experience of breast development and girls' stories about the purchase of a bra. *Journal of Youth and Adolescence, 23,* 539–565.

Brooks-Gunn, J., & Warren, M. (1989). Biological and social contributions to negative affect in young adolescent girls. *Child Development, 60,* 40–55.

Brown, J. A. (2001). Media literacy and critical television viewing in education. In D. G. Singer & J. L. Singer (Eds.), *Handbook of children and the media* (pp. 681–697). Thousand Oaks, CA: Sage.

Brown, J. D., & Walsh-Childers, K. (2002). Effects of media on personal and public health. In J. Bryant & D. Zillmann (Eds.), *Media effects: Advances in theory and research* (2nd ed., pp. 453–488). Mahwah, NJ: Lawrence Erlbaum Associates.

Brown, L. M., & Gilligan, C. (1992). *Meeting at the crossroads.* Cambridge, MA: Harvard University Press.

Brown, L. S., & Burman, E. (1997). Feminist responses to the "false memory" debate. *Feminism & Psychology, 7,* 7–16.

Brownell, K., & Rodin, J. (1994). The dieting maelstrom: Is it possible and advisable to lose weight? *American Psychologist, 49,* 781–791.

Bruch, H. (1973). *Eating disorders: Obesity, anorexia nervosa, and the person within.* New York: Basic Books.

Bruch, H. (1978). *The golden cage: The enigma of anorexia nervosa.* Cambridge, MA: Harvard University Press.

Brumberg, J. (1988). *Fasting girls: The emergence of anorexia nervosa as a modern disease.* Cambridge, MA: Harvard University Press.

Brumberg, J. (1997). *The body project: An intimate history of American girls.* New York: Random House.

Bryant-Waugh, R. J. (2000). Overview of the eating disorders. In B. D. Lask & R. J. Bryant-Waugh (Eds.), *Anorexia nervosa and related disorders in childhood and adolescence* (2nd ed., pp. 27–40). Hove, England: Psychology Press/Taylor & Francis.

Bryant-Waugh, R. J., Cooper, P. J., Taylor, C. L., & Lask, B. D. (1996). The use of the eating disorder examination with children: a pilot study. *International Journal of Eating Disorders, 19,* 391–397.

Buddeberg-Fischer, B., Klaghofer, R., Gnam, G., & Buddeberg, C. (1998). Prevention of disturbed eating behaviour: A prospective intervention study in 14–19-year-old Swiss students. *Acta Pschiatrica Scandinavica, 98,* 146–155.

Buddeberg-Fischer, B., Klaghofer, R., Reed, V., & Buddeberg, C. (2000). Unterrichtsmodule zur gesundheitsförderung: Ergebnisse einer kontrollierten interventionsstudie an zswi gynmnasien [Curriculum module for health promotion: Results of a controlled intervention study in two high schools]. *Soz.-Praventivmed, 45,* 191–202.

Buddeberg-Fischer, B., & Reed, V. (2001). Prevention of disturbed eating behaviors: An intervention program in Swiss high school classes. *Eating Disorders: The Journal of Treatment & Prevention, 9,* 109–124.

Bulik, C. (2001). Eating disorders: Integrating nature and nurture through the study of twins. In M. Nasser, M. Katzman, & R. Gordon (Eds.), *Eating disorders and cultures in transition* (pp. 66–85). New York: Taylor & Francis.

Bulik, C. (2004). Genetic and biological risk factors. In J. K. Thompson (Ed.), *Handbook of eating disorders and obesity* (pp. 3–16). Hoboken, NJ: Wiley.

Bulik, C. M., Sullivan, P. F., Wade, T. D., & Kendler, K. S. (2000). Twin studies of eating disorders: A review. *International Journal of Eating Disorders, 27,* 1–20.

Bulik, C. M., Sullivan, P. F., Weltzin, T. E., & Kaye, W. H. (1995). Temperament in eating disorders. *International Journal of Eating Disorders, 17,* 251–261.

Burgard, D., & Lyons, P. (1994). Alternatives in obesity treatment: Focusing on health for fat women. In P. Fallon, M. A. Katzman, & S. C. Wooley (Eds.), *Feminist perspectives on eating disorders* (pp. 212–230). New York: Guilford.

Byely, L., Archibald, A. B., Graber, J., & Brooks-Gunn, J. (2000). A prospective study of familial and social influences on girls' body image and dieting. *International Journal of Eating Disorders, 28,* 155–164.

Caplan, G. (1964). *Principles of preventive psychiatry.* New York: Basic Books.

Caplan, M. Z., & Weissberg, R. P. (1989). Promoting social competence in early adolescence: Developmental considerations. In B. H. Schneider, G. Attili, J. Nadel, & R. P. Weissberg (Eds.), *Social competence in developmental perspective* (pp. 371–385). Dordrecht: Kluwer.

Carper, J., Fisher, J. O., & Birch, L. (2000). Young girls' emerging dietary restraint and disinhibition are related to parental control in child feeding. *Appetite, 35,* 121–129.

Carter, J. C., Stewart, D. A., Dunn, V., & Fairburn, C. G. (1997). Primary prevention of eating disorders: Might it do more harm than good? *International Journal of Eating Disorders, 22,* 167–173.

Carter, J. C., Stewart, D. A., & Fairburn, C. G. (1998). Primary prevention of eating disorders: The dilemma and its denial. *Eating Disorders: The Journal of Treatment & Prevention, 6,* 213–215.

Carter, W. B. (1990). Health behavior as a rational process: Theory of Reasoned Action and Multiattribute Utility Theory. In K. Glanz, F. M. Lewis, & B. K. Rimer (Eds.), *Health behavior and health education* (pp. 63–91). San Francisco: Jossey-Bass.

Cash, T. F. (1996). The treatment of body image disturbances. In J. K. Thompson (Ed.), *Body image, eating disorders, and obesity: An integrative guide for assessment and treatment* (pp. 83–107). Washington, DC: American Psychological Association.

Cash, T. F. (1997). *The body image workbook: An 8-step program for learning to like your looks.* Oakland, CA: New Harbinger Publications.

Cash, T. F. (2002). A "negative body image": Evaluating epidemiological evidence. In T. Cash & T. Pruzinsky (Eds.), *Body image: A handbook of theory, research, and clinical practice* (pp. 269–276). New York: Guilford.

Cash, T. F., & Hrabosky, J. I. (2004). Treatment of body image disturbances. In J. K. Thompson (Ed.), *Handbook of eating disorders and obesity* (pp. 515–541). Hoboken, NJ: Wiley.

Cash, T. F., & Pruzinsky, T. (Eds.). (2002). *Body image: A handbook of theory, research, and clinical practice.* New York: Guilford.

Cash, T. F., & Strachan, M. D. (2002). Cognitive-behavioral approaches to changing body image. In T. F. Cash & T. Pruzinsky (Eds.), *Body image: A handbook of theory, research, and clinical practice* (pp. 478–486). New York: Guilford.

Caspi, A., & Moffitt, T. E. (1991). Individual differences are accentuated during periods of social change: The sample case of girls at puberty. *Journal of Personality and Social Psychology, 61,* 157–168.

Catalano, R. F., Berglund, M. L., Ryan, J. A. M., Lonczak, H. S., & Hawkins, J. D. (2002). Positive youth development in the United States: Research findings on evaluations of positive youth development programs. *Prevention & Treatment, 5.* Retrieved July 1, 2004, from http://journals.apa.org/prevention/volume5/pre0050015a.html.

Catalano, R., & Dooley, D. (1980). Economic change in primary prevention. In R. H. Price, R. F. Ketterer, B. C. Bader, & J. Monahan (Eds.), *Prevention in mental health: Research, policy, and practice* (pp. 21–40). Beverly Hills, CA: Sage.

REFERENCES

Cattarin, J., & Thompson, J. K. (1994). A three-year longitudinal study of body image, eating disturbance, and general psychological functioning in adolescent females. *Eating Disorders: The Journal of Treatment and Prevention, 2,* 114–125.

Celio, A. A., Winzelberg, A. J., Dev, P., & Taylor, C. B. (2002). Improving compliance in online, structured self-help programs: Evaluation of an eating disorder prevention program. *Journal of Psychiatric Practice, 8,* 14–19.

Celio, A. A., Winzelberg, A. J., Wilfley, D. E., Eppstein, D., Springer, E., Dev, P., & Taylor, C. B. (2000). Reducing risk factors for eating disorders: Comparison of an Internet- and a classroom-delivered psychoeducation program. *Journal of Consulting and Clinical Psychology, 68,* 650–657.

Center for Media Literacy. (n.d.). *Learning for the 21st Century: A report and mile guide for 21st century skills.* Retrieved July 17, 2004, from http://www.medialit.org/reading_room/article580.html.

Centers for Disease Control (CDC). (1996). Guidelines for school health programs to promote lifelong healthy eating. *Mortality & Morbidity Weekly Review, 45* (RR09), 1–33. Retrieved from http://www.cdc.gov/mmwr/PDF/RR/RR4509.pdf.

Centers for Disease Control (CDC). (1997). Guidelines for school and community programs to promote lifelong physical activity among young people. *Mortality & Morbidity Weekly Review, 46* (RR06), 1–36. Retrieved from http://www.cdc.gov/mmwr/preview/mmwrhtml/00046823.

Centers for Disease Control (CDC). (1999). Youth risk behavior surveillance—United States, 1999. *Mortality & Morbidity Weekly Review, 49* (SS05), 1–96. Retrieved from www.cdc.gov/mmwr/preview/mmwrhtml/ss4905a1.htm.

Centers for Disease Control (CDC). (n.d.). *Prevalence of overweight among children and adolescents: United States, 1999–2000.* Retrieved July 16, 2004, from http://www.cdc.gov/nchs/products/pubs/pubd/hestats/overwght99.htm.

Chally, P. (1998). An eating disorders prevention program. *Journal of Child and Adolescent Psychiatric Nursing, 11,* 51–60.

Chase, A. K. (2000). *Eating disorder prevention: An intervention for "at risk" college women.* Unpublished doctoral dissertation, University of Texas, Austin.

Childress, A. C., Brewerton, T. D., Hodges, E. L., & Jarrell, M. P. (1993). The Kids' Eating Disorders Survey (KEDS): A study of middle school students. *Journal of the American Academy of Child and Adolescent Psychiatry, 32,* 843–850.

Chodorow, N. (1978). *The reproduction of mothering.* Berkeley, CA: University of California Press.

Cicchetti, D., & Schneider-Rosen, K. (1986). An organizational approach to childhood depression. In M. Rutter, C. Izard, & P. Read (Eds.), *Depression in young people* (pp. 71–134). New York: Guilford.

Cloninger, C., Svrakic, D., & Przybeck, T. (1993). A psychobiological model of temperament and character. *Archives of General Psychiatry, 50,* 975–989.

Cogan, J. C., & Ernsberger, P. (Eds.). (1999). Dying to be thin in the name of health: Shifting the paradigm. *Journal of Social Issues* [Special Issue], *55,* 187–400.

Cohane, G., & Pope, H. G., Jr. (2001). Body image in boys: A review of the literature. *International Journal of Eating Disorders, 29,* 373–379.

Cohn, L., & Maine, M. (1998). More harm than good (The Last Word). *Eating Disorders: The Journal of Treatment & Prevention, 6,* 93–95.

Coie, J. D., Watt, N. F., West, S. G., Hawkins, J. D., Asarnow, J. R., Markman, H. J., Ramey, S. L., Shure, M. B., & Long, B. (1993). The science of prevention: A conceptual framework and some directions for a national research program. *American Psychologist, 48,* 1013–1022.

Coller, T. G., Neumark-Sztainer, D., Bulfer, J., & Engebretson, J. (1999). Taste of Food, Fun, and Fitness: A community-based program that teaches young girls to feel better about their bodies. *Journal of Nutrition Education, 31,* 283E.

Compas, B. E., & Hammen, C. L. (1994). Child and adolescent depression: Covariation and comorbidity in development. In R. J. Haggerty, L. R. Sherrod, N. Garmezy, & M. Rutter (Eds.), *Stress, risk, and resilience in children and adolescents: Processes, mechanisms, and interventions* (pp. 225–267). Cambridge, UK: Cambridge University Press.

Connors, M. (1996). Developmental vulnerabilities for eating disorders. In L. Smolak, M. Levine, & R. H. Striegel-Moore (Eds.), *The developmental psychopathology of eating disorders: Implica-*

tions for research, prevention, and treatment (pp. 285–310). Mahwah, NJ: Lawrence Erlbaum Associates.
Connors, M. (2001). Relationship of sexual abuse to body image and eating problems. In J. K. Thompson & L. Smolak (Eds.), *Body image, eating disorders, and obesity in youth: Assessment, prevention, and treatment* (pp. 149–168). Washington, DC: American Psychological Association.
Cooper, M. (1997). Bias in interpretation of ambiguous scenarios in eating disorders. *Behavior Research and Therapy, 35,* 619–626.
Cooper, M., & Fairburn, C. G. (1993). Demographic and clinical correlates of selective information processing in patients with bulimia nervosa. *International Journal of Eating Disorders, 13,* 109–116.
Cooper, P. J., Taylor, M. J., Cooper, Z., & Fairburn, C. F. (1987). The development and validation of the Body Shape Questionnaire. *International Journal of Eating Disorders, 6,* 485–494.
Coreil, J., Bryant, C. A., Henderson, J. N., Fortholer, M. S., & Quinn, G. P. (2001). *Social And behavioral foundations of public health.* Thousand Oaks, CA: Sage.
Costin, C. (1997). *Your dieting daughter: Is she dying for attention?* New York: Brunner/Mazel.
Cowen, E. L. (1973). Social and community intervention. *Annual Review of Psychology, 24,* 423–472.
Cowen, E. L. (1983). Primary prevention in mental health: Past, present, and future. In R. D. Felner, L. A. Jason, J. N. Moritsugu, & S. S. Farber (Eds.), *Preventive psychology: Theory, research, and practice* (pp. 11–25). New York: Pergamon.
Cowen, E. L. (1997). On the semantics and operations of primary prevention and wellness enhancement (Or will the real primary prevention please stand up?). *American Journal of Community Psychology, 25,* 245–255.
Cowen, E. L. (2000). Psychological wellness: Some hopes for the future. In D. Cicchetti, J. Rappaport, I. Sandler, & R. P. Weissberg (Eds.), *The promotion of wellness in children and adolescents* (pp. 477–501). Washington, DC: Child Welfare League of America.
Cowen, P. J., Clifford, E. M., Walsh, A. E. S., Williams, C., & Fairburn, C. G. (1996). Moderate dieting causes 5-HT2c receptor supersensitivity. *Psychological Medicine, 26,* 1155–1159.
Crago, M., Shisslak, C. M., & Estes, L. S. (1996). Eating disturbances among American minority groups: A review. *International Journal of Eating Disorders, 19,* 239–248.
Crago, M., Shisslak, C. M., & Ruble, A. (2001). Protective factors in the development of eating disorders. In R. H. Striegel-Moore & L. Smolak (Eds.), *Eating disorders: Innovative directions in research and practice* (pp. 75–90). Washington, DC: American Psychological Association.
Crandall, C. S. (1988). Social contagion of binge eating. *Journal of Personality and Social Psychology, 55,* 588–598.
Crick, N. R., & Bigbee, M. A. (1998). Relational and overt forms of peer victimization: A multi-informant approach. *Journal of Consulting & Clinical Psychology, 66,* 337–347.
Crisp, A. (1980). *Anorexia nervosa: Let me be.* New York: Grune & Stratton.
Crocker, J., Luhtanen, R., Blaine, B., & Broadnax, S. (1994). Collective self-esteem and psychological well-being among White, Black, and Asian college students. *Personality and Social Psychology Bulletin, 20,* 503–513.
Croll, J., Neumark-Sztainer, D., Story, M., & Ireland, M. (2002). Prevalence and risk and protective factors related to disordered eating behaviors among adolescents: Relationship to gender and ethnicity. *Journal of Adolescent Health, 31,* 166–175.
Cuijpers, P. (2002). Effective ingredients of school-based drug prevention programs: A systematic review. *Addictive Behaviors, 27,* 1009–1023.
Cusumano, D. L., & Thompson, J. K. (1997). Body image and body shape ideals in magazines: Exposure, awareness, and internalization. *Sex Roles, 37,* 701–721.
Cusumano, D. L., & Thompson, J. K. (2001). Media influence and body image in 8–11-year-old boys and girls: A preliminary report on the Multidimensional Media Influence Scale. *International Journal of Eating Disorders, 29,* 37–44.
Dalle Grave, R. (2003). School-based prevention programs for eating disorders. *Disease Management and Health Outcomes, 11,* 579–593.
Dalle Grave, R., De Luca, L., & Campello, G. (2001). Middle school primary prevention program for eating disorders: A controlled study with a twelve-month follow-up. *Eating Disorders: The Journal of Treatment & Prevention, 9,* 327–337.

416 REFERENCES

Dalton, J. H., Elias, M. J., & Wandersman, A. (2001). *Community psychology: Linking individuals and communities.* Stamford, CT: Wadsworth/Thomson.

Davis, C., Katzman, D. K., Kaptein, S., Kirsch, C., Brewer, H., Olmsted, M. P., Woodside, D. B., & Kaplan, A. S. (1997). The prevalence of hyperactivity in the eating disorders: Aetiological implications. *Comprehensive Psychiatry, 38,* 321–326.

Davison, K., Markey, C., & Birch, L. (2003). A longitudinal examination of patterns in girls' weight concerns and body dissatisfaction from ages 5 to 9 years. *International Journal of Eating Disorders, 33,* 320–332.

DeBate, R. D., & Thompson, S. H. (2003). *Impacts of a curriculum-based running program: Improvements in self-esteem, body size satisfaction, and eating attitudes/behaviors.* Unpublished manuscript, University of North Carolina, Charlotte.

De Beauvoir, S. (1952). *The second sex.* New York: Vintage.

Dede, C., & Fontana, L. (1995). Transforming health education via new media. In L. M. Harris (Ed.), *Health and the new media: Technologies transforming personal and public health* (pp. 163–183). Mahwah, NJ: Lawrence Erlbaum Associates.

Derzon, J. H., & Lipsey, M. W. (2002). A meta-analysis of the effectiveness of mass communication for changing substance-use knowledge, attitudes, and behavior. In W. B. Crano & M. Burgoon (Eds.), *Mass media and drug prevention: Classic and contemporary theories and research* (pp. 231–258). Mahwah, NJ: Lawrence Erlbaum Associates.

Devlin, M. J., Yanovski, S. Z., & Wilson, G. T. (2000). Obesity: What mental health professionals need to know. *American Journal of Psychiatry, 157,* 854–866.

DiClemente, R. J., Ponton, L. E., & Hansen, W. B. (1996). New directions for adolescent risk prevention and health promotion research and interventions. In R. J. DiClemente, W. B. Hansen, & L. E. Ponton (Eds.), *Handbook of adolescent health risk behavior* (pp. 413–420). New York: Plenum.

Dietz, W. H. (1998). Health consequences of obesity in youth: Childhood predictors of adult disease. *Pediatrics, 101* (Suppl.), 518S–525S.

DiGioacchino, R. F., Keenan, M. F., & Sargent, R. (2000). Assessment of dental practitioners in the secondary and tertiary prevention of eating disorders. *Eating Behaviors, 1,* 79–91.

Dishion, T., & Kavanagh, K. (2000). A multilevel approach to family-centered prevention in schools: Process and outcome. *Addictive Behaviors, 25,* 899–911.

Dohrenwend, B. P. (1998). Overview of evidence for the importance of adverse environmental conditions in causing psychiatric disorders. In B. P. Dohrenwend (Ed.), *Adversity, stress, and psychopathology* (pp. 523–538). New York: Oxford University Press.

Donaldson, S. I., Sussman, S., MacKinnon, D. P., Severson, H. H., Glynn, T., Murray, D. M., & Stone, E. J. (1996). Drug abuse prevention programming: Do we know what content works? *American Behavioral Scientist, 39,* 868–883.

Dornbusch, S., Carlsmith, J., Duncan, P., Gross, R., Martin, J., Ritter, P., & Siegel-Gorelik, B. (1984). Sexual maturation, social class, and the desire to be thin among adolescent females. *Journal of Developmental and Behavioral Pediatrics, 5,* 308–314.

Dounchis, J., Hayden, H., & Wilfley, D. E. (2001). Obesity, body image, and eating disorders in ethnically diverse children and adolescents. In J. K. Thompson & L. Smolak (Eds.), *Body image, eating disorders, and obesity in youth: Assessment, prevention, and treatment* (pp. 67–98). Washington, DC: American Psychological Association.

Doyle, J., & Bryant-Waugh, R. (2000). Epidemiology. In B. Lask & R. Bryant-Waugh (Eds.), *Anorexia nervosa and related eating disorders in childhood and adolescence* (2nd ed., pp. 41–79). East Sussex, UK: Psychology Press.

Drewnowski, A., Yee, D., Kurth, C., & Krahn, D. (1994). Eating pathology and DSM-III-R Bulimia Nervosa: A continuum of behavior. *American Journal of Psychiatry, 151,* 1217–1219.

Dryfoos, J. G. (1997). The prevalence of problem behaviors: Implications for programs. In R. P. Weissberg, T. P. Gullotta, R. L. Hampton, B. A. Ryan, & G. R. Adams (Eds.), *Healthy children 2010: Enhancing children's wellness* (pp. 17–46). Thousand Oaks, CA: Sage.

Durlak, J. A. (1997). Common risk and protective factors in successful prevention programs. *American Journal of Orthopsychiatry, 68,* 512–520.

Eating Disorders Awareness and Prevention, Inc. (1998). *GO GIRLS!™: Giving Our Girls Inspiration and Resources for Lasting Self-esteem.* Seattle, WA: Author. Curriculum guide available from the National Eating Disorders Association (see Appendix A).

Eisenberg, M., Neumark-Sztainer, D., & Story, M. (2003). Associations of weight-based teasing and emotional well-being among adolescents. *Archives of Pediatric and Adolescent Medicine, 157,* 733–738.

Elias, M. J. (1987). Establishing enduring prevention programs: Advancing the legacy of Swampscott. *American Journal of Community Psychology, 15,* 539–553.

Elias, M. J. (1995). Primary prevention as health and social competence promotion. *The Journal of Primary Prevention, 16,* 5–24.

Elias, M. J., Gara, M., Ubriaco, M., Rothbaum, P. A., Clabby, J. F., & Schuyler, T. (1986). Impact of a preventive social problem solving intervention on children's coping with middle-school stressors. *American Journal of Community Psychology, 14,* 259–275.

Elliot, D. L., Goldberg, L., Moe, E. L., DeFrancesco, C. A., Durham, M. B., & Hix-Small, H. (2004, June). *Impact of a high school drug and disordered eating prevention program: Findings following graduation.* Paper presented at the annual meeting of the International Society of Behavioral Nutrition and Physical Activity, Washington, DC.

Elliot, D. L., Goldberg, L., Moe, E. L., DeFrancesco, C. A., Durham, M. B., & Hix-Small, H. (in press). Preventing substance use and disordered eating: Initial outcomes of the ATHENA (Athletes Targeting Health Exercise and Nutrition Alternatives) program. *Archives of Pediatric & Adolescent Medicine.*

Elliot, D. L., Goldberg, L., Moe, E. L., Duncan, T. E., DeFrancesco, C., & Durham, M. (2002). *ATHENA: Deterring drug use and disordered eating.* Paper presented at the Western Section of the American Federation of Clinical Research, Carmel, CA.

Epling, W. F., & Pierce, W. D. (Eds.). (1996). *Activity anorexia: Theory, research, and treatment.* Mahwah, NJ: Lawrence Erlbaum Associates.

Epstein, L. H., Valoski, A., Wing, R. R., & McCurley, J. (1994). Ten-year outcomes of behavioral family-based treatment for childhood obesity. *Health Psychology, 13,* 373–383.

Ernsberger, P. (1989). Obesity is hazardous to your health: Negative. *Debates in Medicine, 2,* 113–123.

Ernsberger, P., & Koletsky, R. J. (1999). Biomedical rationale for a wellness approach to obesity: An alternative to a focus on weight loss. *Journal of Social Issues, 55,* 221–260.

Ewing, R., Schmid, T., Killingsworth, R., Zlot, A., & Raudenbush, S. (2003). Relationship between urban sprawl and physical activity, obesity, and morbidity. *American Journal of Health Promotion, 18,* 47–57.

Fairburn, C. G. (1995). *Overcoming binge eating.* New York: Guilford.

Fairburn, C. G. (1997). Eating disorders. In D. M. Clark & C. G. Fairburn (Eds.), *Science and practice of cognitive behaviour therapy* (pp. 209–241). Oxford, UK: Oxford University Press.

Fairburn, C. G., & Beglin, S. J. (1994). Assessment of eating disorders: Interview or self-report measure. *International Journal of Eating Disorders, 16,* 363–370.

Fairburn, C. G., & Cooper, Z. (1993). The Eating Disorders Examination (12th ed.). In C. G. Fairburn & G. T. Wilson (Eds.), *Binge eating: Nature, assessment, and treatment* (pp. 317–355). New York: Guilford.

Fairburn, C. G., Cowen, P. J., & Harrison, P. J. (1999). Twin studies and the etiology of eating disorders. *International Journal of Eating Disorders, 26,* 349–358.

Fairburn, C. G., Shafran, R., & Cooper, Z. (1998). A cognitive behavioural theory of anorexia nervosa. *Behaviour Research and Therapy, 37,* 1–13.

Fairburn, C. G., & Wilson, G. T. (1993). Binge eating: Definition and classification. In C. G. Fairburn & G. T. Wilson (Eds.), *Binge eating: Nature, assessment, and treatment* (pp. 3–14). New York: Guilford.

Faith, M. S., Pietrobelli, A., Allison, D. B., & Heymsfield, S. B. (1997). Prevention of pediatric obesity: Examining the issues and forecasting research directions. In A. Bendich & R. J. Deckelbaum (Eds.), *Preventive nutrition: The comprehensive guide for health professionals* (pp. 471–486). Totowa, NJ: Humana Press.

Fallon, A. E., & Rozin, P. (1985). Sex differences in perceptions of desirable body shape. *Journal of Abnormal Psychology, 94,* 102–105.

Fallon, P., Katzman, M. A., & Wooley, S. C. (Eds.). (1994). *Feminist perspectives on eating disorders.* New York: Guilford.

REFERENCES

Fassino, S., Abbate-Dage, G., Amianto, F., Leobruni, P., Boggio, S., & Rovera, G. (2002). Temperament and character profile of eating disorders: A controlled study with the Temperament and Character Inventory. *International Journal of Eating Disorders, 32,* 412–425.

Fat is a financial issue. (2000, November 25). *The Economist, 357*(8198), 93–94.

Feingold, A., & Mazzella, R. (1998). Gender differences in body image are increasing. *Psychological Science, 9,* 190–195.

Felner, R. D., & Felner, T. Y. (1989). Primary prevention programs in the educational context: A transactional–ecological framework and analysis. In L. A. Bond & B. E. Compas (Eds.), *Primary prevention and promotion in the schools* (Vol. XII, pp. 13–49). Newbury Park, CA: Sage.

Field, A. E., Austin, S. B., Taylor, C. B., Malpeis, S., Rosner, B., Rockett, H. R., Gillman, M. W., & Colditz, G. A. (2003). Relation between dieting and weight change among preadolescents and adolescents. *Pediatrics, 112,* 900–906.

Field, A. E., Camargo, C. A., Jr., Taylor, C. B., Berkey, C. S., & Colditz, G. A. (1999). Relation of peer and media influences to the development of purging behaviors among preadolescent and adolescent girls. *Archives of Pediatric Adolescent Medicine, 153,* 1184–1189.

Field, A. E., Camargo, C. A., Jr., Taylor, C. B., Berkey, C., Frazier, A. L., Gillman, M. W., & Colditz, G. A. (1999). Overweight, weight concerns, and bulimic behaviors among girls and boys. *Journal of the American Academy of Child and Adolescent Psychiatry, 38,* 754–760.

Field, A. E., Camargo, C. A., Jr., Taylor, C. B., Berkey, C. S., Roberts, S. R., & Colditz, G. A. (2001). Peer, parent, and media influences on development of weight concerns and frequent dieting among preadolescent and adolescent girls and boys. *Pediatrics, 107,* 54–60.

Finkelhor, D., & Browne, A. (1986). Initial and long-term effects: A conceptual framework. In D. Finkelhor (Ed.), *A sourcebook on child sexual abuse* (pp. 180–198). Newbury Park, CA: Sage.

Fishbein, D. (2000). The importance of neurobiological research to the prevention of psychopathology. *Prevention Science, 1,* 89–106.

Fishbein, M., Guenther-Grey, C., Johnson, W., Wolitski, R. J., McAlister, A., Rietmeijer, C. A., O"Reilly, K., & The AIDS Community Demonstration Project. (1997). Using a theory-based community intervention to reduce AIDS risk behaviors: The CDC's AIDS Community Demonstration Projects. In M. E. Goldberg, M. Fishbein, & S. E. Middlestadt (Eds.), *Social marketing: Theoretical and practical perspectives* (pp. 123–146). Mahwah, NJ: Lawrence Erlbaum Associates.

Fisher, J., & Birch, L. (2001). Early experience with food and eating: Implications for the development of eating disorders. In J. K. Thompson & L. Smolak (Eds.), *Body image, eating disorders, and obesity in youth: Assessment, prevention, and treatment* (pp. 23–40). Washington, DC: American Psychological Association.

Flay, B. R. (2000). Approaches to substance use prevention utilizing school curriculum plus social environment change. *Addictive Behaviors, 25,* 861–885.

Flynn, B. S., Worden, J. K., Secker-Walker, R. H., Pirie, P. L., Badger, G. J., Carpenter, J. H., & Geller, B. M. (1994). Mass media and school interventions for cigarette smoking: Effects 2 years after completion. *American Journal of Public Health, 84,* 1148–1150.

Forston, M. T., & Stanton, A. L. (1992). Self-discrepancy theory as a framework for understanding bulimic symptomatology and associated distress. *Journal of Social and Clinical Psychology, 11,* 103–118.

Foster, E. E. (2003). *A group intervention: Increasing body- and self-esteem and decreasing unhealthy dieting behaviors and cognitions.* Unpublished doctoral dissertation, Bowling Green State University, Bowling Green, OH.

Foucault, M. (1979). *Discipline and punish.* New York: Vintage Books.

Fox, N., Henderson, H. A., Rubin, K. H., Calkins, S. D., & Schmidt, L. A. (2001). Continuity and discontinuity of behavioral inhibition and exuberance: Psychophysiological and behavioral influences across the first four years of life. *Child Development, 72,* 1–21.

Franko, D. L. (1998). Secondary prevention of eating disorders in college women at risk. *Eating Disorders: The Journal of Treatment & Prevention, 6,* 29–40.

Franko, D. L. (2004, May). *Innovations in eating disorders prevention: How multimedia tools can enhance your prevention efforts and clinical practice.* Workshop presented at the International Conference on Eating Disorders of the Academy for Eating Disorders, Orlando, FL.

Franko, D. L., Mintz, L. B., Villapiano, M., Green, T. C., Mainelli, D., Folensbee, L., Butler, S. F., Davidson, M. M., Hamilton, E., Little, D., Kearns, M., & Budman, S. H. (2004). *Food, Mood, and*

Attitude: Reducing risk for eating disorders in college women. Manuscript submitted for publication.

Franko, D. L., & Omori, M. (1999). Subclinical eating disorders in adolescent women: a test of the continuity hypothesis and its psychological correlates. *Journal of Adolescence, 22,* 389–396.

Franko, D. L., & Orosan-Weine, P. (1998). The prevention of eating disorders: Empirical, methodological and conceptual considerations. *Clinical Psychology: Science and Practice, 5,* 459–477.

Franzoi, S. L., & Shields, S. A. (1984). The Body Esteem Scale: Multidimensional structure and sex differences in a college population. *Journal of Personality Assessment, 48,* 173–178.

Fredrickson, B., & Roberts, T. (1997). Objectification theory: Toward understanding women's lived experiences and mental health. *Psychology of Women Quarterly, 21,* 173–206.

Fredrickson, B., Roberts, T., Noll, S., Quinn, D., & Twenge, J. (1998). That swimsuit becomes you: Sex differences in self-objectification, restrained eating, and math performance. *Journal of Personality and Social Psychology, 75,* 269–284.

Freedman, D., Dietz, W., Srinivasan, S., & Berenson, G. (1999). The relation of overweight to cardiovascular risk factors among children and adolescents: The Bogalusa Heart Study. *Pediatrics, 103,* 1175–1182.

French, S. A., & Jeffrey, R. (1994). Consequences of dieting to lose weight: Effects on physical and mental health. *Health Psychology, 13,* 195–212.

French, S. A., Leffert, N., Story, M., Neumark-Sztainer, D., Hannan, P., & Benson, P. L. (2001). Adolescent binge/purge and weight loss behaviors: Associations with developmental assets. *Journal of Adolescent Health, 28,* 211–221.

French, S. A., Story, M., Downes, B., Resnick, M., & Blum, R. (1995). Frequent dieting among adolescents: Psychosocial and health behavior correlates. *American Journal of Public Health, 85,* 695–701.

French, S. A., Story, M., Neumark-Sztainer, D., Downes, B., Resnick, M., & Blum, R. (1997). Ethnic differences in psychosocial and health behavior correlates of dieting, purging, and binge eating in a population-based sample of adolescent females. *International Journal of Eating Disorders, 22,* 315–322.

Friedman, S. S. (1999). Discussion groups for girls: Decoding the language of fat. In N. Piran, M. P. Levine, & C. Steiner-Adair (Eds.), *Preventing eating disorders: A handbook of special interventions* (pp. 122–133). Philadelphia: Brunner/Mazel.

Friedman, S. S. (2000). *When girls feel fat: Helping girls through adolescence.* Toronto: HarperCollins.

Friedman, S. S. (2003). *Nurturing GirlPower: Integrating eating disorder prevention/intervention skills into your practice* (updated). Vancouver, BC: Salal Books. Available from Salal Communications, Ltd. (www.salal.com).

Furnham, A., & Calnan, A. (1998). Eating disturbance, self-esteem, reasons for exercising and body weight dissatisfaction in adolescent males. *European Eating Disorders Review, 6,* 58–72.

Gaesser, G. (1996). *Big fat lies: The truth about your weight and your health.* New York: Fawcett Columbine.

Gardner, R. (2001). Assessment of body image disturbance in children and adolescents. In J. K. Thompson & L. Smolak (Eds.), *Body image, eating disorders, and obesity in youth: Assessment, prevention, and treatment* (pp. 193–214). Washington, DC: American Psychological Association.

Gardner, R., Sorter, R., & Friedman, B. (1997). Developmental changes in children's body images. *Journal of Social Behavior and Personality, 12,* 1019–1036.

Garfinkel, P. E., & Garner, D. M. (1982). *Anorexia nervosa: A multidimensional perspective.* New York: Brunner/Mazel.

Garmezy, N. (1983). Stressors of childhood. In N. Garmezy & M. Rutter (Eds.), *Stress, coping, and development in children* (pp. 43–84). New York: McGraw-Hill.

Garner, D. M. (1985). Iatrogenesis in anorexia nervosa and bulimia nervosa. *International Journal of Eating Disorders, 4,* 701–726.

Garner, D. M. (1991). *Eating Disorders Inventory–2 manual.* Odessa, FL: Psychological Assessment Resources.

Garner, D. M., & Garfinkel, P. E. (1980). Socio-cultural factors in the development of anorexia nervosa. *Psychological Medicine, 10,* 647–656.

REFERENCES

Garner, D., Olmsted, M. P., Polivy, J., & Garfinkel, P. (1984). Comparison between weight-preoccupied women and anorexia nervosa. *Psychosomatic Medicine, 46,* 255–266.

Garner, D. M., Vitousek, K., & Pike, K. (1997). Cognitive-behavioral therapy for anorexia nervosa. In D. M. Garner & P. E. Garfinkel (Eds.), *Handbook of treatment for eating disorders* (2nd ed., pp. 94–144). New York: Guilford.

Garner, D. M., & Wooley, S. C. (1991). Confronting the failure of behavioral and dietary treatments for obesity. *Clinical Psychology Review, 11,* 729–780.

Garvin, V., & Striegel-Moore, R. H. (2001). Health services research for eating disorders in the United States: A status report and a call to action. In R. H. Striegel-Moore & L. Smolak (Eds.), *Eating disorders: Innovative directions in research and practice* (pp. 135–152). Washington, DC: American Psychological Association.

Garvin, V., Striegel-Moore, R. H., Kaplan, A., & Wonderlich, S. (2001). The potential of professionally developed self-help interventions for the treatment of eating disorders. In R. H. Striegel-Moore & L. Smolak (Eds.), *Eating disorders: Innovative directions in research and practice* (pp. 153–172). Washington, DC: American Psychological Association.

Geller, J., Zaitsoff, S., & Srikameswaran, S. (2002). Beyond shape and weight: Exploring the relationship between nonbody determinants of self-esteem and eating disorder symptoms in adolescent females. *International Journal of Eating Disorders, 32,* 344–351.

Gill, T. P. (1997). Key issues in the prevention of obesity. *British Medical Journal, 53,* 359–388.

Gilligan, C. (1982). *In a different voice.* Cambridge, MA: Harvard University Press.

Goldberg, L., & Elliot, D. L. (1999). *The ATLAS Program: Background information for instructors—drug prevention, sports nutrition, exercise training.* Unpublished curriculum, Oregon Health & Sciences University. Contact D. L. Elliot, MD, 3181 SW Sam Jackson Park Road, Portland, OR 97201 (elliotd@oshu.edu).

Goldberg, L., & Elliot, D. L. (2000). Prevention of anabolic steroid use. In C. E. Yesalis (Ed.), *Anabolic steroids in sports and exercise* (2nd ed., pp. 117–136). Champaign, IL: Human Kinetics.

Goldberg, L., Elliot, D. L., Clarke, G. N., MacKinnon, D. P., Moe, E. L., Zoref, L., Green, C., Wolf, S. L., Greffrath, E., Miller, D. J., & Lapin, A. (1996). Effects of a multidimensional anabolic steroid prevention intervention. *Journal of the American Medical Association, 276,* 1555–62.

Goldberg, L., MacKinnon, D. P., Elliot, D. L., Moe, E. L., Clarke, G., & Cheong, J. (2000). The Adolescents Training and Learning to Avoid Steroids Program: Preventing drug use and promoting healthy behaviors. *Archives of Pediatrics & Adolescent Medicine, 154,* 332–338.

Goldberg, M. E., Fishbein, M., & Middlestadt, S. E. (Eds.). (1997). *Social marketing: Theoretical and practical perspectives.* Mahwah, NJ: Lawrence Erlbaum Associates.

Gordon, R. A. (2000). *Eating disorders: Anatomy of a social epidemic* (2nd ed.). Malden, MA: Blackwell.

Gortmaker, S. L., Peterson, K., Wiecha, J., Sobol, A. M., Dixit, S., Fox, M. K., & Laird, N. (1999). Reducing obesity via a school-based interdisciplinary intervention among youth: Planet Health. *Archives of Pediatric & Adolescent Medicine, 153,* 409–418.

Graber, J. A., Brooks-Gunn, J., Paikoff, R., & Warren, M. P. (1994). Prediction of eating problems: An 8-year study of adolescent girls. *Developmental Psychology, 30,* 823–834.

Graber, J. A., Brooks-Gunn, J., & Warren, M. P. (1999). The vulnerable transition: Puberty and the development of eating pathology and negative mood. *Women's Health Issues, 9,* 107–114.

Graber, J., Petersen, A., & Brooks-Gunn, J. (1996). Pubertal processes: Methods, measures, and models. In J. Graber, J. Brooks-Gunn, & A. Petersen (Eds.), *Transitions through adolescence: Interpersonal domains and context* (pp. 23–54). Mahwah, NJ: Lawrence Erlbaum Associates.

Greenberg, M. T., Domitrovich, C., & Bumbarger, B. (2001). The prevention of mental disorders in school-aged children: Current state of the field. *Prevention & Treatment, 4* (article 1), retrieved March 7, 2002, from journal.apa.org/preventon/volume4/pre004001a.html.

Gresko, R. B., & Rosenvinge, J. H. (1998). The Norwegian school-based prevention model: Development and evaluation. In W. Vandereycken & G. Noordenbos (Eds.), *The prevention of eating disorders* (pp. 75–98). London: Athlone.

Grodner, M. (1991). Using the Health Belief Model for bulimia prevention. *Journal of American College Health, 40,* 107–112.

Groesz, L. M., Levine, M. P., & Murnen, S. K. (2002). The effect of experimental presentation of thin media images on body satisfaction: A meta-analytic review. *International Journal of Eating Disorders, 31,* 1–16.

Grogan, S., Williams, Z., & Conner, M. (1996). The effects of viewing same-gender photographic models on body-esteem. *Psychology of Women Quarterly, 20,* 569–575.

Guo, S., Roche, A., Chumlea, W., Gardner, J., & Siervogel, R. (1994). The predictive value of childhood body mass index values for overweight at age 35 y. *American Journal of Clinical Nutrition, 59,* 810–819.

Gurney, V. W. (1997). *An eating disturbances intervention program for college students.* Unpublished doctoral dissertation, Ohio University, Athens, OH.

Gurney, V. W., & Halmi, K. (2001). An eating disorder curriculum for primary care providers. *International Journal of Eating Disorders, 30,* 209–212.

Gustafson-Larson, A., & Terry, R. (1992). Weight-related behaviors and concerns of fourth-grade children. *Journal of the American Dietetic Association, 92,* 818–822.

Hamilton, C. (2000). Continuity and discontinuity of attachment from infancy through adolescence. *Child Development, 71,* 690–694.

Hansen, W. B. (1992). School-based substance abuse prevention: A review of the state of the art in curriculum, 1980–1990. *Health Education Research, 7,* 403–430.

Hansen, W. B. (2002). Program evaluation strategies for substance abuse prevention. *The Journal of Primary Prevention, 22,* 409–436.

Harned, M. (2000). Harassed bodies: An examination of the relationships among women's experiences of sexual harassment, body image, and eating disturbances. *Psychology of Women Quarterly, 24,* 336–348.

Harrison, K. (1997). Does interpersonal attraction to thin media personalities promote eating disorders? *Journal of Broadcasting & Electronic Media, 41,* 478–500.

Harrison, K., & Cantor, J. (1997). The relationship between media consumption and eating disorders. *Journal of Communication, 47*(1), 40–66.

Harter, S. (1986). *Manual: Self-perception profile for adolescents.* Denver, CO: University of Colorado.

Hawkins, J. D., Catalano, R., & Arthur, M. (2002). Promoting science-based prevention in communities. *Addictive Behaviors, 27,* 951–976.

Hay, P., & Fairburn, C. (1998). The validity of the DSM-IV scheme for classifying bulimic disorders. *International Journal of Eating Disorders, 23,* 7–15.

Hayward, C., Killen, J., Wilson, D., Hammer, L., Litt, I., Kraemer, H., Haydel, K., Varady, A., & Taylor, C. B. (1997). Psychiatric risk associated with early puberty in adolescent girls. *Journal of the American Academy of Child and Adolescent Psychiatry, 36,* 255–262.

Healy, C. (1998). Health promoting schools: Learning from the European project. *Health Education, 1,* 216–226.

Heatherton, T. F., & Polivy, J. (1992). Chronic dieting and eating disorders: A spiral model. In J. H. Crowther, D. L. Tennenbaum, S. E. Hobfoll, & M. A. P. Stephens (Eds.), *The etiology of bulimia nervosa: The individual and familial context* (pp. 133–155). Washington, DC: Hemisphere.

Heinberg, L. J., Thompson, J. K., & Matzon, J. (2001). Body image dissatisfaction as a motivator for healthy lifestyle change: Is some distress beneficial? In R. H. Striegel-Moore & L. Smolak (Eds.), *Eating disorders: Innovations in research, treatment, and prevention* (pp. 215–232). Washington, DC: American Psychological Association.

Heinberg, L. J., Thompson, J. K., & Stormer, S. (1995). Development and validation of the Sociocultural Attitudes Towards Appearance Questionnaire. *International Journal of Eating Disorders, 17,* 81–89.

Heinze, V., Wertheim, E. H., & Kashima, Y. (2000). An evaluation of the importance of message source and age of recipient in a primary prevention program for eating disorders. *Eating Disorders: The Journal of Treatment & Prevention, 8,* 131–145.

Heller, K. (1996). Coming of age of prevention science: Comments on the 1994 National Institute of Mental Health-Institute of Medicine prevention reports. *American Psychologist, 51,* 1123–1127.

Herzog, D. B., & Delinsky, S. (2001). Classification of eating disorders. In R. H. Striegel-Moore & L. Smolak (Eds.), *Eating disorders: Innovations in research, treatment, and prevention* (pp. 31–50). Washington, DC: American Psychological Association.

REFERENCES

Herzog, D. B., Greenwood, D. N., Dorer, D. J., Flores, A. T., Ekeblad, E. R., Richards, A., Blais, M. A., & Keller, M. B. (2000). Mortality in eating disorders: A descriptive study. *International Journal of Eating Disorders, 28,* 20–26.

Herzog, W., Deter, H. C., & Vandereycken, W. (Eds.). (1992). *The course of eating disorders: Long-term follow-up studies of anorexia and bulimia nervosa.* Berlin: Springer-Verlag.

Hewlings, S. J. (2000). *An eating disorder prevention program for preadolescent children.* Unpublished doctoral dissertation, Florida State University, Tallahassee.

Higgins, E. T. (1987). Self-discrepancy: A theory relating self and affect. *Psychological Review, 84,* 319–340.

Higgins, L. C., & Gray, W. (1998). Changing the body image concern and eating behaviour of chronic dieters: The effects of a psychoeducational intervention. *Psychology and Health, 13,* 1045–1060.

Hill, A. J., & Robinson, A. (1991). Dieting concerns have a functional effect on the behaviour of nine-year-old girls. *British Journal of Clinical Psychology, 30,* 265–267.

Hill, K., & Pomeroy, C. (2001). Assessment of physical status of children and adolescents with eating disorders and obesity. In J. K. Thompson & L. Smolak (Eds.), *Body image, eating disorders, and obesity in youth: Assessment, prevention, and treatment* (pp. 171–192). Washington, DC: American Psychological Association.

Hobbs, R. (1998). The seven great debates in the media literacy movement. *Journal of Communication,* Winter, 16–32.

Hoek, H., & van Hoeken, D. (2003). Review of the prevalence and incidence of eating disorders. *International Journal of Eating Disorders, 34,* 383–396.

Hoff, H. (2002a, March). *Changing our culture: Eating disorder prevention strategies inspired and implemented by Lori Irving.* Presentation at the conference Partners in Eating Disorders Research and Practice: A Dedication to Lori Irving, Vancouver, WA.

Hoff, H. (2002b). National Eating Disorders Association *Listen to Your Body* Campaign. Unpublished NEDA document. Contact NEDA (see Appendix A).

Holden, E. W., & Black, M. (1999). Theory and concepts of prevention science as applied to clinical psychology. *Clinical Psychology Review, 19,* 391–401.

Hotelling, K. (1999). An integrated prevention/intervention program for the university setting. In N. Piran, M. P. Levine, & C. Steiner-Adair (Eds.), *Preventing eating disorders: A handbook of interventions and special challenges* (pp. 208–221). Philadelphia: Brunner/Mazel.

Huon, G. F. (1995). The Stroop color-naming task in eating disorders: A review of the research. *Eating Disorders: The Journal of Treatment & Prevention, 3,* 124–132.

Huon, G., Roncolato, W., Ritchie, J., & Braganza, C. (1997). Prevention of diet-induced disorders: Findings and implications of a pilot study. *Eating Disorders: The Journal of Treatment & Prevention, 5,* 280–295.

Ikeda, J. (1998). *If my child is overweight, what should I do about it?* [Publication 21455] Oakland, CA: Division of Agriculture and Natural Resources, University of California. Available from 1–800–994–8849.

Ikeda, J. P., & Mitchell, R. A. (2001). Dietary approaches to the treatment of pediatric overweight. *Pediatric Clinics of North America, 48,* 955–968.

Ikeda, J., Mitchell, R., & Crawford, P. (2000). *Overweight among children in California: A fact sheet for schools and communities.* Berkeley, CA: Department of Nutritional Services, University of California Cooperative Extension. Available by calling 1–800–994–8849.

Ikeda, J., & Naworski, P. (1992). *Am I fat? Helping young children accept differences in body size.* Santa Cruz, CA: ETR Associates.

Irving, L. M. (1990). Mirror images: Effects of the standard of beauty on the self- and body-esteem of women exhibiting varying levels of bulimic symptoms. *Journal of Social and Clinical Psychology, 9,* 230–242.

Irving, L. M. (1999). A bolder model of prevention: Science, practice, and activism. In N. Piran, M. P. Levine, & C. Steiner-Adair (Eds.), *Preventing eating disorders: A handbook of interventions and special challenges* (pp. 63–83). Philadelphia: Brunner/Mazel.

Irving, L. M. (2000). Promoting size acceptance in elementary school children: The EDAP Puppet Program. *Eating Disorders: The Journal of Treatment and Prevention, 8,* 221–232.

Irving, L. M., & Berel, S. R. (2001). Comparison of media-literacy programs to strengthen college women's resistance to media images. *Psychology of Woman Quarterly, 25,* 103–111.

REFERENCES

Irving, L. M., DuPen, J., & Berel, S. (1998). A media literacy program for high school females. *Eating Disorders: The Journal of Treatment and Prevention, 6,* 119–131.

Irving, L. M., & Levine, M. P. (2000, September). *GO GIRLS^{TM}! An update on media literacy and prevention.* Presentation at the Sixth Annual Conference of Eating Disorders Awareness & Prevention, Inc., Scottsdale, Arizona.

Irving, L. M., Levine, M. P., & Piran, N. (2003). Primary prevention of disordered eating behavior in adults. In T. P. Gullotta & M. Bloom (Eds.), *The encyclopedia of primary prevention and health promotion* (pp. 428–435). New York: Kluwer Academic/Plenum.

Irving, L. M., & Neumark-Sztainer, D. (2002). Integrating the prevention of eating disorders and obesity: Feasible or futile? *Preventive Medicine, 34,* 299–309.

Irving, L. M., Wall, M., Neumark-Sztainer, D., & Story, M. (2002). Steroid use among adolescents: Findings from Project EAT. *Journal of Adolescent Health, 30,* 243–252.

Jackman, L. P., Williamson, D. A., Netemeyer, R. G., & Anderson, D. A. (1995). Do weight-preoccupied women misinterpret ambiguous stimuli related to body size? *Cognitive Therapy and Research, 19,* 341–355.

Jacobi, C., Hayward, C., de Zwaan, M., Kraemer, H. C., & Agras, W. S. (2004). Coming to terms with risk factors for eating disorders: Application of risk terminology and suggestions for a general taxonomy. *Psychological Bulletin, 130,* 19–65.

Janz, N., & Becker, M. H. (1984). The Health Belief Model: A decade later. *Health Education Quarterly, 11,* 1–47.

Jasper, K. (1993). Monitoring and responding to media messages. *Eating Disorders: The Journal of Treatment & Prevention, 1,* 109–114.

Jerome, L. W. (1987). *Primary intervention for bulimia: The evaluation of a media presentation for an adolescent population.* Unpublished masters thesis, Kent State University, Kent, OH.

Jerome, L. W. (1991). *Primary intervention for bulimia: The evaluation of a media presentation for an adolescent population.* Unpublished doctoral dissertation, Kent State University, Kent, OH.

Johnson, C., & Connors, M. (1987). *The etiology and treatment of bulimia nervosa: A biopsychosocial perspective.* New York: Basic Books.

Johnson, C., Powers, P. S., & Dick, R. (1999). Athletes and eating disorders: The National Collegiate Athletic Association Study. *International Journal of Eating Disorders, 26,* 179–188.

Joja, O. (2001). History and current state of treatment for eating disorders in Romania. *European Eating Disorders Review, 9,* 374–380.

Jones, D. C., Vigfusdottir, T. H., & Lee, Y. (2004). Body image and the appearance culture among adolescent girls and boys: An examination of friend conversations, peer criticism, appearance magazines, and the internalization of appearance ideals. *Journal of Adolescent Research, 19,* 323–339.

Kaminski, P. L., & McNamara, K. (1996). A treatment for college women at risk for bulimia: A controlled evaluation. *Journal of Counseling & Development, 74,* 288–294.

Kaplan, A. S., & Garfinkel, P. E. (Eds.). (1993). *Medical issues and the eating disorders: The interface.* New York: Brunner/Mazel.

Kaplan, R. M. (2000). Two pathways to prevention. *American Psychologist, 55,* 382–396.

Kater, K. J. (1998). *Healthy body images: Teaching kids to eat, and love their bodies, too!* Curriculum available from the National Eating Disorders Association, 603 Stewart Street, Suite 803, Seattle, WA. 98101. [www.nationaleatingdisorders.org]

Kater, K. (2004). *Real kids come in all sizes: 10 essential lessons to build your child's body esteem.* New York: Broadway Books.

Kater, K., Rohwer, J., & Levine, M. (2000). An elementary school project for developing healthy body image and reducing risk factors for unhealthy and disordered eating. *Eating Disorders: The Journal of Treatment & Prevention, 8,* 3–16.

Kater, K. J., Rohwer, J., & Londre, K. (2002). Evaluation of an upper elementary school program to prevent body image and weight concerns. *Journal of School Health, 72,* 199–204.

Kaye, W. H. (1995). Neurotransmitters and anorexia nervosa. In K. D. Brownell & C. G. Fairburn (Eds.), *Eating disorders and obesity: A comprehensive handbook* (pp. 255–260). New York: Guilford.

Kaye, W. H. (1997). Neurobiology and genetics: Anorexia nervosa, obsessional behavior, and serotonin. *Psychopharmacology Bulletin, 33,* 335–344.

REFERENCES

Kaye, W. H. (2000, October). *The new biology of eating disorders: Implications for treatment*. Keynote address at the conference Eating Disorders: New Directions for Treatment and Prevention, sponsored by The Ophelia Project and St. Vincent Health System, Erie, PA.

Kaye, W. H., Barbarich, N., Putnam, K., Gendall, K., Fernstrom, J., Fernstrom, M., McConaha, C., & Kishore, A. (2003). Anxiolytic effects of acute tryptophan depletion in anorexia nervosa. *International Journal of Eating Disorders, 33*, 257–267.

Kaye, W. H., Gendall, K., & Strober, M. (1998). Serotonin neuronal function and selective serotonin reuptake inhibitor treatment in anorexia and bulimia nervosa. *Biological Psychiatry, 44*, 825–838.

Kaye, W., & Strober, M. (1999). The neurobiology of eating disorders. In D. S. Charney, E. J. Nestler, & B. S. Bunney (Eds.), *Neurobiology of mental illness* (pp. 891–906). New York: Oxford University Press.

Kazdin, A. E., Kraemer, H. C., Kessler, R. C., Kupfer, D. J., & Offord, D. R. (1997). Contributions of risk-factor research to developmental psychopathology. *Clinical Psychology Review, 17*, 375–406.

Kelly, J. (2002a). *Dads and daughters: How to inspire, understand and support your daughter when she's growing up so fast*. New York: Broadway Books.

Kelly, J. (2002b, April 23). *DAD's victory: ASKO dumps sick appliance ad*. Message posted to Dads and Daughters electronic mailing list (http://www.dadsanddaughters.org).

Kelton-Locke, S. (2001, January/February). Revisiting the question: Can helping hurt? *The California Therapist, 56*–58.

Kendall-Tackett, K. A., Williams, L. M., & Finkelhor, D. (1993). Impact of sexual abuse on children: A review and synthesis of recent empirical studies. *Psychological Bulletin, 113*, 164–180.

Kessler, M., & Albee, G. W. (1975). Primary prevention. *Annual Review of Psychology, 26*, 557–591.

Kilbourne, J. (1994). Still killing us softly: Advertising and the obsession with thinness. In P. Fallon, M. Katzman, & S. Wooley (Eds.), *Feminist perspectives on eating disorders* (pp. 395–418). New York: Guilford Press.

Kilbourne, J. (1995). *Slim hopes: Advertising & the obsession with thinness* [video]. Available from the Media Education Foundation, 28 Center Street, Northampton, MA 01060 (www.mediaed.org).

Killen, J. D. (1996). Development and evaluation of a school-based eating disorder symptoms prevention program. In L. Smolak, M. P. Levine, & R. H. Striegel-Moore (Eds.), *The developmental psychopathology of eating disorders: Implications for research, prevention, and treatment* (pp. 313–339). Mahwah, NJ: Lawrence Erlbaum Associates.

Killen, J. D., Taylor, C. B., Hammer, L. D., Litt, I., Wilson, D. M., Rich, T., Hayward, C., Simmonds, B., Kraemer, H., & Varady, A. (1993). An attempt to modify unhealthful eating attitudes and weight regulation practices of young adolescent girls. *International Journal of Eating Disorders, 13*, 369–384.

Killen, J. D., Taylor, C. B., Hayward, C., Haydel, K., Wilson, D. M., Hammer, L. D., Kraemer, H., Blair-Greiner, A., & Strachowski, D. (1996). Weight concerns influence the development of eating disorders: A 4-year prospective study. *Journal of Consulting and Clinical Psychology, 64*, 936–940.

Killen, J. D., Taylor, C. B., Hayward, C., Wilson, D. M., Haydel, K., Hammer, L. D., Simmonds, B., Robinson, T. N., Litt, I., Varady, A., & Kraemer, H. (1994). Pursuit of thinness and onset of eating disorder symptoms in a community sample of adolescent girls: A three-year prospective analysis. *International Journal of Eating Disorders, 16*, 227–288.

Kirby, D. (1999). *Evidence-based programs: Effective curricula and their common characteristics*. Retrieved July 15, 2004, from the Resource Center for Adolescent Pregnancy Prevention Website: http://www.etro.org/recapp/programs/effectiveprograms.

Klump, K. L., McGue, M., & Iacono, W. G. (2000). Age differences in genetic and environmental influences on eating attitudes and behaviors in preadolescent and adolescent female twins. *Journal of Abnormal Psychology, 109*, 239–251.

Klump, K. L., McGue, M., & Iacono, W. G. (2003). Differential heritability of eating attitudes and behaviors in prepubertal versus pubertal twins. *International Journal of Eating Disorders, 33*, 287–292.

Klump, K. L., Wonderlich, S., Lehoux, P., Bulik, C. M., & Lilenfeld, L. R. R. (2002). Nonshared environment and eating disorders: A review. *International Journal of Eating Disorders, 31*, 118–135.

REFERENCES

Kohler, C. L., Grimley, D., & Reynolds, K. (1999). Theoretical approaches guiding the development and implementation of health promotion programs. In J. M. Raczynski & R. J. DiClemente (Eds.), *Handbook of health promotion and disease prevention* (pp. 23–49). New York: Kluwer Academic/Plenum.

Kotler, P., Roberto, N., & Lee, N. (2002). *Social marketing: Strategies for changing public behavior* (2nd ed.). Thousand Oaks: Sage.

Kowalski, R. (2000). "I was only kidding!": Victims' and perpetrators' perceptions of teasing. *Personality and Social Psychology Bulletin, 26,* 231–241.

Kraemer, H. C., Kazdin, A. E., Offord, D. R., Kessler, R. C., Jensen, P. S., & Kupfer, D. J. (1997). Coming to terms with the terms of risk. *Archives of General Psychiatry, 54,* 337–343.

Kumanyika, S. (1995). Obesity in minority populations: An epidemiologic assessment. *Obesity Research, 2,* 166–182.

Kumar, R., O'Malley, P. M., Johnston, L. D., Schulenberg, J. E., & Bachman, J. G. (2002). Effects of school-level norms on student substance use. *Prevention Science, 3,* 105–124.

Kumpfer, K. L. (1999). Factors and processes contributing to resilience: The resilience framework. In M. D. Glantz & J. L. Johnson (Eds.), *Resilience and development: Positive life adaptations* (pp. 179–224). New York: Kluwer Academic/Plenum.

Kusel, A. B. (1999). *Primary prevention of eating disorders through media literacy training of girls.* Unpublished doctoral dissertation, California School of Professional Psychology, San Diego.

Labre, M. (2002). Adolescent boys and the muscular male body ideal. *Journal of Adolescent Health, 30,* 233–242.

Lamertz, C., Jacobi, C., Yassouridis, A., Arnold, K., & Henkel, A. (2002). Are obese adolescents and young adults at higher risk for mental disorders? A community survey. *Obesity Research, 11,* 1152–1160.

Larkin, J., Rice, C., & Russell, V. (1999). Sexual harassment and the prevention of eating disorders: Educating young women. In N. Piran, M. P. Levine, & C. Steiner-Adair (Eds.), *Preventing eating disorders: A handbook of interventions and special challenges* (pp. 194–207). Philadelphia, PA: Brunner/Mazel.

Lask, B. (2000). Eating disturbances in childhood and adolescence. *Current Paediatrics, 10,* 254–258.

Latzer, Y., & Shatz, S. (1999). Comprehensive community prevention of disturbed attitudes to weight control: A three-level intervention program. *Eating Disorders: The Journal of Treatment & Prevention, 7,* 3–31.

LeCroy, C. W., & Daley, J. (2001). *Empowering adolescent girls: Examining the present and building skills for the future with the Go Grrrls Program.* New York: W. W. Norton.

Lee, S., Ho, T., & Hsu, L. (1993). Fat phobic and non-fat phobic anorexia nervosa: A comparative study of 70 Chinese patients in Hong Kong. *Psychological Medicine, 23,* 999–1017.

Lee, S., Lee, A., Ngai, E., Lee, D., & Wing, Y. (2001). Rationales for food refusal in Chinese patients with anorexia nervosa. *International Journal of Eating Disorders, 29,* 224–229.

Leffert, N., Benson, P. L., Scales, P. C., Sharma, A. R., Drake, D. R., & Blyth, D. A. (1998). Developmental assets: Measurement and prediction of risk behaviors among adolescents. *Applied Developmental Science, 2,* 209–230.

Leichner, P., Arnett, J., Rallo, J. S., Srikameswaran, S., & Vulcano, B. (1986). An epidemiologic study of maladaptive eating attitudes in a Canadian school age population. *International Journal of Eating Disorders, 5,* 969–982.

Leit, R. A., Gray, J. J., & Pope, H. G., Jr. (2002). The media's representation of the ideal male body: A cause for muscle dysmorphia. *International Journal of Eating Disorders, 31,* 334–338.

Lemery, K., Goldsmith, H., Klinnert, M., & Mrazek, D. (1999). Developmental models of infant and child temperament. *Developmental Psychology, 35,* 189–204.

Leon, G., Fulkerson, J., Perry, C., & Early-Zald, M. (1995). Prospective analysis of personality and behavioral vulnerabilities and gender influences in the later development of disordered eating. *Journal of Abnormal Psychology, 104,* 140–149.

Lerner, R. M. (1990). Plasticity, person–context relations, and cognitive training in the aged years: A developmental contextual perspective. *Developmental Psychology, 26,* 911–915.

REFERENCES

Lerner, R. M., Fisher, C. B., & Weinberg, R. A. (2000). Toward a science for and of the people: Promoting civil society through the application of developmental science. *Child Development, 71,* 11-20.

Levine, M. P. (1987). *How schools can help combat student eating disorders.* Washington, DC: National Education Association.

Levine, M. P. (1994). "Beauty Myth" and the Beast: What men can do and be to help prevent eating disorders. *Eating Disorders: The Journal of Treatment and Prevention, 2,* 101-113.

Levine, M. P. (1996). Researching the future of primary prevention. *The Renfrew Perspective, 2*(1), 6-7.

Levine, M. P. (1999). Prevention of eating disorders, eating problems and negative body image. In R. Lemberg (Ed.), *Eating disorders: A reference sourcebook* (pp. 64-72). Phoenix: Oryx Press.

Levine, M. P., & Harrison, K. (2004). The role of mass media in the perpetuation and prevention of negative body image and disordered eating. In J. K. Thompson (Ed.), *Handbook of eating disorders and obesity* (pp. 695-717). New York: Wiley.

Levine, M. P., & Hill, L. (1991). *A 5 Day Lesson Plan Book on Eating Disorders: Grades 7-12.* Published now by The National Eating Disorder Association (see Appendix A), and also available from Gurze Books at 1-800-756-7533 or www.gurze.com.

Levine, M. P., & Piran, N. (1999). Prevention of eating disorders: Reflections, conclusions, and future directions. In N. Piran, M. P. Levine, & C. Steiner-Adair (Eds.), *Preventing eating disorders: A handbook of interventions and special challenges* (pp. 319-329). Philadelphia: Brunner/Mazel.

Levine, M. P., & Piran, N. (2001). The prevention of eating disorders: Towards a participatory ecology of knowledge, action, and advocacy. In R. H. Striegel-Moore & L. Smolak (Eds.), *Eating disorders: New directions for research and practice* (pp. 233-253). Washington, DC: American Psychological Association.

Levine, M. P., & Piran, N. (2004). The role of body image in the prevention of eating disorders. *Body Image, 1,* 57-70.

Levine, M. P., & Piran, N. (in press). Treatment and prevention of eating disorders in adolescence. In T. P. Gullotta & G. Adams (Eds.), *The handbook of dysfunctional behavior in adolescence: Theory, practice, and prevention.* New York: Kluwer/Academic.

Levine, M. P., Piran, N., & Irving, L. M. (2003). Primary prevention of disordered eating behavior in adolescents. In T. P. Gullotta & M. Bloom (Eds.), *The encyclopedia of primary prevention and health promotion* (pp. 423-428). New York: Kluwer Academic/Plenum.

Levine, M. P., Piran, N., & Stoddard, C. (1999). Mission more probable: Media literacy, activism, and advocacy as primary prevention. In N. Piran, M. P. Levine, & C. Steiner-Adair (Eds.), *Preventing eating disorders: A handbook of interventions and special challenges* (pp. 3-25). Philadelphia: Brunner/Mazel.

Levine, M. P., & Smolak, L. (1992). Toward a model of the developmental psychopathology of eating disorders: The example of early adolescence. In J. H. Crowther, D. L. Tennenbaum, S. E. Hobfoll, & M. A. P. Stephens (Eds.), *The etiology of bulimia nervosa: The individual and familial context* (pp. 59-80). Washington, DC: Hemisphere.

Levine, M. P., & Smolak, L. (1996). Media as a context for the development of disordered eating. In L. Smolak, M. P. Levine, & R. H. Striegel-Moore (Eds.), *The developmental psychopathology of eating disorders: Implications for research, prevention, and treatment* (pp. 235-257). Mahwah, NJ: Lawrence Erlbaum Associates.

Levine, M. P., & Smolak, L. (1998). The mass media and disordered eating: Implications for primary prevention. In W. Vandereycken & G. Noordenbos (Eds.), *The prevention of eating disorders* (pp. 23-56). London: Athlone.

Levine, M. P., & Smolak, L. (2001). Primary prevention of body image disturbances and disordered eating in childhood and early adolescence. In J. K. Thompson & L. Smolak (Eds.), *Body image, eating disorders, and obesity in youth: Assessment, prevention, and treatment* (pp. 237-260). Washington, DC: American Psychological Association.

Levine, M. P., & Smolak, L. (2002). Ecological and activism approaches to prevention. In T. F. Cash & T. Pruzinsky (Eds.), *Body images: A handbook of theory, research, and clinical practice* (pp. 497-505). New York: Guilford.

Levine, M. P., Smolak, L., & Hayden, H. (1994). The relation of sociocultural factors to eating attitudes and behaviors among middle school girls, *Journal of Early Adolescence, 14,* 471-490.

REFERENCES

Levine, M. P., Smolak, L., Schermer, F., & Etling, C. (1995). *Eating smart, eating for me: Nutrition education program for the 4th and 5th grades.* Unpublished manuscript, Kenyon College, Ohio.

Levinson, D. (1986). A conception of adult development. *American Psychologist, 41,* 3–13.

Lewis, M., Fiering, C., & Rosenthal, S. (2000). Attachment over time. *Child Development, 71,* 707–720.

Lilenfeld, L. R., & Kaye, W. H. (1998). Genetic studies of anorexia and bulimia nervosa. In H. W. Hoek, J. L. Treasure, & M. A. Katzman (Eds.), *Neurobiology in the treatment of eating disorders* (pp. 169–194). Chichester, UK: John Wiley.

Littleton, H. L., & Ollendick, T. (2003). Negative body image and disordered eating behavior in children and adolescents: What places youth at risk and how can these problems be prevented? *Clinical and Child Family Psychology Review, 6,* 51–66.

Loftus, E. (1997). Memory for a past that never was. *Current Directions in Psychological Science, 6,* 60–65.

Lowe, M., Gleaves, D., DiSimone-Weiss, R., Furgueson, C., Gayda, C., Kolshy, P., Neal-Walden, T., Nelsen, L., & McKinney, S. (1996). Restraint, dieting, and the continuum model of bulimia nervosa. *Journal of Abnormal Psychology, 105,* 508–517.

Lucas, A., Crowson, C., O'Fallon, M., & Melton, L. (1999). The ups and downs of anorexia nervosa. *International Journal of Eating Disorders, 26,* 397–405.

Luthar, S. S., Cicchetti, D., & Becker, B. (2000). The construct of resilience: A critical evaluation and guidelines for future work. *Child Development, 71,* 543–562.

MacKinnon, D. P., Goldberg, L., Clarke, G. N., Elliot, D. L., Cheong, J., Lapin, A., Moe, E. L., & Krull, J. L. (2001). Mediating mechanisms in a program to reduce intentions to use anabolic steroids and improve exercise self-efficacy and dietary behavior. *Prevention Science, 2,* 15–27.

MacKinnon, D. P., & Lockwood, C. M. (2003). Advances in statistical methods for substance abuse prevention research. *Prevention Science, 4,* 155–171.

Macrina, D. M. (1999). Historical and conceptual perspectives on health promotion. In J. M. Raczynski & R. J. DiClemente (Eds.), *Handbook of health promotion and disease prevention* (pp. 11–20). New York: Kluwer Academic/Plenum.

Maine, M. (1991). *Father hunger: Fathers, daughters and food.* Carlsbad, CA: Gürze Books.

Maine, M. (2000). *BodyWars: Making peace with women's bodies—An activist's guide.* Carlsbad, CA: Gürze Books.

Mallick, M. J. (1983). Health hazards of obesity and weight control in children: A review of the literature. *American Journal of Public Health, 73,* 78–82.

Maloney, M., McGuire, J., Daniels, S., & Specker, B. (1989). Dieting behavior and eating attitudes in children. *Pediatrics, 84,* 482–489.

Mann, T., Abdollahi, P. A., Chee, N., Obagi, S., Bruhl, C., Nikkhou, N., & Shukiban, L. (1999, August). *A dissonance approach to eating disorder prevention: Why it should work even though it didn't.* Paper presented at the annual conference of the American Psychological Association, Boston.

Mann, T., & Burgard, D. (1998). Eating disorder prevention programs: What we don't know can hurt us. *Eating Disorders: The Journal of Treatment & Prevention, 6,* 101–103.

Mann, T., Nolen-Hoeksema, S., Huan, K., Burgard, D., Wright, A., & Hanson, K. (1997). Are two interventions worse than none? Joint primary and secondary prevention of eating disorders in college females. *Health Psychology, 16,* 1–11.

Manson, J. E., Willett, W. C., Stampfer, M. J., Golditz, G. A., Hunter, D. J., Hankinson, S. E., Hennekens, C. H., & Speizer, F. E. (1995). Body weight and mortality among women. *New England Journal of Medicine, 333,* 677–685.

Marcus, M., Moulton, M., & Greeno, C. (1995). Binge eating onset in obese patients with binge eating disorders. *Addictive Behaviors, 20,* 747–755.

Marsh, H. M. (1999). Cognitive discrepancy models: Actual, ideal, potential, and future self-perspectives of body image. *Social Cognition, 17,* 46–75.

Martin, G. C., Wertheim, E. H., Prior, M., Smart, D., Sanson, A., & Oberklaid, F. (2000). Longitudinal study of the role of childhood temperament in the later development of eating concerns. *International Journal of Eating Disorders, 27,* 150–162.

Martin, M. C., & Kennedy, P. F. (1993). Advertising and social comparison: Consequences for female preadolescents and adolescents. *Psychology & Marketing, 10,* 513–530.

Martin, M. C., & Kennedy, P. F. (1994). Social comparison and the beauty of advertising models: The role of motives for comparison. *Advances in Consumer Research, 21,* 365–371.

Martz, D. M., & Bazzini, D. G. (1999). Eating disorders prevention programming may be failing: Evaluation of two, one-shot programs. *Journal of College Student Development, 40,* 32–42.

Martz, D. M., Graves, K. D., & Sturgis, E. T. (1997). A pilot peer-leader eating disorders prevention program for sororities. *Eating Disorders: The Journal of Treatment & Prevention, 6,* 294–308.

Masten, A. S., & Coatsworth, J. D. (1995). Competence, resilience, and psychopathology. In D. Cicchetti & D. Cohen (Eds.), *Developmental psychology, Vol. 2: Risk, disorder, and adaptation* (pp. 715–722). New York: Wiley.

Maton, K. (2000). Making a difference: The social ecology of social transformation. *American Journal of Community Psychology, 28,* 25–57.

McCreary, D. R., & Sasse, D. K. (2000). An exploration of the drive for muscularity in adolescent boys and girls. *Journal of American College Health, 48,* 297–304.

McKinley, N. M. (1998). Gender differences in undergraduates' body esteem: The mediating effect of objectified body consciousness and actual/ideal weight discrepancy. *Sex Roles, 39,* 113–123.

McKinley, N. M. (1999). Women and objectified body consciousness: Mothers' and daughters' body experience in cultural, developmental, and familial context. *Developmental Psychology, 35,* 760–769.

McKinley, N. M. (2002). Feminist perspectives and objectified body consciousness. In T. F. Cash & T. Pruzinsky (Eds.), *Body images: A handbook of theory, research, and clinical practice* (pp. 55–62). New York: Guilford.

McKinley, N. M., & Hyde, J. (1996). The Objectified Body Consciousness Scale: Development and validation. *Psychology of Women Quarterly, 20,* 181–215.

McLoyd, V. (1999). Cultural influences in a multicultural society: Conceptual and methodological issues. In A. Masten (Ed.), *Cultural processes in child development: The Minnesota Symposia on Child Psychology* (Vol. 29, pp. 123–136). Mahwah, NJ: Lawrence Erlbaum Associates.

McVey, G. L. (2004). Eating disorders. In L. Rapp-Paglicci, C. Dulmus, & J. Wodarski (Eds.), *Handbook of preventive interventions for children and adolescents* (pp. 275–300). New York: John Wiley.

McVey, G. L., & Davis, R. (2002). A program to promote positive body image: A 1-year follow-up evaluation. *Journal of Early Adolescence, 22,* 96–108.

McVey, G. L., Davis, R., Tweed, S., & Shaw, B. F. (2004). Evaluation of a school-based program designed to improve body image satisfaction, global self-esteem, and eating attitudes and behaviors: A replication study. *International Journal of Eating Disorders, 36,* 1–11.

McVey, G. L., Lieberman, M., Voorberg, N., Wardrope, D., & Blackmore, E. (2003a). School-based peer support groups: A new approach to the prevention of eating disorders. *Eating Disorders: The Journal of Treatment and Prevention, 11,* 169–185.

McVey, G. L., Lieberman, M., Voorberg, N., Wardrope, D., Blackmore, E., & Tweed, S. (2003b). Replication of a peer support prevention program designed to reduce disordered eating: Is a life skills approach sufficient for all middle school students? *Eating Disorders: The Journal of Treatment and Prevention, 11,* 187–195.

McVey, G. L., Tweed, S., & Blackmore, E. (2004). *Evaluation of a comprehensive school-based program designed to increase healthy eating, active living and self-acceptance in middle school students.* Manuscript submitted for publication. [contact gail.mcvey@sickkids.ca]

Mendelson, B., & White, D. (1993). *Manual for the Body Esteem Scale–Children.* Montreal, Canada: Center for Research in Human Development, Concordia University.

Merikangas, K. R., & Avenevoli, S. (2000). Implications of genetic epidemiology for the prevention of substance use disorders. *Addictive Behaviors, 25,* 807–820.

Mickalide, A. D. (1990). Sociocultural factors influencing weight among males. In A. E. Andersen (Ed.), *Males with eating disorders* (pp. 30–39). New York: Brunner/Mazel.

Milkie, M. A. (1999). Social comparisons, reflected appraisals, and mass media: The impact of pervasive beauty images on Black and White girls' self-concepts. *Social Psychology Quarterly, 62,* 190–210.

Miller, J. (1976). *Toward a new psychology of women.* Boston: Beacon Press.

Miller, W. C. (1999). Fitness and fatness in relation to health: Implications for a paradigm shift. *Journal of Social Issues, 55,* 207–219.

Mills, A., Osborn, B., & Neitz, E. (2003). *Shapesville.* Carlstad, CA: Gürze Books.
Minke, K. M. (2000). Preventing school problems & promoting school success through family–school–community collaboration. In K. M. Minke & G. C. Bear (Eds.), *Preventing school problems—Promoting school success: Strategies and programs that work* (pp. 377–420). Bethesda, MD: National Association of School Psychologists.
Mintz, L., & Betz, N. (1988). Prevalence and correlates of eating disordered behaviors among undergraduate women. *Journal of Counseling Psychology, 35,* 463–471.
Mitchell, J. (2001). Psychopharmacology of eating disorders: Current knowledge and future directions. In R. H. Striegel-Moore & L. Smolak (Eds.), *Eating disorders: Innovative directions in research and practice* (pp. 197–212). Washington, DC: American Psychological Association.
Moran, J. R., & Reaman, J. A. (2002). Critical issues for substance abuse prevention targeting American Indian youth. *The Journal of Primary Prevention, 22,* 201–233.
Moreno, A. B., & Thelen, M. H. (1993). A preliminary prevention program for eating disorders in a junior high school population. *Journal of Youth & Adolescence, 22,* 109–124.
Moriarty, D., Shore, R., & Maxim, N. (1990). Evaluation of an eating disorders curriculum. *Evaluation and Program Planning, 13,* 407–413.
Mrazek, P. J., & Haggerty, R. J. (Eds.). (1994). *Reducing risks for mental disorders: Frontiers for prevention intervention research* (report of the Institute of Medicine's Committee on Prevention of Mental Disorders). Washington, DC: National Academy Press.
Muñoz, R. F., Mrazek, P. J., & Haggerty, R. J. (1996). Institute of Medicine report on prevention of mental disorders: Summary and commentary. *American Psychologist, 51,* 1116–1122.
Murnen, S. K., & Smolak, L. (2000). The experience of sexual harassment among grade-school students: Early socialization of female subordination? *Sex Roles, 43,* 1–17.
Murnen, S. K., Smolak, L., Mills, J. A., & Good, L. (2003). Thin, sexy women and strong, muscular men: Grade-school children's responses to objectified images of women and men. *Sex Roles, 49,* 427–437.
Murray, S. H., Touyz, S. W., & Beumont, P. J. V. (1996). Awareness and perceived influence of body ideals in the media: A comparison of eating disorder patients and the general community. *Eating Disorders: The Journal of Treatment & Prevention, 4,* 33–46.
Muse, A., Stein, D., & Abbess, G. (2003). Eating disorders in adolescent boys: A review of the adolescent and young adult literature. *Journal of Adolescent Health, 33,* 427–435.
Mussell, M. P., Binford, R. B., & Fulkerson, J. A. (2000). Eating disorders: Summary of risk factors, prevention programming, and prevention research. *The Counseling Psychologist, 28,* 764–796.
Must, A. (1996). Morbidity and mortality associated with elevated body weight in children and adolescents. *American Journal of Clinical Nutrition, 63,* 445s–447s.
Muth, J., & Cash, T. (1997). Body-image attitudes: What difference does gender make? *Journal of Applied Social Psychology, 27,* 1438–1452.
Mutterperl, J. A., & Sanderson, C. A. (2002). Mind over matter: Internalization of the thinness norm as a moderator of responsiveness to norm misperception education in college women. *Health Psychology, 21,* 519–523.
National Center for Education Statistics. (n.d.). *Dropout rates in the United States: 1999—Hispanic dropout rates by immigration status.* Retrieved July 14, 2004 from http://nces.ed.gov/pubs2001/dropout/StatusRates3.asp.
National Center for Health Statistics. (2000). *Growth charts.* Accessed May 31, 2000 at www.cdc.gov/nchs.
National Center for Health Statistics. (2004). *Prevalence of overweight and obesity among adults: United States, 1999–2002.* Retrieved December 30, 2004, from http://www.cdc.gov/nchs/products/pubs/pubd/hestats/obese/obse99.htm.
National Heart Lung and Blood Institute/National Institute of Health. (1998). *Practical guide to the identification, evaluation and treatment of overweight and obesity in adults* [on-line]. Available: http://www.nhlbi.nih.gov/guidelines/obesity/practgde.pdf.
National Task Force on the Prevention and Treatment of Obesity. (2000). Dieting and the development of eating disorders in overweight and obese adults. *Archives of Internal Medicine, 160,* 2581–2589.
Nebel, M. (1995). *Prevention of disordered eating among college women: A clinical intervention.* Unpublished doctoral dissertation, University of Arizona, Tucson.

REFERENCES

Netemeyer, S. B., & Williamson, D. A. (2001). Assessment of eating disturbance in children and adolescents with eating disorders and obesity. In J. K. Thompson & L. Smolak (Eds.), *Body image, eating disorders, and obesity in youth: Assessment, prevention, and treatment* (pp. 215–234). Washington, DC: American Psychological Association.

Neumark-Sztainer, D. (1992). *The weigh to eat! A program for the prevention of eating disturbances among adolescents.* Contact Dr. Neumark-Sztainer, Division of Epidemiology, School of Public Health, University of Minnesota, Minneapolis, MN 55455.

Neumark-Sztainer, D. (1995). Excessive weight preoccupation: Normative but not harmless. *Nutrition Today, 30,* 68–74.

Neumark-Sztainer, D. (1996). School-based programs for preventing eating disturbances. *Journal of School Health, 66,* 64–71.

Neumark-Sztainer, D. (1999). The weight dilemma: A range of philosophical perspectives. *International Journal of Obesity, 23* (Suppl. 2), S31-S37.

Neumark-Sztainer, D. (2003). Obesity and eating disorder prevention: An integrated approach? *Adolescent Medicine: State of the Art Reviews, 14,* 159–173.

Neumark-Sztainer, D., Butler, R., & Palti, H. (1995). Eating disturbances among adolescent girls: Evaluation of a school-based primary prevention program. *Journal of Nutrition Education, 27,* 24–30.

Neumark-Sztainer, D., Croll, J., Story, M., Hannan, P. J., French, S. A., & Perry, C. (2002). Ethnic/racial differences in weight-related concerns and behaviors among adolescent girls and boys: Findings from Project EAT. *Journal of Psychosomatic Research, 53,* 963–974.

Neumark-Sztainer, D., Falkner, N., Story, M., Perry, C., Hannan, P. J., & Mulert, S. (2002). Weight-teasing among adolescents: Correlations with weight status and disordered eating behaviors. *International Journal of Obesity & Related Metabolic Disorders, 26,* 123–131.

Neumark-Sztainer, D., Sherwood, N., Coller, T., & Hannan, P. J. (2000). Primary prevention of disordered eating among pre-adolescent girls: Feasibility and short-term impact of a community-based intervention. *Journal of the American Dietetic Association, 100,* 1466–1473.

Neumark-Sztainer, D., Story, M., & Faibisch, L. (1997). Perceived stigmatization among overweight African-American and Caucasian adolescent girls. *Journal of Adolescent Health, 23,* 1–7.

Neumark-Sztainer, D., Story, M., Falkner, N. H., Beuhring, T., & Resnick, M. D. (1999). Sociodemographic and personal characteristics of adolescents engaged in weight loss and weight/muscle gain behaviors: Who is doing what? *Preventive Medicine, 28,* 40–50.

Neumark-Sztainer, D., Story, M., & French, S. A. (1996). Covariations of unhealthy weight loss behaviors and other high-risk behaviors among adolescents. *Archives of Pediatric and Adolescent Medicine, 150,* 304–308.

Neumark-Sztainer, D., Story, M., Hannan, P. J., & Rex, J. (2003). New Moves: A school-based obesity prevention program for adolescent girls. *Preventive Medicine, 37,* 41–51.

Neumark-Sztainer, D., Story, M., & Harris, T. (1999). Perceptions of secondary school staff toward the implementation of school-based activities to prevent weight-related disorders. *American Journal of Health Promotion, 13,* 153–156.

Nicholls, D., Chater, R., & Lask, B. (2000). Children into DSM don't go: A comparison of classification systems for eating disorders in childhood and early adolescence. *International Journal of Eating Disorders, 28,* 317–324.

Nichter, M. (2000). *Fat talk: What girls and their parents say about dieting.* Cambridge, MA: Harvard University Press.

Nichter, M., Vukovic, N., & Parker, S. (1999). The Looking Good, Feeling Good Program: A multi-ethnic intervention for healthy body image, nutrition, and physical activity. In N. Piran, M. Levine, & C. Steiner-Adair (Eds.), *Preventing eating disorders: A handbook of interventions and special challenges* (pp. 175–193). Philadelphia: Brunner/Mazel.

Nicolino, J. C., Martz, D. M., & Curtin, L. (2001). Evaluation of a cognitive-behavioral therapy intervention to improve body image and decrease dieting in college women. *Eating Behaviors, 2,* 353–362.

Nielsen, S. (2002). Eating disorders in females with Type 1 diabetes: An update of a meta-analysis. *European Eating Disorders Review, 10,* 241–254.

Nielsen, S., Møller-Madsen, S., Isager, T., Jørgensen, J., Pagsberg, K., & Theander, S. (1998). Standardized mortality in eating disorders—A quantitative summary of previously published and new evidence. *Journal of Psychosomatic Research, 44,* 413–434.

Noll, S., & Fredrickson, B. (1998). A mediational model linking self-objectification, body shame, and disordered eating. *Psychology of Women Quarterly, 22,* 623–636.

O'Dea, J. (2000). School-based interventions to prevent eating disorders: First do no harm. *Eating Disorders: The Journal of Treatment and Prevention, 8,* 123–131.

O'Dea, J. (2002a). Body Basics: A nutrition education program for adolescents about food, nutrition, growth, body image, and weight control. *Journal of the American Dietetic Association, 102*(Suppl. 3), S68-S70.

O'Dea, J. (2002b). Can body image education programs be harmful to adolescent females? *Eating Disorders: The Journal of Treatment & Prevention, 10,* 1–13.

O'Dea, J. (2002c). The new self-esteem approach for the prevention of body image and eating problems in children and adolescents. *Health Weight Journal, 16,* (November/December), 89–93.

O'Dea, J., & Abraham, S. (2000). Improving the body image, eating attitudes and behaviors of young male and female adolescents: A new educational approach which focuses on self-esteem. *International Journal of Eating Disorders, 28,* 43–57.

O'Dea, J., & Maloney, D. (2000). Preventing eating and body image problems in children and adolescents using the Health Promoting Schools Framework. *Journal of School Health, 70,* 18–21.

Offord, D. (2000). Selection of levels of prevention. *Addictive Behaviors, 25,* 833–842.

Offord, D., Kraemer, H., Kazdin, A., Jensen, P., & Harrington, R. (1998). Lowering the burden of suffering from child psychiatric disorder: Trade-offs among clinical, targeted, and universal interventions. *Journal of the American Academy of Child and Adolescent Psychiatry, 37,* 686–694.

Ogg, E. C., Millar, H. R., Pusztai, E. E., & Thom, A. S. (1997). General practice consultation patterns preceding diagnosis of eating disorders. *International Journal of Eating Disorders, 22,* 89–93.

Olmsted, M. P., Daneman, D., Rydall, A. C., Lawson, M. L., & Rodin, G. M. (2002). The effects of psychoeducation on disturbed eating attitudes and behavior in young women with Type 1 diabetes mellitus. *International Journal of Eating Disorders, 32,* 230–239.

Outwater, A. D. (1990). *An intervention project to improve body image and self-esteem in 6th-grade boys and girls as a potential prevention against eating disorders.* Unpublished doctoral dissertation, The Union Institute, Cincinnati, OH.

Overton, W. (1985). Scientific methodologies and the competence-moderator-performance issue. In E. Neimark, R. DeLisi, & J. Newman (Eds.), *Moderators of competence* (pp. 15–41). Hillsdale, NJ: Lawrence Erlbaum Associates.

Papazian, R. (1991). *Never say diet.* Retrieved July 17, 2001, from the web site of the US Food & Drug Administration: http://www.fda.gov/bbs/topics/consumer/CON00111.html.

Parkinson, K., Tovée, M., & Cohen-Tovée, E. (1998). Body shape perceptions of preadolescent and young adolescent children. *European Eating Disorders Review, 6,* 126–135.

Pasqualoni, E., Ginetti, S., Guardini, S., Sartirana, M., & Dalle Grave, R. (2002, May). *Prevenzione primaria dei disturbi dell'alimentazione nella cuola media inferiore: Uno studeo aperto* [Primary prevention of eating disorders in middle schools: An open study]. Paper presented at the Conference "Promozione della Salute nella Regione Veneto" sponsored by the Italian Association of Eating Disorders and Weight Problems, Verona, Italy.

Paxton, S. J. (1993). A prevention program for disturbed eating and body dissatisfaction in adolescent girls: A 1 year follow-up. *Health Education Research: Theory & Practice, 8,* 43–51.

Paxton, S. J. (1999). Peer relations, body image, and disordered eating in adolescent girls: Implications for prevention. In N. Piran, M. P. Levine, & C. Steiner-Adair (Eds.), *Preventing eating disorders: A handbook of interventions and special challenges* (pp. 134–147). Philadelphia: Brunner/Mazel.

Paxton, S. J., Schutz, H. K., Wertheim, E. H., & Muir, S. L. (1999). Friendship clique and peer influences on body image concerns, dietary restraint, extreme weight-loss behaviors, and binge eating in adolescent girls. *Journal of Abnormal Psychology, 108,* 255–266.

Paxton, S. J., Wertheim, E. H., Pilawski, A., Durkin, S., & Holt, T. (2002). Evaluations of dieting prevention messages by adolescent girls. *Preventive Medicine, 35,* 474–491.

Peirce, K. (1990). A feminist theoretical perspective on the socialization of teenage girls through *Seventeen* magazine. *Sex Roles, 23,* 491–500.

REFERENCES

Pentz, M. A. (2000). Institutionalizing community-based prevention through policy change. *Journal of Community Psychology, 28,* 257–270.

Pentz, M. A., Dwyer, J., MacKinnon, D. P., Flay, B. R., Hansen, W. B., Wang, E. Y., & Johnson, C. A. (1989). A multicommunity trial for primary prevention of adolescent drug abuse: Effects on drug use prevalence. *Journal of the American Medical Association, 261*(22), 3259–3266.

Perry, C. L. (1999). *Creating health behavior change: How to develop community-wide programs for youth.* Thousand Oaks, CA: Sage.

Petersen, A. C., Sargiani, P., & Kennedy, R. E. (1991). Adolescent depression: Why more girls? *Journal of Youth and Adolescence, 20,* 247–271.

Petersen, A. C., Shulenberg, J. E., Abramowitz, R. H., Offer, D., & Jarcho, H. D. (1984). A Self-Image Questionnaire for Young Adults (SIQYA): Reliability and validity studies. *Journal of Youth and Adolescence, 13,* 93–111.

Peterson, A., Mann, S., Kealey, K., & Marek, P. (2000). Experimental design and methods for school-based randomized trials: Experience from the Hutchinson Smoking Prevention Project (HSPP). *Controlled Clinical Trials, 21,* 144–165.

Phelps, L., Dempsey, M., Sapia, J., & Nelson, L. (1999). The efficacy of a school-based eating disorder prevention program: Building physical self-esteem and personal competencies. In N. Piran, M. P. Levine, & C. Steiner-Adair (Eds.), *Preventing eating disorders: A handbook of interventions and special challenges* (pp. 163–174). Philadelphia: Brunner/Mazel.

Phelps, L., Sapia, J., Nathanson, D., & Nelson, L. (2000). An empirically supported eating disorder prevention program. *Psychology in the Schools, 37,* 443–452.

Phinney, J. (1996). When we talk about American ethnic groups, what do we mean? *American Psychologist, 51,* 918–927.

Phinney, J., & Chavera, V. (1995). Parental ethnic socialization and adolescent coping with problems related to ethnicity. *Journal of Research on Adolescence, 5,* 31–54.

Piaget, J. (1967). *Six psychological studies.* New York: Vintage.

Pierce, J. P., Lee, L., & Gilpin, E. A. (1994). Smoking initiation by adolescent girls, 1944 through 1988: An association with targeted advertising. *Journal of the American Medical Association, 271,* 608–611.

Pike, K. (1995). Bulimic symptomatology in high school girls. *Psychology of Women Quarterly, 19,* 373–396.

Piran, N. (1995). Prevention: Can early lessons lead to a delineation of an alternative model? A critical look at prevention with schoolchildren. *Eating Disorders: The Journal of Treatment & Prevention, 3,* 28–36.

Piran, N. (1998). A participatory approach to the prevention of eating disorders in a school. In W. Vandereycken & G. Noordenbos (Eds.), *The prevention of eating disorders* (pp. 173–186). London: Athlone.

Piran, N. (1999a). Eating disorders: A trial of prevention in a high risk school setting. *Journal of Primary Prevention, 20,* 75–90.

Piran, N. (1999b). On the move from tertiary to secondary and primary prevention: Working with an elite dance school. In N. Piran, M. P. Levine, & C. Steiner-Adair (Eds.), *Preventing eating disorders: A handbook of interventions and special challenges* (pp. 256–269). Philadelphia: Brunner/Mazel.

Piran, N. (1999c). The reduction of preoccupation with body weight and shape in schools: A feminist approach. In N. Piran, M. P. Levine, & C. Steiner-Adair (Eds.), *Preventing eating disorders: A handbook of interventions and special challenges* (pp. 148–159). Philadelphia: Brunner/Mazel.

Piran, N. (1999d, February). *The whole-school approach to the prevention of eating disorders.* Second Annual Conference for Educators, Harvard Eating Disorders Center, Boston.

Piran, N. (2001). Re-inhabiting the body from the inside out: Girls transform their school environment. In D. L. Tolman & M. Brydon-Miller (Eds.), *From subjects to subjectivities: A handbook of interpretative and participatory methods* (pp. 218–238). New York: New York University Press.

Piran, N. (2002). Embodiment: A mosaic of inquiries in the area of body weight and shape preoccupation. In S. M. Abbey (Ed.), *Ways of knowing in and through the body: Diverse perspectives on embodiment* (pp. 211–214). Welland, Ontario: Soleil Publishing.

Piran, N. (2004). Teachers: On "being" (rather than "doing") prevention. *Eating Disorders: The Journal of Treatment & Prevention, 12,* 1–9.

REFERENCES

Piran, N., Carter, W., Thompson, S., & Pajouhandeh, P. (2002). Powerful girls: A contradiction in terms? Young women speak about growing up in a girl's body. In S. M. Abbey (Ed.), *Ways of knowing in and through the body: Diverse perspectives on embodiment* (pp. 206–210). Welland, Ontario: Soleil Publishing.

Piran, N., Levine, M. P., Irving, L. M., & the EDAP/NEDA Staff. (2000, May). *GO GIRLS!^{TM} Preventing negative body image through media literacy.* Paper/workshop presented at the Summit 2000 (Children, Youth, and the Media Beyond the Millennium) conference, Toronto.

Piran, N., Levine, M. P., & Steiner-Adair, C. (Eds.). (1999). *Preventing eating disorders: A handbook of interventions and special challenges.* Philadelphia: Brunner/Mazel.

Pi-Sunyer, F. X. (1999). Comorbidities of overweight and obesity: Current evidence and research issues. *Medicine and Science in Sports and Exercise, 31* (Suppl.), S602-S608.

Polivy, J., & Herman, C. P. (1985). Dieting and bingeing: A causal analysis. *American Psychologist, 40,* 193–201.

Pomeroy, C. (2004). Assessment of medical status and physical factors. In J. K. Thompson (Ed.), *Handbook of eating disorders and obesity* (pp. 81–111). New York: Wiley.

Pope, H. G., Jr., Olivardia, R., Gruber, A., & Borowiecki, J. (1999). Evolving ideals of male body image as seen through action toys. *International Journal of Eating Disorders, 26,* 65–72.

Pope, H. G., Jr., Phillips, K. A., & Olivardia, R. (2000). *The Adonis Complex: The secret crisis of male body obsession.* New York: The Free Press.

Porter, J., Morrell, T., & Moriarty, D. (1986). Primary prevention of anorexia nervosa: Evaluation of a pilot project for early and pre-adolescents. *The Canadian Association for Health, Physical Education and Recreation Journal, 52,* 21–26.

Posavac, H. D., Posavac, S. S., & Posavac, E. J. (1998). Exposure to media images of female attractiveness and concern with body weight among young women. *Sex Roles, 38*(3/4), 187–201.

Posavac, H. D., Posavac, S. S., & Weigel, R. G. (2001). Reducing the impact of media images on women at risk for body image disturbance: Three targeted interventions. *Journal of Social and Clinical Psychology, 20,* 324–340.

Power, C., Lake, J. K., & Cole, T. J. (1997). Measurement and long-term health risks of child and adolescent fatness. *International Journal of Obesity, 21,* 507–526.

Pratt, B. M., & Woolfenden, S. R. (2002). Interventions for preventing eating disorders in children and adolescents (Cochrane Review). *The Cochrane Library, Issue 2.* Oxford: Update Software (http://www.update-software.com/abstracts/mainindex.html).

Presnell, K., & Stice, E. (2003). An experimental test of the effect of weight-loss dieting on bulimic pathology: Tipping the scales in a different direction. *Journal of Abnormal Psychology, 112,* 166–170.

Prevention Research Steering Committee (D. Reiss, Chair). (1993). *The prevention of mental disorders: A national research agenda.* Washington, DC: Author.

Price, R. H. (1983). The education of a prevention psychologist. In R. D. Felner, L. A. Jason, J. N. Moritsugu, & S. S. Farber (Eds.), *Preventive psychology: Theory, research, and practice* (pp. 290–296). New York: Pergamon.

Puhl, R., & Brownell, K. (2001). Obesity, bias, and discrimination. *Obesity Research, 8,* 788–805.

Rabak-Wagener, J., Eickhoff-Shemek, J., & Kelly-Vance, L. (1998). The effect of media analysis on attitudes and behaviors regarding body image among college students. *Journal of American College Health, 47,* 29–35.

Raevuori, A. (2002). Temperament, character and eating disorders. *European Eating Disorders Review, 10,* 146–150.

Ransley, J. (1999). Eating disorders and adolescents: What are the issues for secondary schools? *Health Education, 1,* 35–42.

Reed, D. L., Thompson, J. K., Brannick, M. T., & Sacco, W. P. (1991). Development and validation of the Physical Appearance State and Trait Anxiety Scale (PASTAS). *Journal of Anxiety Disorders, 5,* 323–332.

Reger, B., Wootan, M. G., & Booth-Butterfield, S. (1999). Using mass media to promote healthy eating: A community-based demonstration project. *Preventive Medicine, 29,* 414–421.

Reiss, D., & Price, R. H. (1996). National research agenda for prevention research: The National Institute of Mental Health report. *American Psychologist, 51,* 1109–1115.

REFERENCES

Rende, R. (1996). Liability to psychopathology: A quantitative genetic perspective. In L. Smolak, M. P. Levine, & R. H. Striegel-Moore (Eds.), *The developmental psychopathology of eating disorders: Implications for research, prevention, and treatment* (pp. 59–76). Mahwah, NJ: Lawrence Erlbaum Associates.

Ricciardelli, L. A., & McCabe, M. P. (2001a). Children's body image concerns and eating disturbance: A review of the literature. *Clinical Psychology Review, 21,* 325–344.

Ricciardelli, L. A., & McCabe, M. P. (2001b). Self-esteem and negative affect as moderators of sociocultural influences on body dissatisfaction, strategies to decrease weight, and strategies to increase muscles among adolescent boys and girls. *Sex Roles, 44,* 189–207.

Ricciardelli, L. A., & McCabe, M. P. (2004). A biopsychosocial model of disordered eating and the pursuit of muscularity in adolescent boys. *Psychological Bulletin, 130,* 179–205.

Ricciardelli, L. A., McCabe, M. P., & Banfield, S. (2000). Body image and body change methods in adolescent boys. Role of parents, friends, and the media. *Journal of Psychosomatic Research, 49,* 189–197.

Rice, R. E., & Atkin, C. K. (Eds.). (2001). *Public communication campaigns* (3rd ed.). Thousand Oaks, CA: Sage.

Rice, R. E., & Atkin, C. K. (2002). Communication campaigns: Theory, design, implementation, and evaluation. In J. Bryant & D. Zillmann (Eds.), *Media effects: Advances in theory and research* (2nd ed., pp. 427–451). Mahwah, NJ: Lawrence Erlbaum Associates.

Rice, R. E., & Katz, J. E. (Eds.). (2001). *The Internet and health communication: Experiences and expectations.* Thousand Oaks, CA: Sage.

Richards, P. S., Baldwin, B. M., Frost, H. A., Clark-Sly, J. B., Berrett, M. E., & Hardman, R. K. (2000). What works for treating eating disorders: Conclusions of 28 outcome reviews. *Eating Disorders: The Journal of Treatment & Prevention, 8,* 189–206.

Richman, R. D. (1993). *Primary prevention of eating disorders: A pilot program.* Unpublished masters thesis, Simon Fraser University, Burnaby, British Columbia.

Richman, R. D. (1997). *Preventing eating disorders; promoting healthy attitudes and behaviors: A school-based program.* Unpublished doctoral dissertation, Simon Fraser University, Burnaby, British Columbia.

Rieger, E., Touyz, S., Swain, R., & Beumont, P. (2001). Cross-cultural research on anorexia nervosa: Assumptions regarding the role of body weight. *International Journal of Eating Disorders, 29,* 205–215.

Robinson, T. N., & Killen, J. D. (2001). Obesity prevention for children and adolescents. In J. K. Thompson & L. Smolak (Eds.), *Body image, eating disorders, and obesity in youth* (pp. 261–292). Washington, DC: American Psychological Association.

Robison, J. (2003). Health at Every Size: Antidote for the "obesity epidemic." *Healthy Weight Journal,* January/February, 4–7.

Rocco, P. L., Ciano, R. P., & Balestrieri, M. (2001). Psychoeducation in the prevention of eating disorders: An experimental approach in adolescent schoolgirls. *British Journal of Medical Psychology, 74,* 359–367.

Rodin, J., Silberstein, L. R., & Striegel-Moore, R. H. (1985). Women and weight: A normative discontent. In T. B. Sonderegger (Ed.), *Nebraska symposium on motivation: Vol. 32. Psychology and gender* (pp. 267–307). Lincoln: University of Nebraska Press.

Roosa, M. W., Dumka, L. E., Gonzales, N. A., & Knight, G. P. (2002). Cultural/ethnic issues and the prevention scientist in the 21st century. *Prevention & Treatment, 5,* Article 0005a. Retrieved April 1, 2002, from http://journals.apa.org/prevention/Volume5/pre0050005a.html.

Rosen, J. C. (1989, April–June). Prevention of eating disorders. *Newsletter of the National Anorexic Aid Society, 12,* 1–3. Available from the National Eating Disorders Association, 603 Stewart Street, Suite 803, Seattle, WA 98101.

Rosen, J. C., Saltzberg, E., & Srebnik, D. (1989). Cognitive behavior therapy for negative body image. *Behavior Therapy, 20,* 393–404.

Rosen, K. (1996). The principles of developmental psychopathology: Illustration from the study of eating disorders. In L. Smolak, M. P. Levine, & R. H. Striegel-Moore (Eds.), *The developmental psychopathology of eating disorders: Implications for research, prevention, and treatment* (pp. 3–30). Mahwah, NJ: Lawrence Erlbaum Associates.

Rosenthal, R., & Rosnow, R. L. (1991). *Essentials of behavioral research: Methods and data analysis* (2nd ed.). New York: McGraw-Hill.

Rosenvinge, J. H., & Børresen, R. (1999). Preventing eating disorders—Time to change programmes or paradigms? Current update and further recommendations. *European Eating Disorders Review, 7,* 5–16.

Rosenvinge, J. H., & Westjordet, M. Ø (2004). Is information about eating disorders experienced as harmful? A consumer perspective on primary prevention. *Eating Disorders: The Journal of Treatment & Prevention, 12,* 11–20.

Rosner, B., Prineas, R., Loggie, J., & Daniels, S. (1998). Percentiles for body mass index in U.S. children 5 to 17 years of age. *Journal of Pediatrics, 132,* 211–222.

Roth, J. L., & Brooks-Gunn, J. (2003). Youth development programs: Risk, prevention, and policy. *Journal of Adolescent Health, 32,* 170–182.

Roth, J. L., Brooks-Gunn, J., Murray, L., & Foster, W. (1998). Promoting healthy adolescents: Synthesis of youth development program evaluations. *Journal of Research on Adolescence, 8,* 423–459.

Rothblum, E. D. (1994). "I'll die for the revolution but don't ask me not to diet": Feminism and the continuing stigma of obesity. In P. Fallon, M. A. Katzman, & S. C. Wooley (Eds.), *Feminist perspectives on eating disorders* (pp. 53–76). New York: Guilford.

Russell, G. F. M. (2004). Thoughts on the 25th anniversary of bulimia nervosa. *European Eating Disorders Review, 12,* 139–152.

Ryff, C. D. (1989). Happiness is everything, or is it? Explorations of the meaning of psychological well-being. *Journal of Personality and Social Psychology, 57,* 1069–1081.

Sameroff, A., & Chandler, M. (1975). Reproductive risk and the continuum of caretaking casualty. In F. Horowitz (Ed.), *Review of child development research* (Vol. 4, pp. 197–244). Chicago: University of Chicago Press.

Sanderson, C. A., Darley, J. M., & Messinger, C. S. (2002). "I'm not as thin as you think I am": The development and consequences of feeling discrepant from the thinness norm. *Personality and Social Psychology Bulletin, 28,* 172–183.

Sanderson, C. A., & Holloway, R. M. (2003). Who benefits from what? Drive for thinness as a moderator of responsiveness to different eating disorders prevention messages. *Journal of Applied Social Psychology, 33,* 1837–1861.

Santonastaso, P., Zanetti, T., Ferrara, S., Olivetto, M. C., Magnavita, N., & Favaro, A. (1999). A preventive intervention program in adolescent schoolgirls: A longitudinal study. *Psychotherapy and Psychosomatics, 68,* 46–50.

Sawrer, D. (2001). Plastic surgery in children and adolescents. In J. K. Thompson & L. Smolak (Eds.), *Body image, eating disorders, and obesity in youth: Assessment, prevention, and treatment* (pp. 341–366). Washington, DC: American Psychological Assocation.

Schmidt, U., & Treasure, J. (1997). Eating disorders and the dental practitioner. *European Journal of Prosthodontic Restoration Dentistry, 5,* 161–167.

Schuman, M., Contento, I., Graber, J. A., & Brooks-Gunn, J. (1994). *The formative evaluation of a curriculum designed to promote healthy eating behavior in adolescent girls.* Paper presented at the annual meeting of the Society for Nutrition Education, Portland, OR.

Schur, E., Sanders, M., & Steiner, H. (2000). Body dissatisfaction and dieting in young children. *International Journal of Eating Disorders, 27,* 74–82.

Schwitzer, A. M., Bergholz, K., Dore, T., & Salimi, L. (1998). Eating disorders among college women: Prevention, education, and treatment responses. *Journal of American College Health, 46,* 199–207.

Scott, E., & Sobczak, C. (2002). *Body aloud! Helping children and teens find their own solutions to eating and body image problems.* Berkeley, CA: The Body Positive.

Seaver, A., McVey, G., Fullerton, Y., & Stratton, L. (1997). *"Every BODY is a Somebody": An active learning program to promote healthy body image, positive self-esteem, healthy eating and an active lifestyle for adolescent females: Teachers Guide.* Body Image Coalition of Peel, Brampton, Ontario, Canada. For information, contact gail.mcvey@sickkids.ca.

Shaw, J., & Waller, G. (1995). The media's impact on body image: Implications for prevention and treatment. *Eating Disorders: The Journal of Treatment & Prevention, 3,* 115–123.

Sheffield, C. (1995). Sexual terrorism. In J. Freeman (Ed.), *Women: A feminist perspective* (pp. 1–21). Mountain View, CA: Mayfield.

Shepard, R. E. (2000). *The Body and Soul Program: Evaluation of a peer educator-led eating disorders education and prevention program*. Unpublished doctoral dissertation, The University of Oregon, Eugene, OR.

Sheridan, C. (1996). The losing game. On *One Sure Thing* [CD]. Evanston, IL: Waterbug Records.

Shiltz, T. J. (1997). *Eating concerns support group curriculum grades 7–12*. Greenfield, WI: Community Recovery Press.

Shisslak, C. M., & Crago, M. (2001). Risk and protective factors in the development of eating disorders. In J. K. Thompson & L. Smolak (Eds.), *Body image, eating disorders, and obesity in youth: Assessment, prevention, and treatment* (pp. 103–126). Washington, DC: American Psychological Association.

Shisslak, C. M., Crago, M., & Estes, L. S. (1995). The spectrum of eating disturbances. *International Journal of Eating Disorders, 18*, 209–219.

Shisslak, C. M., Crago, M., Estes, L. S., & Gray, N. (1996). Content and method of developmentally appropriate prevention programs. In L. Smolak, M. P. Levine, & R. H. Striegel-Moore (Eds.), *The developmental psychopathology of eating disorders: Implications for research, prevention, and treatment* (pp. 341–363). Mahwah, NJ: Lawrence Erlbaum Associates.

Shisslak, C. M., Crago, M., & Neal, M. E. (1990). Prevention of eating disorders among adolescents. *American Journal of Health Promotion, 5*, 100–106.

Shisslak, C. M., Crago, M., Renger, R., & Clark-Wagner, A. (1998). Self-esteem and the prevention of eating disorders. *Eating Disorders: The Journal of Treatment & Prevention, 6*, 105–117.

Shisslak, C. M., Renger, R., Sharpe, T., Crago, M., McKnight, K., Gray, N., Bryson, S., Estes, L. S., Parnaby, O., Killen, J. D., & Taylor, C. B. (1999). Development and evaluation of the McKnight Risk Factor Survey for assessing potential risk and protective factors for disordered eating in preadolescent and adolescent girls. *International Journal of Eating Disorders, 25*, 195–214.

Silverman, J. G., Raj, A., Mucci, L. A., & Hathaway, J. E. (2001). Dating violence against adolescent girls and associated substance use, unhealthy weight control, sexual risk behavior, pregnancy, and suicidality. *Journal of the American Medical Association, 286*, 572–579.

Silverstein, B., & Perlick, D. (1995). *The cost of competence: Why inequality causes depression, eating disorders, and illness in women*. New York: Oxford University Press.

Smith, J. E., Wolfe, B. L., & Laframboise, D. E. (2001). Body image treatment for a community sample of obligatory and nonobligatory exercisers. *International Journal of Eating Disorders, 30*, 375–388.

Smolak, L. (1996). Methodological implications of a developmental psychopathology approach to the study of eating problems. In L. Smolak, M. P. Levine, & R. H. Striegel-Moore (Eds.), *The developmental psychopathology of eating disorders: Implications for research, prevention, and treatment* (pp. 31–56). Hillsdale, NJ: Lawrence Erlbaum Associates.

Smolak, L. (1999). Elementary school curricula for the primary prevention of eating problems. In N. Piran, M. P. Levine, & C. Steiner-Adair (Eds.), *Preventing eating disorders: A handbook of interventions and special challenges* (pp. 85–104). Philadelphia: Brunner/Mazel.

Smolak, L. (2002). Body image development in childhood. In T. F. Cash & T. Pruzinsky (Eds.), *Body image: A handbook of theory, research, and clinical practice* (pp. 65–73). New York: Guilford.

Smolak, L. (2004). Body image in childhood and adolescence: Where do we go from here? *Body Image, 1*, 15–28.

Smolak, L., Harris, B., Levine, M. P., & Shisslak, C. M. (2001). Teachers: The forgotten influence on the success of prevention programs. *Eating Disorders: The Journal of Treatment and Prevention, 9*, 261–266.

Smolak, L., & Levine, M. P. (1994a). Critical issues in the developmental psychopathology of eating disorders. In L. Alexander & D. B. Lumsden (Eds.), *Understanding eating disorders* (pp. 37–60). Washington, DC: Taylor & Francis.

Smolak, L., & Levine, M. P. (1994b). Psychometric properties of the Children's Eating Attitudes Test. *International Journal of Eating Disorders, 16*, 275–282.

Smolak, L., & Levine, M. P. (1996). Developmental transitions at middle school and college. In L. Smolak, M. P. Levine, & R. H. Striegel-Moore (Eds.), *The developmental psychopathology of eating disorders: Implications for research, prevention, and treatment* (pp. 207–233). Hillsdale, NJ: Lawrence Erlbaum Associates.

Smolak, L., & Levine, M. P. (2001a). A two-year follow-up of a primary prevention program for negative body image and unhealthy weight regulation. *Eating Disorders: Journal of Treatment and Prevention, 9,* 313–326.

Smolak, L., & Levine, M. P. (2001b). Body image in children. In J. K. Thompson & L. Smolak (Eds.), *Body image, eating disorders, and obesity in youth: Assessment, prevention, and treatment* (pp. 41–66). Washington, DC: American Psychological Association.

Smolak, L., Levine, M. P., & Gralen, S. (1993). The impact of puberty and dating on eating problems among middle school girls. *Journal of Youth and Adolescence, 22,* 355–368.

Smolak, L., Levine, M. P., & Schermer, F. (1998a). A controlled evaluation of an elementary school primary prevention program for eating problems. *Journal of Psychosomatic Research, 44,* 339–353.

Smolak, L., Levine, M. P., & Schermer, F. (1998b). Lessons from lessons: An evaluation of an elementary school prevention program. In W. Vandereycken & G. Noordenbos (Eds.), *The prevention of eating disorders* (pp. 137–172). London: Athlone.

Smolak, L., Levine, M. P., & Schermer, F. (1999). Parental input and weight concerns among elementary school children. *International Journal of Eating Disorders, 25,* 263–271.

Smolak, L., Levine, M. P., & Striegel-Moore, R. H. (Eds.). (1996). *The developmental psychopathology of eating disorders: Implications for research, prevention, and treatment.* Hillsdale, NJ: Lawrence Erlbaum Associates.

Smolak, L., Levine, M. P., & Thompson, J. K. (2001). The use of the Sociocultural Attitudes Toward Appearance Questionnaire with middle school boys and girls. *International Journal of Eating Disorders, 29,* 216–223.

Smolak, L., & Munstertieger, B. (2002). The relationship of gender and voice to depression and eating disorders. *Psychology of Women Quarterly, 26,* 234–241.

Smolak, L., & Murnen, S. K. (2001). Gender and eating problems. In R. H. Striegel-Moore & L. Smolak (Eds.), *Eating disorders: Innovations in research, treatment, and prevention* (pp. 91–110). Washington, DC: American Psychological Association.

Smolak, L., & Murnen, S. K. (2002). A meta-analytic examination of the relationship between sexual abuse and eating problems. *International Journal of Eating Disorders, 31,* 136–150.

Smolak, L., & Murnen, S. K. (2004). A feminist approach to eating disorders. In J. K. Thompson (Ed.), *Handbook of eating disorders and obesity* (pp. 590–605). Hoboken, NJ: Wiley.

Smolak, L., Murnen, S. K., & Ruble, A. E. (2000). Female athletes and eating disorders: A meta-analysis. *International Journal of Eating Disorders, 27,* 371–381.

Smolak, L., & Striegel-Moore, R. H. (2001). Challenging the myth of the golden girl: Ethnicity and eating disorders. In R. H. Striegel-Moore & L. Smolak (Eds.), *Eating disorders: Innovations in research, treatment, and prevention* (pp. 111–132). Washington, DC: American Psychological Association.

Spiller, B. B. (2000). *The development and evaluation of an eating disorder prevention program for college age women.* Unpublished doctoral dissertation, The University of Tennessee at Knoxville.

Springer, E. A., Winzelberg, A. J., Perkins, R., & Taylor, C. B. (1999). Effects of a body image curriculum for college students on improved body image. *International Journal of Eating Disorders, 26,* 13–20.

Spurrell, E., Wilfley, D. E., Tanofsky, M., & Brownell, K. (1997). Age of onset of binge eating: Are there different pathways to binge eating? *International Journal of Eating Disorders, 21,* 55–65.

Steen, S. N., Wadden, T. A., Foster, G. D., & Andersen, R. E. (1996). Are obese adolescent boys ignoring an important health risk? *International Journal of Eating Disorders, 20,* 281–286.

Stein, N. (1995). Sexual harassment in school: The public performance of gendered violence. *Harvard Educational Review, 65,* 145–162.

Stein, N. (1999). *Classrooms and courtrooms: Facing sexual harassment in K–12 schools.* New York: Teachers College Press.

Stein, N. (2001). Sexual harassment meets zero tolerance: Life in K–12 schools. In W. Ayers, B. Dohrn, & R. Ayers (Eds.), *Zero tolerance: Resisting the drive for punishment. A handbook for parents, students, educators and citizens* (pp. 130–137). New York: New Press.

Stein, S., Chalhoub, N., & Hodes, M. (1998). Very early-onset bulimia nervosa: Report of two cases. *International Journal of Eating Disorders, 24,* 323–327.

Steiner-Adair, C. (1986). The body politic: Normal female adolescent development and the development of eating disorders. *Journal of the American Academy of Psychoanalysis, 14,* 95–114.

REFERENCES

Steiner-Adair, C. (1994). The politics of prevention. In P. Fallon, M. A. Katzman, & S. C. Wooley (Eds.), *Feminist perspectives on eating disorders* (pp. 381–394). New York: Guilford.

Steiner-Adair, C., Sjostrom, L., Franko, D. L., Pai, S., Tucker, R., Becker, A. E., & Herzog, D. B. (2002). Primary prevention of eating disorders in adolescent girls: Learning from practice. *International Journal of Eating Disorders, 32,* 401–411.

Steiner-Adair, C., & Vorenberg, A. P. (1999). Resisting weightism: Media literacy for elementary school children. In N. Piran, M. P. Levine, & C. Steiner-Adair (Eds.), *Preventing eating disorders: A handbook of interventions and special challenges* (pp. 105–121). Philadelphia: Brunner/Mazel.

Stevenson, J. F., & Mitchell, R. E. (2003). Community-level collaboration for substance abuse prevention. *The Journal of Primary Prevention, 23,* 371–404.

Stewart, A. (1998). Experience with a school-based eating disorders prevention programme. In W. Vandereycken & G. Noordenbos (Eds.), *The prevention of eating disorders* (pp. 99–136). London: Athlone.

Stewart, D. A., Carter, J. C., Drinkwater, J., Hainsworth, J., & Fairburn, C. G. (2001). Modification of eating attitudes and behavior in adolescent girls: A controlled study. *International Journal of Eating Disorders, 29,* 107–118.

Stice, E. (1994). Review of the evidence for a sociocultural model of bulimia nervosa and an exploration of the mechanisms of action. *Clinical Psychology Review, 14,* 633–661.

Stice, E. (1998a). Modeling of eating pathology and social reinforcement of the thin-ideal predict onset of bulimic symptoms. *Behaviour Research and Therapy, 36,* 931–944.

Stice, E. (1998b). Relations of restraint and negative affect to bulimic pathology: A longitudinal test of three competing models. *International Journal of Eating Disorders, 23,* 243–260.

Stice, E. (2001a). A prospective test of the dual-pathway model of bulimic pathology: Mediating effects of dieting and negative affect. *Journal of Abnormal Psychology, 110,* 124–135.

Stice, E. (2001b). Risk factors for eating pathology: Recent advances and future directions. In R. H. Striegel-Moore & L. Smolak (Eds.), *Eating disorders: New directions for research and practice* (pp. 51–74). Washington, DC: American Psychological Association.

Stice, E. (2002). Risk and maintenance factors for eating pathology: A meta-analytic review. *Psychological Bulletin, 128,* 825–848.

Stice, E., & Agras, W.S. (1998). Predicting onset and cessation of bulimic behaviors during adolescence: A longitudinal grouping analysis. *Behavior Therapy, 29,* 257–276.

Stice, E., & Agras, W. S. (1999). Subtyping of bulimic women along dietary restraint and negative affect dimensions. *Journal of Consulting and Clinical Psychology, 67,* 460–469.

Stice, E., & Bearman, S. K. (2001). Body image and eating disturbances prospectively predict increases in depressive symptoms in adolescent girls: A growth curve analysis. *Developmental Psychology, 37,* 597–607.

Stice, E., Cameron, R. P., Hayward, C., Taylor, C. B., & Killen, J. D. (1999). Naturalistic weight-reduction efforts prospectively predict growth in relative weight and onset among female adolescents. *Journal of Consulting and Clinical Psychology, 67,* 967–974.

Stice, E., Chase, A., Stormer, S., & Appel, A. (2001). A randomized trial of a dissonance-based eating disorder prevention program. *International Journal of Eating Disorders, 29,* 247–262.

Stice, E., Hayward, C., Cameron, R., Killen, J. D., & Taylor, C. B. (2000). Body image and eating related factors predict onset of depression in female adolescents: A longitudinal study. *Journal of Abnormal Psychology, 109,* 438–444.

Stice, E., & Hoffman, E. (2004). Eating disorder prevention programs. In J. K. Thompson (Ed.), *Handbook of eating disorders and obesity* (pp. 33–57). Hoboken, NJ: Wiley.

Stice, E., Killen, J., Hayward, C., & Taylor, C. B. (1998). Age of onset for binge eating and purging during adolescence: A four-year survival analysis. *Journal of Abnormal Psychology, 107,* 671–675.

Stice, E., Mazotti, L., Weibel, D., & Agras, W.S. (2000). Dissonance prevention program decreases thin-ideal internalization, body dissatisfaction, dieting, negative affect, and bulimic symptoms: A preliminary experiment. *International Journal of Eating Disorders, 27,* 206–217.

Stice, E., Nemeroff, C., & Shaw, H. E. (1996). A test of the dual pathway model of bulimia nervosa: Evidence for restrained-eating and affect-regulation mechanisms. *Journal of Social and Clinical Psychology, 15,* 340–363.

Stice, E., & Ragan, J. (2001). A preliminary controlled evaluation of an eating disturbance psychoeducational intervention for college students. *International Journal of Eating Disorders, 31,* 159–171.

Stice, E., Schupak-Neuberg, E., Shaw, H. E., & Stein, R. I. (1994). Relation of media exposure to eating disorder symptomatology: An examination of mediating mechanisms. *Journal of Abnormal Psychology, 103,* 836–840.

Stice, E., & Shaw, H. E. (2003). Prospective relations of body image, eating, and affective disturbances to smoking onset in adolescent girls: How Virginia Slims. *Journal of Consulting and Clinical Psychology, 71,* 129–135.

Stice, E., & Shaw, H. E. (2004). Eating disorder prevention programs: A meta-analytic review. *Psychological Bulletin, 130,* 206–227.

Stice, E., Trost, A., & Chase, A. (2003). Healthy weight control and dissonance-based eating disorder prevention programs: Results from a controlled trial. *International Journal of Eating Disorders, 33,* 10–21.

Stormer, S. M., & Thompson, J. K. (1995, November). *The effect of media images and sociocultural beauty ideals on college-age women: A proposed psychoeducational program.* Paper presented at the annual meeting of the Association for the Advancement of Behavior Therapy, Washington, DC.

Stormer, S. M., & Thompson, J. K. (1998, November). *An evaluation of a media-focused psychoeducational programs for body image disturbance.* Paper presented at the annual meeting of the Association for the Advancement of Behavior Therapy, Washington, DC.

Story, M. (1999). School-based approaches to preventing and treating obesity. *International Journal of Obesity, 23* (Suppl. 2), S43-S51.

Strasburger, V. C., & Donnerstein, E. (2000). Children, adolescents, and the media in the 21st century. *Adolescent Medicine, 11,* 51–68.

Strauman, T. J., & Glenberg, A. M. (1994). Self-concept and body-image disturbance: Which self-beliefs predict body size overestimation? *Cognitive Therapy and Research, 18,* 105–125.

Strauman, T. J., Vookles, J., Berenstein, V., Chaiken, S., & Higgins, E. T. (1991). Self-discrepancies and vulnerability to body dissatisfaction and disordered eating. *Journal of Personality and Social Psychology, 61,* 946–956.

Striegel-Moore, R. H. (1993). Etiology of binge eating: A developmental perspective. In C. Fairburn & G. T. Wilson (Eds.), *Binge eating: Nature, assessment, and treatment* (pp. 144–172). New York: Guilford.

Striegel-Moore, R. H., Cachelin, F., Dohm, F., Pike, K., Wilfley, D. E., & Fairburn, C. G. (2001). Comparison of binge eating disorder and bulimia nervosa in a community sample. *International Journal of Eating Disorders, 29,* 157–165.

Striegel-Moore, R. H., Silberstein, L., & Rodin, J. (1986). Toward an understanding of risk factors for bulimia. *American Psychologist, 41,* 246–263.

Striegel-Moore, R. H., & Smolak, L. (2000). The influence of ethnicity on eating disorders in women. In R. M. Eisler & M. Hersen (Eds.), *Handbook of gender, culture, and health* (pp. 227–253). Mahwah, NJ: Lawrence Erlbaum Associates.

Striegel-Moore, R. H., & Smolak, L. (2001). Conclusion: Imagining the future. In R. H. Striegel-Moore & L. Smolak (Eds.), *Eating disorders: New directions for research and practice* (pp. 271–278). Washington, DC: American Psychological Association.

Striegel-Moore, R. H., & Smolak, L. (2002). Gender, ethnicity, and eating disorders. In C. G. Fairburn & K. Brownell (Eds.), *Eating disorders and obesity: A comprehensive handbook* (2nd ed., pp. 251–255). New York: Guilford.

Striegel-Moore, R. H., & Steiner-Adair, C. (1998). Primary prevention of eating disorders: Further considerations from a feminist perspective. In W. Vandereycken & G. Noordenbos (Eds.), *The prevention of eating disorders* (pp. 1–22). London: Athlone.

Striegel-Moore, R., Wilfley, D. E., Pike, K., Dohm, F., & Fairburn, C. G. (2000). Recurrent binge eating in black American women. *Archives of Family Medicine, 9,* 83–87.

Strober, M. (1990). Family-genetic studies of eating disorders. *Journal of Clinical Psychiatry, 52,* 9–12.

REFERENCES

Strober, M., Freeman, R., Lampert, C., Diamond, J., & Kaye, W. H. (2000). Controlled family study of anorexia and bulimia nervosa: Evidence of shared liability and transmission of partial syndromes. *American Journal of Psychiatry, 157,* 393–401.

Strong, K. G., & Huon, G. F. (1998). An evaluation of a structural model for studies of the initiation of dieting among adolescent girls. *Journal of Psychosomatic Research, 44,* 315–326.

Strong, K. O. (2000). *Media effects on eating disorders in preadolescent and adolescent females: A program for primary prevention.* Unpublished doctoral dissertation, Azusa Pacific University, Azusa, California.

Szymanski, M. L., & Cash, T. F. (1995). Body-image disturbances and self-discrepancy theory: Expansion of the Body-Image Ideals Questionnaire. *Journal of Social & Clinical Psychology, 14,* 134–146.

Tanofsky-Kraff, M., Hayden, H. A., Cavazos, P. A., & Wilfley, D. E. (2003). Pediatric obesity treatment and prevention. In R. Andersen (Ed.), *Obesity: Etiology, assessment, treatment, and prevention* (pp. 155–176). Champaign, IL: Human Kinetics.

Tantleff-Dunn, S., & Gokee, J. L. (2002). Interpersonal influences on body image development. In T. F. Cash & T. Pruzinsky (Eds.), *Body image: A handbook of theory, research, and clinical practice* (pp. 108–116). New York: Guilford Press.

Tantleff-Dunn, S., & Thompson, J. K. (1998). Body image and appearance-related feedback: Recall, judgment, and affective response. *Journal of Social and Clinical Psychology, 17,* 319–340.

Tavris, C. (1992). *The mismeasure of woman.* New York: Simon & Schuster.

Taylor C. B., Cameron R., Newman M., & Junge, J. (2002). Issues related to combining risk factor reduction and clinical treatment for eating disorders in defined populations. *The Journal of Behavioral Health Services and Research, 29,* 81–90.

Taylor, C. B., Winzelberg, A. J., & Celio, A. A. (2001). The use of interactive media to prevent eating disorders. In R. H. Striegel-Moore & L. Smolak (Eds.), *Eating disorders: Innovative directions in research and practice* (pp. 255–270). Washington, DC: American Psychological Association.

Taylor, J. M., Gilligan, C., & Sullivan, A. M. (1995). *Between voice and silence: Women and girls, race and relationship.* Cambridge MA: Harvard University Press.

Taylor, S. E. (2003). *Health psychology* (5th ed.). Boston: McGraw-Hill.

The Consortium on the School-Based Promotion of Social Competence. (1994). The school-based promotion of social competence: Theory, research, practice, and policy. In R. J. Haggerty, L. R. Sherrod, N. Garmezy, & M. Rutter (Eds.), *Stress, risk, and resilience in children and adolescents: Processes, mechanisms, and interventions* (pp. 268–316). Cambridge, UK: Cambridge University Press.

The McKnight Investigators. (2003). Risk factors for the onset of eating disorders in adolescent girls: Results of the McKnight Longitudinal Risk Factor Study. *American Journal of Psychiatry, 160,* 248–254.

The world's priorities. (n.d.). Retrieved July 17, 2001 from www.thirdworldtraveler.com.

Then, D. (1992, August). *Women's magazines: Messages they convey about looks, men and careers.* Paper presented at the annual convention of the American Psychological Association, Washington, DC.

Thompson, B. (1994). *A hunger so wide and so deep: American women speak out on eating problems.* Minneapolis: University of Minnesota Press.

Thompson, J. K., & Heinberg, L. J. (1999). The media's influence on body image disturbance and eating disorders: We've reviled them, now can we rehabilitate them? *Journal of Social Issues, 55,* 339–353.

Thompson, J. K., Heinberg, L. J., Altabe, M., & Tantleff-Dunn, S. (1999). *Exacting beauty: Theory, assessment, and treatment of body image disturbance.* Washington, DC: American Psychological Association.

Thompson, J. K., & Stice, E. (2001). Internalization of the thin-ideal: Mounting evidence for a new risk factor for body image disturbance and eating pathology. *Current Directions in Psychological Science, 10,* 181–183.

Thompson, S., Corwin, S., & Sargent, R. (1997). Ideal body size beliefs and weight concerns of fourth-grade children. *International Journal of Eating Disorders, 21,* 279–284.

Thomsen, S. R., Weber, M. M., & Brown, L. B. (2002). The relationship between reading beauty and fashion magazines and the use of pathogenic dieting methods among adolescent females. *Adolescence, 37,* 1–18.

Tiggemann, M. (2001). Effect of gender composition of school on body concerns in adolescent women. *International Journal of Eating Disorders, 29,* 239–243.

Tiggemann, M., & Lynch, J. (2001). Body image across the life span in adult women: The role of self-objectification. *Developmental Psychology, 37,* 243–253.

Tiggemann, M., & Slater, A. (2001). A test of objectification theory in former dancers and non-dancers. *Psychology of Women Quarterly, 25,* 57–64.

Tilgner, L., Wertheim, E. H., & Paxton, S. J. (2004). Effect of social desirability on adolescent girls' responses to an eating disorders prevention program. *International Journal of Eating Disorders, 35,* 211–216.

Tobler, N. S., Roona, M. R., Ochshorn, P., Marshall, D. G., Streke, A. V., & Stackpole, K. M. (2000). School-based adolescent prevention programs: 1998 meta-analysis. *The Journal of Primary Prevention, 20,* 27–336.

Toledo, T., & Neumark-Sztainer, D. (1999). *Weighting for You!*: Training for high school faculty and staff in the prevention and detection of weight-related disorders among adolescents. *Journal of Nutrition Education, 31,* 283A.

Troiano, R. P., & Flegal, K. M. (1998). Overweight children and adolescents: Description, epidemiology, and demographics. *Pediatrics, 101* (Suppl.), 497–504.

Troiano, R. P., Flegal, K. M., Kuczmarski, R. J., Campbell, S. M., & Johnson, C. L. (1995). Overweight prevalence and trends for children and adolescents: The National Health and Nutrition Examination Surveys, 1963 to 1991. *Archives of Pediatric & Adolescent Medicine, 149,* 1085–1091.

Troiano, R. P., Frongillo, E. A., Jr., Sobal, J., & Levitsky, D. A. (1996). The relationship between body weight and mortality: A quantitative analysis of combined information from existing studies. *International Journal of Obesity, 20,* 63–75.

Trotta, L. (2001). Children's advocacy groups: A history and analysis. In D. G. Singer & J. L. Singer (Eds.), *Handbook of children and the media* (pp. 699–719). Thousand Oaks, CA: Sage.

United States Bureau of the Census. (1999*). Statistical abstract for the United States* (119th ed.). Washington, DC: Government Printing Office.

United States Department of Health and Human Services [Office on Women's Health]. (1999). *BodyWise eating disorders information packet for middle school personnel.* Available from www.4woman.gov/BodyImage/bodywise/bodywise.htm or call National Women's Health Information Center: 1–800–994-WOMAN.

United States Department of Health and Human Services. (2001). Nutrition and overweight. In *Healthy people 2010* (Vol. II, No. 19). Retrieved July 15, 2004, from http://www.healthypeople.gov/Document/tableof contents.htm#Volume2/.

United States Office of the Surgeon General (1999). *Mental health: A report of the Surgeon General.* Retrieved July 17, 2004 from www.surgeongeneral.gov/library/reports.htm/.

Utter, J., Neumark-Sztainer, D., Wall, M., & Story, M. (2003). Reading magazine articles about dieting and associated weight control behaviors among adolescents. *Journal of Adolescent Health, 32,* 78–82.

Valdez, R., Gregg, E., & Williamson, D. (2002). Effects of weight loss on morbidity and mortality. In C. G. Fairburn & K. D. Brownell (Eds.), *Eating disorders and obesity: A comprehensive handbook* (2nd ed., pp. 490–494). New York: Guilford.

Vandereycken, W., & Noordenbos, G., (Eds.). (1998). *Prevention of eating disorders.* London: Athlone.

van Hoeken, D., Lucas, A. R., & Hoek, H. W. (1998). Epidemiology. In H. W. Hoek, J. Treasure, & M. A. Katzman (Eds.), *Neurobiology in the treatment of eating disorders* (pp. 97–126). London: John Wiley & Sons.

Van Strien, T., Frijters, J., Bergers, G., & Defares, P. (1986). The Dutch Eating Behavior Questionnaire (DEBQ) for assessment of restrained, emotional, and external eating behavior. *International Journal of Eating Disorders, 5,* 295–315.

Varnado-Sullivan, P. J., Zucker, N., Williamson, D. A., Reas, D., Thaw, J., & Netemeyer, S. B. (2001). Development and implementation of the Body Logic Program for adolescents: A two-stage prevention program for eating disorders. *Cognitive and Behavioral Practice, 8,* 248–259.

Villena, J., & Castillo, M. (1999). La prevención primaria de los trastornos de alimentación[The primary prevention of eating disorders]. *Annuario de Psicologia, 30*, 131–143.

Vincent, M., & McCabe, M. P. (2000). Gender differences among adolescents in family and peer influences on body dissatisfaction, weight loss, and binge eating behaviors. *Journal of Youth and Adolescence, 29*, 205–221.

Vitiello, B., & Lederhendler, I. (2000). Research on eating disorders: Current status and future prospects. *Biological Psychiatry, 47*, 777–786.

Vitousek, K. B., & Hollon, S. D. (1990). The investigation of schematic content and processing in eating disorders. *Cognitive Therapy and Research, 14*, 191–214.

Wade, T. D., Davidson, S., & O'Dea, J. (2003). A preliminary controlled evaluation of a school-based media literacy and self-esteem program for reducing eating disorder risk factors. *International Journal of Eating Disorders, 33*, 371–383.

Wallack, L., & Dorfman, L. (2001). Putting policy into health communication: The role of media advocacy. In R. E. Rice & C. K. Atkin (Eds.), *Public communication campaigns* (3rd ed., pp. 389–401). Thousand Oak, CA: Sage.

Wallack, L., Dorfman, L., Jernigan, D., & Themba, M. (1993). *Media advocacy and public health: Power for prevention.* Newbury Park, CA: Sage.

Wandersman, A., & Florin, P. (2003). Community interventions and effective prevention. *American Psychologist, 58*, 441–448.

Waters, E., Merrick, S., Treboux, D., Crowell, J., & Albersheim, L. (2000). Attachment security in infancy and early adulthood: A twenty-year longitudinal study. *Child Development, 71*, 684–689.

Wechsler, H., Devereaux, R. S., Davis, M., & Collins, J. (2000). Using the school environment to promote physical activity and healthy eating. *Preventive Medicine, 31*(2, pt. 2), S121–S137.

Weiner, R. (1999). Working with physicians toward the goal of primary and secondary prevention. In N. Piran, M. P. Levine, & C. Steiner-Adair (Eds.), *Preventing eating disorders: A handbook of interventions and special challenges* (pp. 285–303). Philadelphia: Brunner/Mazel.

Weiss, K. R. (2001). *An evaluation of a primary prevention program for disordered eating in adolescent girls: Examining responses of high- and low-risk girls.* Unpublished doctoral dissertation, La Trobe University, Victoria, Australia.

Weissberg, R. P., Barton, H. A., & Shriver, T. P. (1997). The social-competence promotion program for young adolescents. In G. W. Albee & T. P. Gullotta (Eds.), *Primary prevention works* (pp. 268–290). Thousand Oaks, CA: Sage.

Weissberg, R. P., & Greenberg, M. (1998). School and community competence-enhancement and prevention programs. In I. E. Siegel & K. Renninger (Eds.), *Handbook of child psychology. Vol. 4, Child psychology in practice* (5th ed., pp. 877–954). New York: Wiley.

Weissberg, R. P., Kumpfer, K. L., & Seligman, M. E. P. (Eds.). (2003). Prevention that works for children and youth [Special issue]. *American Psychologist, 58*(6/7).

Wenter, D. L., Ennett, S. T., Ribisl, K. M., Vincus, A. A., Rohrbach, L., Ringwalt, C. L., & Jones, S. M. (2002). Comprehensiveness of substance use prevention programs in U.S. middle schools. *Journal of Adolescent Health, 30*, 455–462.

Wertheim, E. H., Paxton, S. J., Schultz, H. K., & Muir, S. I. (1997). Why do adolescent girls watch their weight? An interview study of the sociocultural pressures to be thin. *Journal of Psychosomatic Research, 42*, 345–355.

Whitaker, A., Davies, M., Shaffer, D., Johnson, J., Abrams, S., Walsh, T., & Kalikow, K. (1989). The struggle to be thin: A survey of anorexic and bulimia symptoms in a non-referred adolescent population. *Psychological Medicine, 19*, 143–163.

Wichstrøm, L. (1999). The emergence of gender differences in depressed mood during adolescence: The role of intensified gender socialization. *Developmental Psychology, 35*, 232–245.

Wilfley, D. E., & Saelens, B. E. (2002). Epidemiology and causes of obesity in children. In C. G. Fairburn & K. D. Brownell (Eds.), *Eating disorders and obesity: A comprehensive handbook* (2nd ed., pp. 429–432). New York: Guilford.

Williamson, D. A. (May, 2003). *Categorical versus dimensional classification of eating disorders: An examination of the evidence.* Paper presented at the International Conference on Eating Disorders of the Academy for Eating Disorders, Denver, CO.

Williamson, D. A., Stewart, T. M., White, M. A., & York-Crowe, E. (2002). An information-processing perspective on body image. In T. F. Cash & T. Pruzinsky (Eds.), *Body image: A handbook of theory, research, and clinical practice* (pp. 38–46). New York: Guilford.

Williamson, I., & Hartley, P. (1998). British research into the increased vulnerability of young gay men to eating disturbance and body dissatisfaction. *European Eating Disorders Review, 6,* 160–170.

Wilson, G. T., Fairburn, C. G., & Agras, W. S. (1997). Cognitive-behavioral therapy for bulimia nervosa. In D. M. Garner & P. E. Garfinkel (Eds.), *Handbook of treatment for eating disorders* (2nd ed., pp. 67–93). New York: Guilford.

Winett, R. A. (1998). Prevention: A proactive-developmental-ecological perspective. In T. H. Ollendick & M. Hersen (Eds.), *Handbook of child psychopathology* (3rd ed., pp. 637–671). New York: Plenum.

Winzelberg, A. J., Eppstein, D., Eldredge, K. L., Wilfley, D. E., Dasmahapatra, R., Dev, P., & Taylor, C. B. (2000). Effectiveness of an internet-based program for reducing risk factors for eating disorders. *Journal of Consulting and Clinical Psychology, 68,* 346–350.

Winzelberg, A. J., Taylor, C. B., Sharpe, T., Eldredge, K. L., Dev, P., & Constantinou, P. S. (1998). Evaluation of a computer-mediated eating disorder intervention program. *International Journal of Eating Disorders, 24,* 339–349.

Wiseman, C. V., Sunday, S. R., Bortolotti, F., & Halmi, K. (2001, November). *Primary prevention of eating disorders: A tale of two countries.* Paper presented at the meeting of the Eating Disorders Research Society, Albuquerque, NM.

Withers, G. F., Twigg, K., Wertheim, E. H., & Paxton, S. J. (2002). A controlled evaluation of an eating disorders primary prevention videotape using the Elaboration Likelihood Model of persuasion. *Journal of Psychosomatic Research, 53,* 1021–1027.

Withers, G. F., & Wertheim, E. H. (2004). Applying the Elaboration Likelihood Model of persuasion to a videotape-based eating disorders primary prevention program for adolescent girls. *Eating Disorders: The Journal of Treatment & Prevention, 12,* 103–124.

Wolf, N. (1991). *The beauty myth: How images of beauty are used against women.* New York: William Morrow.

Wolf-Bloom, M. S. (1998). *Using media literacy training to prevent body dissatisfaction and subsequent eating problems in early adolescent girls.* Unpublished doctoral dissertation, University of Cincinnati.

Wonderlich, S. (2002). Personality and eating disorders. In K. D. Brownell & C. G. Fairburn (Eds.), *Handbook of obesity and eating disorders* (2nd ed., pp. 204–209). New York: Guilford.

Wonderlich, S., & Mitchell, J. E. (2001). The role of personality in the onset of eating disorders and treatment implications. *Psychiatric Clinics of North America, 24,* 249–258.

Wood, C., Becker, J., & Thompson, J. K. (1996). Body image dissatisfaction in preadolescent children. *Journal of Applied Developmental Psychology, 17,* 85–100.

Woodside, D., & Garfkinkel, P. (1992). Age of onset in eating disorders. *International Journal of Eating Disorders, 12,* 31–36.

Wooley, S. C. (1994). Sexual abuse and eating disorders: The concealed debate. In P. Fallon, M. Katzman, & S. C. Wooley (Eds.), *Feminist perspectives on eating disorders* (pp. 171–211). New York: Guilford.

World Health Organization (1999, June 17). *Introduction to The European Network of Health Promoting Schools.* Retrieved from http://www.who.dk/enhps/page/intenglish.html.

Wroblewska, A.-M. (1997). Androgenic-anabolic steroids and body dysmorphia in young men. *Journal of Psychosomatic Research, 42,* 225–234.

Yuker, H. E., & Allison, D. B. (1994). Obesity: Sociocultural perspectives. In L. Alexander-Mott & D. B. Lumsden (Eds.), *Understanding eating disorders: Anorexia nervosa, bulimia nervosa, and obesity* (pp. 243–270). Washington, DC: Taylor & Francis.

Zabinski, M. F., Celio, A. A., Jacobs, M. J., Manwaring, J., & Wilfley, D. E. (2003). Internet-based prevention of eating disorders. *European Eating Disorders Review, 11,* 183–197.

Zabinski, M. F., Pung, M., Wilfley, D., Eppstein, D., Winzelberg, A., Celio, A., & Taylor, C. B. (2001). Reducing risk factors for eating disorders: Targeting at-risk women with a computerized psychoeducational program. *International Journal of Eating Disorders, 29,* 401–408.

Zeckhausen, D., & Boyd, B. (Illustrator). (2003). *Full mouse, empty mouse.* Atlanta, GA: Eating Disorders Information Network (EDIN; see www.edin-ga.org for information about this children's book and 5-day companion lesson plan).

Author Index

A

Abascal, L., 203, 212, 340, 354
Abbate-Dage, G., 47
Abbess, G., 56
Abdollahi, P. A., 215
Abood, D. A., 207, 210
Abraham, S., 17, 80, 142, 143, 144, 146, 147, 148, 189, 190, 198, 221, 239, 248, 250, 275, 322, 341, 364
Abramowitz, R. H., 408
Abrams, S., 55, 56
Ackard, D., 57
Agras, W. S., 40, 83, 96, 98, 102, 105, 106, 107, 109, 127, 215, 341
Albee, G. W., 3, 4, 5, 6, 9, 10, 11, 12, 13, 17, 134, 135, 139, 141
Albersheim, L., 82
Allen, J., 95
Allison, D. B., 38, 40, 60, 64
Altabe, M., 13, 14, 45, 51, 54, 67, 68, 101, 102, 114, 115, 116, 117, 119, 122, 123, 124, 153, 240, 241, 254, 283, 291, 306, 307, 308, 315, 345
Altman, T., 82

Amianto, F., 47
Andersen, A. E., 12, 58, 59
Andersen, R. E., 56
Anderson, D. A., 122
Anderson, I. M., 50
Anderson-Fye, E. P., 283
Anesbury, T., 255
Antoniadis, A., 15
Appel, A., 101, 211, 213, 214, 215, 364
Archibald, A. B., 114
Arnett, J., 56
Arnold, K., 40
Arthur, M., 79, 237, 238, 239, 269, 272, 273, 275, 278, 281, 298, 300, 302
Ary, D. V., 236, 266, 268, 284, 384
Asarnow, J. R., 353
Atkin, C. K., 327, 328
Atkins, D., 21
Attie, I., 33, 98
Austin, E. W., 311, 314, 316
Austin, S. B., 61, 132, 179, 180, 181, 192, 197, 198, 211, 250, 259, 335, 337, 339, 340, 349, 351, 356, 361, 364, 367
Avenevoli, S., 388

445

B

Bachman, J. G., 233
Badger, G. J., 235, 328
Baglioni, A., 278
Bahrke, M., 59
Baker, D., 114
Baker, E., 274
Baldwin, B. M., 12
Balestriere, M., 202, 204
Bandura, A., 108, 109, 110, 111, 112, 124, 125–126, 132, 133, 146
Banfield, S., 242
Baranowski, M. J., 189, 193, 222
Baranowski, T., 108, 109, 124, 126, 133
Barbarich, N., 49, 50
Barlow, S. E., 37, 39, 60
Barton, H. A., 133, 141, 251, 376
Bates, J., 48, 76
Battle, E. K., 67
Bazzini, D. G., 206, 208, 222
Bearman, S. K., 91, 106, 211, 214, 368
Beck, A. T., 117, 119, 132
Becker, A. E., 163, 164, 174, 175, 190, 194, 198, 283, 308
Becker, B., 11
Becker, J., 141
Becker, M. H., 324, 365
Beglin, S. J., 407
Belensky, M. F., 150
Benedikt, R., 114
Bennett, W. B., 249
Benson, P. L., 138 139, 141, 281
Berel, S., 311, 312, 313, 314, 316, 317, 323, 407
Berenson, G., 37
Berenstein, V., 122, 123
Berg, F. M., 12, 60, 61, 62, 65, 66, 68, 69, 259, 286, 368, 402
Berg, M. L., 48
Bergen, A., 50
Bergers, G., 92, 346, 407
Bergholz, K., 353
Bergin, A. E., 222
Berglund, M. L., 104
Berkey, C., 33, 40, 55, 65, 242, 258, 308

Berrett, M. E., 12
Betz, N., 213
Beuhring, T., 55, 58
Beumont, P., 24, 308
Bigbee, M. A., 241
Biglan, A., 236, 266, 268, 284, 384, 386
Bilukha, O. O., 308
Binford, R. B., 179
Birch, L., 92, 98, 254, 283
Black, C., 236, 266, 268, 284, 384
Black, D. R., 207, 210
Black, M., 12
Blackmore, E., 174, 190, 193, 233, 250, 275, 294, 295, 297, 300, 342
Blaine, B., 246
Blair-Greiner, A., 33, 347
Blais, M. A., 285
Bloom, M., 4, 5, 6, 135
Blum, R., 135–136, 246, 377
Blume, J., 396
Blyth, D. A., 138, 141, 281
Boggio, S., 47
Booth-Butterfield, S., 238
Bordo, S., 54, 67, 153, 154, 173, 262, 291
Borowiecki, J., 155, 243
Borresen, R., 16, 179, 222, 223
Bortolotti, F., 202, 204
Botta, R. A., 308
Botvin, G. J., 92, 108, 139, 141, 228, 230, 231, 232, 233, 239, 240, 242, 244, 248, 249, 250, 258, 274
Boutelle, K. N., 65
Boyd, B., 266, 396, 397
Braet, C., 92
Braganza, C., 185, 186, 188, 222
Brannick, M. T., 408
Brewer, H., 287
Brewerton, T. D., 49, 50, 51, 346, 407
Brisman, J., 403
Broadnax, S., 246
Bronfenbrenner, U., 14, 74, 75, 94, 278, 280, 376
Brooks-Gunn, J., 33, 40, 89, 90, 98, 114, 137–138, 191, 196, 386
Brown, J. A., 309, 310
Brown, J. B., 203, 212, 340, 354

AUTHOR INDEX

Brown, J. D., 327
Brown, L. B., 308
Brown, L. M., 104, 157, 160
Brown, L. S., 99
Browne, A., 83
Brownell, K., 27, 64, 65, 66, 67
Bruch, H., 24, 31, 33, 73
Bruhl, C., 215
Brumberg, J., 24, 99
Bruning, J., 203, 212, 354
Bryant, C. A., 331, 332
Bryant-Waugh, R., 25, 29, 30, 255, 346, 403, 407
Bryson, S., 26, 27, 82, 408
Buddeberg, C., 200, 201
Buddeberg-Fischer, B., 200, 201
Budman, S. H., 206, 211, 212, 213, 217, 262, 333, 340
Bulfer, J., 185, 186
Bulik, C., 43, 44, 45, 47, 52, 104
Bumbarger, B., 136
Burgard, D., 62, 65, 67, 86, 205, 206, 208, 210, 292, 353
Burman, E., 99
Butler, R., 124, 125, 126, 128, 131, 132, 133, 201, 204, 205, 221, 250, 261, 317, 366
Butler, S. F., 206, 211, 212, 213, 217, 262, 333, 340
Byely, L., 114

C

Cachelin, F., 27, 28
Calkins, S. D., 48
Calnan, A., 58
Calvo Sagardoy, R., 399
Camargo, C. A., Jr., 33, 40, 55, 65, 242, 258, 304
Cameron, R., 40, 66, 91, 106, 212, 301, 346, 349, 351
Campbell, S. M., 61, 285
Campello, G., 189, 192, 194, 196
Cantor, J., 308
Caplan, G., 7, 8, 9
Caplan, M. Z., 140

Carlsmith, J., 242
Carnine, D., 386
Carpenter, J. H., 235, 328
Carper, J., 92
Carter, J., 92, 127, 130, 132, 133, 189, 191, 194, 208, 222, 353
Carter, W., 54, 365
Cash, T., 52, 55, 67, 109, 116, 117, 119, 120, 121, 123, 150, 155, 157, 211, 213, 214, 218, 219, 222, 223, 254, 259, 261, 272, 338
Caspi, A., 89
Castillo, M., 191
Catalano, R., 79, 104, 237, 238, 239, 260, 272, 273, 275, 278, 281, 284, 298, 300, 302, 337
Cattarin, J., 98
Cavazos, P. A., 60, 66
Celio, A., 206, 207, 210, 211, 217, 222, 250, 262, 333, 340, 341, 344, 351, 354, 355, 355, 364
Chaiken, S., 122, 123
Chalhoub, N., 25
Chally, P., 181, 372
Chandler, M., 75
Chase, A., 101, 211, 213, 214, 215, 218, 364, 368
Chater, R., 29
Chavera, V., 246
Chee, N., 215
Cheong, J., 57, 58, 59, 241, 243, 324, 325, 326, 363
Childress, A. C., 346, 407
Chodorow, N., 149
Chumlea, W., 37
Ciano, R. P., 202, 204
Cicchetti, D., 11, 73
Clabby, J. F., 140
Clarke, G., 51, 58, 59, 241, 243, 324, 324, 325, 326, 363
Clark-Sly, J. B., 12
Clark-Wagner, A., 131, 148
Clifford, E. M., 49
Clinchy, B. M., 150
Clonninger, D., 47
Coatsworth, J. D., 135

Cohane, G., 242
Cohen-Tovée, E., 151
Cohn, L., 58, 59, 208
Coie, J. D., 353
Colditz, G. A., 33, 40, 55, 65, 242, 258, 308, 349, 351
Cole, T. J., 60
Coller, T., 163, 164, 175, 181, 185, 186, 250, 260, 261, 317, 318, 319, 336
Collins, J., 290
Compas, B. E., 135, 136
Conner, M., 308
Connors, M., 34, 46, 73, 82, 83, 98, 102, 152, 155, 345
Constantinou, P. S., 206, 211
Contento, I., 191, 196
Cooper, M., 121, 122
Cooper, P. J., 346, 407
Cooper, Z., 116, 132, 346, 407
Cordes, H., 402
Coreil, J., 331, 332
Corwin, S., 151
Costin, C., 272, 403
Cowen, E. L., 4, 5, 6, 8, 9, 10, 11, 12, 13, 14, 18, 134, 135, 352, 362
Cowen, P. J., 44, 45, 49, 50, 104
Crago, M., 11, 20, 25, 26, 27, 31, 78, 82, 102, 105, 131, 148, 179, 202, 253, 336, 372, 408
Crandall, C. S., 82
Crawford, P., 65, 66
Crick, N. R., 241
Crisp, A., 24, 31
Crocker, J., 246
Croll, J., 57, 243
Crosby, R. D., 48
Crowell, J., 82
Crowson, C., 87
Cuijpers, P., 238, 239, 240, 242, 250, 258
Curtin, L., 206, 208
Cusumano, D. L., 291, 308

D

Daley, J., 295
Dalle Grave, R., 179, 189, 192, 193, 196, 397
Dalton, J. H., 147, 383
Daneman, D., 216, 344
Daniels, S., 26, 39, 256, 346, 407
Darley, J. M., 258, 259
Dasmahapatra, R., 206, 211
Davidson, M. M., 206, 211, 212, 213, 217, 262, 333, 340
Davidson, S., 181, 190, 205, 311, 318, 322, 323
Davies, M., 55, 56
Davis, C., 287
Davis, M., 290
Davis, R., 146, 186, 189, 193, 194, 199, 200, 300, 398
Davison, K., 98
de Beauvoir, S., 150
De Luca, L., 189, 192, 194, 196, 397
DeBate, R. D., 185, 186, 188
Dede, C., 333
Defares, P., 92, 346, 407
DeFrancesco, C., 326, 345
Delinsky, S., 20, 23, 24, 26, 28
Dempsey, M., 53, 146, 196, 209, 213
Derzon, J. H., 328
Dev, P., 203, 206–207, 210, 211, 212, 262, 340, 354, 355
Devereaux, R. S., 290
Devlin, M. J., 38, 66
de Zwaan, M., 96, 98, 102, 105, 106, 107
Diamond, J., 43
Dick, R., 57
DiClemente, R. J., 136
Dietz, W., 37, 39, 60, 61
DiGioacchino, R. F., 338
Dishion, T., 234, 235, 300, 302, 354
DiSimone-Weiss, R., 35
Dixit, S., 61, 197, 250, 251, 259, 286, 288, 340, 367, 397
Dohm, F., 27, 28
Dohrenwend, B. P., 135
Domitrovich, C., 136
Donaldson, S. I., 230, 232, 258
Donnerstein, E., 334
Dooley, D., 337
Dore, T., 353
Dorer, D. J., 285

AUTHOR INDEX 449

Dorfman, L., 307, 329
Dornbusch, S., 242
Dounchis, J., 25, 151
Downes, B., 135–136, 246
Doyle, J., 255
Drake, D. R., 138
Drewnowski, A., 213
Drinkwater, J., 127, 130, 132, 133, 189, 194
Dryfoos, J. G., 138
Dumka, L. E., 244, 248
Duncan, P., 242
Duncan, T., 236, 266, 268, 284, 326, 384
Dunn, V., 191, 194, 222
DuPen, J., 312, 313, 314, 316, 323, 407
Durham, M., 326, 345
Durkin, S., 365
Durlak, J. A., 136, 137
Dusenbury, L., 274
Dwyer, J., 235, 328

E

Early-Zald, M., 33, 56, 103
Eickhoff-Shemek, J., 318, 323
Eisenberg, M., 240, 243, 246, 283
Ekeblad, E. R., 285
Eldredge, K. L., 206, 211
Elias, M. J., 135, 139, 140, 147, 383
Elliot, D. L., 57, 58, 59, 241, 243, 324, 325, 326, 345, 350, 363, 398
Emery, G., 117, 119, 132
Engebreston, J., 185, 186
Ennett, S. T., 237
Eppstein, D., 206, 207, 211, 217, 262
Epstein, L. H., 66
Ernsberger, P., 36, 38, 64
Estes, L., 20, 25, 26, 27, 31, 78, 82, 105, 179, 253, 336, 408
Etling, C., 183, 187
Ewing, R., 287

F

Faibisch, L., 65
Fairburn, C., 26, 27, 28, 44, 45, 49, 50, 104, 109, 116, 117, 119, 121, 127, 130, 132, 133, 136, 189, 191, 194, 208, 222, 272, 282, 346, 353, 407
Faith, M. S., 60
Falkner, N., 55, 58
Fallon, A. E., 408
Fassino, S., 47
Favaro, A., 133, 201, 204, 205, 221, 250, 261, 341
Feingold, A., 52
Felner, R. D., 14, 15
Felner, T. Y., 14, 15
Fernstrom, J., 49, 50
Fernstrom, M., 49, 50
Ferrara, S., 133, 201, 204, 205, 221, 250, 261, 341
Field, A. E., 33, 40, 55, 65, 192, 197, 198, 211, 242, 250, 258259, 308, 340, 349, 351, 364, 367
Fiering, C., 82
Finkelhor, D., 83
Fishbein, D., 51, 52
Fishbein, M., 331
Fisher, C. B., 138
Fisher, J., 92, 254, 283
Flay, B. R., 233, 234, 235, 239, 304, 328, 386
Flegal, K. M., 61, 285
Flores, A. T., 285
Florin, P., 386
Flynn, B. S., 235, 328
Folensbee, L., 206, 211, 212, 213, 217, 262, 333, 340
Fontana, L., 333
Forston, M. T., 123
Fortholer, M. S., 331, 332
Foster, E. E., 218
Foster, G. D., 56
Foster, W., 137–138
Foucault, M., 54, 153
Fox, M. K., 61, 197, 250, 251, 259, 286, 288, 340, 376, 397
Fox, N., 48
Franko, D. L., 35, 163, 164, 174, 175, 179, 181, 190, 194, 198, 206, 211, 212, 213, 216, 217, 262, 333, 340
Franzoi, S. L., 407
Frazier, A. L., 33, 40, 55, 65, 242, 258

Fredrickson, B., 76, 152, 153, 155, 156, 157, 172, 175, 291, 408
Freedman, D., 37
Freeman, R., 43
French, S. A., 57, 135–136, 138, 139, 243, 246, 258
Friedman, B., 25
Friedman, S. S., 53, 159, 162, 164, 174, 260, 278, 279, 341, 342, 343, 397, 402
Frijters, J., 92, 346, 407
Frongillo, E. A., Jr., 38, 63, 64
Frost, H. A., 12
Fulkerson, J., 33, 56, 103, 179
Fullerton, Y., 146, 193, 239, 294, 398
Furgueson, C., 35
Furnham, A., 58

G

Gaesser, G., 66
Gara, M., 140
Gardner, J., 37
Gardner, R., 25, 345
Garfinkel, P., 34, 35, 83, 87, 169, 261, 346, 407
Garmezy, N., 78, 104
Garner, D., 34, 35, 38, 40, 66, 83, 116, 119, 157, 169, 222, 346, 407
Garvin, V., 21, 28, 77, 78, 272
Gayda, C., 35
Geller, B. M., 235, 328
Geller, J., 105, 277, 291
Gendall, K., 47, 49, 50
Gill, T. P., 61
Gilligan, C., 104, 149, 157, 159, 160
Gillman, M. W., 33, 40, 55, 65, 242, 258, 349, 351
Gilpin, E. A., 331
Ginetti, S., 192, 196
Gleaves, D., 35
Glenberg, A. M., 123
Glynn, T., 230, 232, 258
Gnam, G., 200, 201
Gokee, J. L., 288, 290
Goldberg, L., 57, 58, 59, 241, 243, 324, 325, 326, 345, 350, 363, 398
Goldberger, N. R., 150

Golditz, G. A., 38
Goldsmith, H., 48
Gonzales, N. A., 244, 248
Good, L., 105, 157, 158, 175, 291
Gordon, R. A., 12, 14, 31, 36, 51, 77, 112, 116
Gortmaker, S. L., 61, 192, 197, 198, 211, 250, 251, 259, 286, 288, 340, 364, 367, 396, 397, 398
Graber, J., 40, 89, 90, 114, 191, 196
Gralen, S., 98
Graves, K. D., 207, 209
Gray, J. J., 291, 308
Gray, N., 26, 27, 82, 179, 253, 408
Gray, W., 219, 222
Green, C., 58, 241, 324
Green, T. C., 206, 211, 212, 213, 217, 262, 333, 340
Greenberg, M., 134, 136, 140, 141, 153
Greeno, C., 28
Greenwood, D. N., 285
Greffrath, E., 58, 241, 324
Gregg, E., 287
Gresko, R. B., 376
Griffin, K. W., 228, 230, 231, 232, 233, 239, 242, 244
Grimley, D., 16, 126, 365
Grodner, M., 365
Groesz, L. M., 13, 102, 114, 152, 157, 306, 308, 311
Grogan, S., 308
Gross, R., 242
Gruber, A., 155, 243
Guardini, S., 192, 196
Guenther-Grey, C., 331
Gullota, T. P., 3, 5, 10, 12, 13, 134, 135, 139, 141
Guo, S., 37
Gurin, J., 249
Gurney, V. W., 206, 208, 337
Gustafson-Larson, A., 151

H

Haggerty, R. J., 6, 7, 8, 10
Hainsworth, J., 127, 130, 132, 133, 189, 194

AUTHOR INDEX 451

Halmi, K., 202, 204, 337
Hamilton, C., 82
Hamilton, E., 206, 211, 212, 213, 217, 262, 333, 340
Hammen, C. L., 135, 136, 137
Hammer, L., 33, 40, 89, 92, 103, 189, 193, 199, 344, 347, 366, 408
Hankinson, S. E., 38
Hannan, P., 57, 138, 139, 163, 164, 175, 181, 250, 260–261, 292, 317, 318, 319, 336, 368
Hansen, W. B., 136, 227, 228, 229, 230, 232, 235, 239, 245, 248, 264, 265, 266, 270, 273, 274, 328
Hanson, K., 56, 205, 206, 208, 210, 353
Hardman, R. K., 12
Harned, M., 99, 152, 158, 175
Harrington, R., 338, 339, 344, 348, 350, 351, 352, 353
Harris, B., 174
Harris, T., 270, 299
Harrison, K., 113, 114, 306, 307, 308
Harrison, P. J., 44, 45, 104
Harter, S., 318, 408
Hartley, P., 57
Hathaway, J. E., 240
Hawkins, J. D., 79, 104, 237, 238, 239, 269, 272, 273, 275, 278, 281, 289, 298, 300, 302, 353
Hawley, D., 48
Hay, P., 28
Haydel, K., 33, 40, 89, 103, 347, 408
Hayden, H., 25, 26, 60, 66, 114, 151, 278, 294, 308
Hayward, C., 33, 35, 40, 66, 89, 91, 92, 96, 98, 102, 103, 105, 106, 107, 189, 193, 199, 301, 344, 346, 347, 349, 351, 366, 408
Healy, C., 371
Heatherton, T. F., 346
Heinberg, L. J., 13, 14, 45, 51, 54, 60, 67, 68, 86, 101, 102, 114, 115, 116, 117, 119, 122, 123, 124, 152, 240, 241, 254, 283, 291, 306, 307, 308, 315, 345, 408
Heinze, V., 190, 191, 195, 202, 205, 365

Heller, K., 4, 16
Henderson, H. A., 48
Henderson, J. N., 331, 332
Henkel, A., 40
Hennekens, C. H., 38
Herman, C. P., 346
Herrin, M., 403
Herrling, S., 95
Herzog, D. B., 20, 23, 24, 26, 28, 163, 164, 174, 175, 190, 194, 198, 285
Hetherington, M. M., 189, 193, 222
Hewlings, S. J., 184, 187
Heymsfield, S. B., 60
Higgins, E. T., 122, 123
Higgins, L. C., 219, 222
Hill, A. J., 92
Hill, K., 21, 285
Hill, L., 132, 280, 290, 398
Hix-Small, H., 326, 345
Ho, T., 24, 33
Hobbs, R., 309, 310
Hodes, M., 25
Hodges, E. L., 346, 407
Hoek, H., 6, 20, 21, 25, 52, 56, 87, 97, 259, 387
Hoff, H., 329, 330
Hoffman, E., 179, 213, 221, 222, 266, 335, 344
Holbrook, T., 58, 59
Holden, E. W., 12
Holderness, C., 90
Hollon, S. D., 116, 118, 119, 132
Holloway, R. M., 207, 208, 222, 366
Holt, T., 365
Hotelling, K., 353
Hrabosky, J. I., 213, 214, 218
Hsu, L., 24, 33
Huan, K., 86, 205, 206, 208, 210, 353
Hunter, D. J., 38
Huon, G., 114, 121, 185, 186, 188, 222
Hyde, J., 156, 408

I

Iacono, W. G., 45, 46
Ikeda, J., 65, 66, 67, 254, 397, 402

Ireland, M., 57, 243
Irving, L., 17, 36, 39, 60, 61, 68, 69, 101, 184, 187, 188, 209, 213, 247, 254, 259, 307, 309, 310, 311, 312, 313, 314, 316–317, 318, 319, 320, 321, 323, 342, 351, 368, 369, 389, 397, 407
Isager, T., 285

J

Jackman, L. P., 122
Jacobi, C., 40, 96, 98, 102, 105, 106, 107
Jacobs, M. J., 210
James-Ortiz, S., 274
Janz, N., 324, 365
Jarcho, H. D., 408
Jarrell, M. P., 346, 407
Jasper, K., 311, 396
Jeffrey, R., 258
Jensen, P., 16, 86, 92, 95, 102, 107, 338, 339, 344, 348, 350, 351, 352, 353
Jernigan, D., 307, 329
Jerome, L. W., 201, 204
Johnson, C., 34, 46, 57, 61, 73, 82, 83, 235, 285, 328
Johnson, J., 55, 56
Johnson, K., 311, 316
Johnson, W., 331
Johnston, L. D., 233
Joja, O., 308
Jones, D. C., 243, 308, 356
Jones, S. M., 237
Jorgensen, J., 285
Junge, J., 212

K

Kalikow, K., 55, 56
Kaminski, P. L., 181, 218
Kaplan, A., 272, 287
Kaplan, R. M., 3
Kaptein, S., 287
Kashima, Y., 190, 191, 195, 202, 205, 365
Kater, K., 67, 184, 185, 187, 188, 239, 250, 251, 257, 336, 397, 402
Katzman, D. K., 287
Kavanagh, K., 234, 235, 300, 302, 354
Kaye, W., 43, 44, 46, 47, 49, 50, 51, 78, 285
Kazdin, A., 10, 11, 16, 86, 92, 85, 102, 107, 338, 339, 344, 348, 350, 351, 352, 353
Kealey, K., 266, 267, 268, 269
Kearns, M., 206, 211, 212, 213, 217, 262, 333, 340
Keenan, M. F., 338
Keller, M. B., 285
Kelly, J., 55, 60, 68, 307, 309, 389, 402
Kelly-Vance, L., 318, 323
Kelton-Locke, S., 202
Kendall-Tackett, K. A., 83
Kendler, K. S., 43, 44
Kennedy, P. F., 308
Kennedy, R. E., 13
Kerner, J., 274
Kessler, M., 6, 9
Kessler, R. C., 10, 11, 16, 86, 92, 95, 102, 107
Kilbourne, J., 154, 211, 213, 405
Killen, J., 9, 17, 26, 27, 33, 35, 40, 61, 62, 66, 82, 89, 91, 92, 95, 103, 106, 110, 111, 124, 125, 128, 133, 139, 189, 193, 199, 210, 282, 301, 335, 344, 346, 347, 349, 351, 364, 366, 408
Killingsworth, R., 287
Kirby, D., 239
Kirsch, C., 287
Kishore, A., 49, 50
Klaghofer, R., 200, 201
Klinnert, M., 48
Klump, K. L., 44, 45, 46
Knight, G. P., 244, 248
Kohler, C. L., 16, 126, 365
Koletsky, R. J., 36
Kolshy, P., 35
Konek, J., 398
Kopstein, A., 59
Kosharek, S., 403

AUTHOR INDEX

Kotler, P., 320, 331, 332
Kowalski, R., 240
Kraemer, H., 10, 11, 16, 33, 40, 86, 89, 92, 95, 96, 98, 102, 103, 105, 106, 107, 189, 193, 199, 338, 339, 344, 347, 348, 350, 351, 352, 353, 366, 408
Krahn, D., 213
Krull, J. L., 324, 326
Kuczmarski, R. J., 61, 285
Kumanyika, S., 39
Kumar, R., 233
Kumpfer, K. L., 137
Kupermine, G., 95
Kupfer, D. J., 10, 11, 16, 86, 92, 95, 102, 107
Kurth, C., 213
Kusel, A. B., 312, 313, 317

L

Labre, M., 242
Laframboise, D. E., 218
Laird, N., 61, 197, 250, 251, 259, 286, 288, 340, 367, 397
Lake, J. K., 60
Lambert, M. J., 222
Lamertz, C., 40
Lampert, C., 43
Lapin, A., 58, 241, 324, 326
Larkin, J., 90, 152, 158, 159, 171, 240, 246
Lask, B., 29, 346, 403, 407
Latzer, Y., 353, 354
Lawson, M. L., 216, 344
LeCroy, C. W., 295
Lederhendler, I., 51
Lee, A., 24
Lee, D., 24
Lee, L., 331
Lee, N., 320, 331, 332
Lee, S., 24, 33
Lee, Y., 243, 308, 356
Leffert, N., 138, 139, 141, 281
Lehoux, P., 44, 45
Leichner, P., 56

Leit, R. A., 291, 308
Lemery, K., 48
Leobruni, P., 47
Leon, G., 33, 56, 103
Lerner, R. M., 75, 138
Levine, M. P., 6, 9, 12, 13, 15, 17, 29, 31, 32, 34, 36, 45, 53, 54, 55, 59, 60, 67, 74, 76, 80, 82, 87, 90, 92, 98, 102, 103, 108, 110, 111, 113, 114, 116, 124, 132, 133, 135, 141, 145, 146, 148, 150, 151, 152, 155, 157, 164, 165, 171, 174, 179, 181, 183, 184, 185, 186, 187, 188, 197, 200, 209, 213, 221, 222, 235, 240, 241, 242, 243, 249, 250, 252, 253, 254, 255, 257, 258, 278, 280, 290, 293, 294, 306, 307, 308, 309, 310, 311, 313, 318, 319, 320, 321, 330, 333, 342, 346, 361, 369, 372, 397, 398, 408
Levinson, D., 89
Levitsky, D. A., 38, 63, 64
Lewis, M., 82
Lieberman, M., 190, 193, 250, 275, 295, 342
Lilenfeld, L. R., 43, 44, 45, 46
Lipsey, M. W., 328
Litt, I., 33, 40, 89, 92, 103, 189, 193, 199, 344, 366, 408
Little, D., 206, 211, 212, 213, 217, 262, 333, 340
Littleton, H. L., 179, 188
Lockwood, C. M., 386
Loftus, E., 99
Loggie, J., 39
Lonczak, H. S., 104
Londre, K., 184, 185, 250
Long, B., 353
Love, A., 114
Lowe, M., 35
Lubker, B. B., 15
Lucas, A., 6, 52, 87
Luhtanen, R., 246
Luthar, S. S., 11
Lynch, J., 157, 170
Lyons, P., 62, 65, 67, 292

M

MacKinnon, D. P., 57, 58, 59, 230, 232, 235, 241, 243, 258, 324, 325, 326, 328, 363, 386
Macrina, D. M., 6
Magnavita, N., 133, 201, 204, 205, 221, 250, 261, 341
Maine, M., 17, 53, 55, 60, 68, 208, 241, 307, 389, 402, 405
Mainelli, D., 206, 211, 212, 213, 217, 262, 333, 340
Mallick, M. J., 69
Maloney, D., 147, 148, 198, 239, 240, 276, 370
Maloney, M., 26, 256, 346, 407
Malpeis, S., 349, 351
Manley, K., 397
Mann, S., 266, 267, 268, 269
Mann, T., 86, 205, 206, 208, 210, 215, 353
Manson, J. E., 38
Manwaring, J., 210
Marcus, M., 28
Marek, P., 266, 267, 268, 269
Markey, C., 98
Markman, H. J., 353
Marsh, H. M., 123
Marshall, D. G., 79, 220, 228, 229, 231, 232, 233, 234, 239, 240, 243, 248, 250, 267, 284, 294, 338
Martin, G. C., 48
Martin, J., 242
Martin, M. C., 308
Martz, D. M., 206, 207, 208, 209, 222
Masten, A. S., 135
Maton, K., 284, 298, 302, 304, 305
Matsumoto, N., 403
Matzon, J., 60, 86
Maxim, N., 191, 202, 204
Mazotti, L., 215, 341
Mazzella, R., 52
McAlister, A., 331
McCabe, M. P., 102, 152, 156, 242, 283, 289, 308, 344
McConaha, C., 49, 50

McCreary, D. R., 58, 59
McCurley, J., 66
McGue, M., 45, 46
McGuire, J., 26, 256, 346, 407
McKinley, N. M., 152, 156, 157, 172, 408
McKinney, S., 35
McKnight, K., 26, 27, 82, 408
McLoyd, V., 153
McNamara, K., 181, 218
McNeeley, C., 377
McVey, G., 146, 174, 179, 186, 189, 190, 193, 194, 199, 200, 233, 239, 242, 250, 275, 294, 295, 297, 300, 398
Melton, L., 87
Menassa, B., 397
Mendelson, B., 407
Merikangas, K. R., 388
Merrick, S., 82
Messinger, C. S., 258, 259
Mickalide, A. D., 57
Milkie, M. A., 308
Millar, H. R., 338
Miller, D. J., 58, 241, 324
Miller, J., 149
Miller, W. C., 287
Mills, A., 254, 396
Mills, J. A., 105, 157, 158, 175, 291
Minke, K. M., 284, 298, 299, 300, 302, 303, 305
Mintz, L., 206, 211, 212, 213, 217, 262, 333, 340
Mitchell, J., 47, 78, 104
Mitchell, R. A., 65, 66, 67
Mitchell, R. E., 386
Moe, E. L., 57, 58, 59, 241, 243, 324, 325, 326, 345, 363
Moffit, T. E., 89
Moller-Madsen, S., 285
Moran, J. R., 239, 244, 245, 247, 248
Moran, R., 403
Moreno, A. B., 189, 194, 195, 340
Moriarty, D., 182, 191, 202, 204
Morrell, T., 182, 191
Moulton, M., 28
Mrazek, D., 48
Mrazek, P. J., 6, 7, 8, 10, 386

Mucci, L. A., 240
Muir, S. L., 114, 283, 290
Muñoz, R. F., 6, 8, 10
Munstertieger, B., 106, 161, 243
Murnen, S. K., 6, 11, 13, 17, 47, 48, 51, 52, 53, 55, 77, 79, 80, 83, 90, 91, 92, 98, 99, 102, 103, 105, 114, 152, 154, 157, 158, 159, 165, 171, 175, 240, 241, 243, 257, 262, 277, 278, 279, 283, 291, 306, 308, 311, 331, 345
Murray, D. M., 230, 232, 258
Murray, L., 137–138
Murray, S. H., 308
Muse, A., 56
Mussell, M. P., 179
Must, A., 37
Muth, J., 52, 150
Mutterperl, J. A., 207, 208, 258

N

Natenshon, A., 403
Nathanson, D., 191, 196, 202, 204, 207, 209, 213
Naworski, P., 66, 254, 397
Neal, M. E., 202, 372
Neal-Walden, T., 35
Nebel, M., 206, 209
Neitz, E., 254, 396
Nelsen, L., 35
Nelson, L., 53, 146, 191, 196, 202, 204, 207, 209, 213
Nemeroff, C., 86
Netemeyer, R. G., 122
Netemeyer, S. B., 25, 189, 196, 197, 297, 300, 345
Neumark-Sztainer, D., 12, 15, 36, 39, 55, 57, 58, 60, 61, 62, 65, 68, 69, 79, 110, 124, 125, 126, 128, 131, 132, 133, 136, 138, 139, 163, 164, 175, 181, 185, 186, 201, 204, 205, 218, 221, 240, 243, 243, 246, 247, 250, 258, 259, 260–261, 261, 270, 276, 278, 283, 285, 292, 299, 317, 319, 336, 351, 363, 366, 368, 372, 398
Newman, D., 90
Newman, L., 396
Newman, M., 212
Newsholme, E. A., 50
Ngai, E., 24
Nicholls, D., 29
Nichter, M., 4, 25, 54, 81, 111, 152, 202, 205, 247, 248, 249, 258, 262, 283, 290, 308, 339, 399
Nicolino, J. C., 206, 208
Nielsen, S., 216, 285
Nikkhou, N., 215
Nolen-Hoeksema, S., 86, 205, 206, 208, 210, 353
Noll, S., 156, 157, 408
Nonnemaker, J., 377

O

Obagi, S., 215
Oberklaid, F., 48
Ochshorn, P., 79, 220, 228, 229, 231, 232, 233, 234, 239, 240, 243, 248, 250, 267, 284, 294, 338
O'Dea, J., 17, 80, 142, 143, 144, 145, 146, 147, 148, 181, 189, 190, 198, 205, 221, 222, 239, 240, 248, 250, 275, 276, 311, 318, 322, 323, 341, 364, 370, 388, 389, 397
O'Fallon, M., 87
Offer, D., 408
Offord, D., 10, 11, 16, 86, 92, 95, 102, 107, 338, 339, 344, 348, 350, 351, 352, 353
Ogg, E. C., 338
Olivardia, R., 55, 58, 59, 155, 242, 243, 262, 283, 291, 315, 324, 345
Olivetto, M. C., 133, 201, 204, 205, 221, 250, 261, 341
Ollendick, T., 179, 188
Olmsted, M. P., 34, 35, 216, 287, 344
O'Malley, P. M., 233
Omori, M., 35

AUTHOR INDEX

O'Reilly, K., 331
Orosan-Weine, P., 179
Osborn, B., 254, 396
Outwater, A. D., 186, 189, 196, 197
Overton, W., 75

P

Pagsberg, K., 285
Pai, S., 163, 164, 174, 175, 190, 194, 198
Paikoff, R., 40
Pajouhandeh, P., 54
Palti, H., 124, 125, 126, 128, 131, 132, 133, 201, 204, 205, 221, 250, 261, 317, 366
Papazian, R., 154
Parcel, G., 108, 109, 124, 126, 133
Parker, S., 81, 202, 205, 247, 248, 399
Parkinson, K., 151
Parnaby, O., 26, 27, 408
Parry-Billings, M., 50
Pasqualoni, E., 192, 196
Paxton, S. J., 114, 152, 190, 191, 195, 200, 201, 283, 290, 323, 365
Peirce, K., 319
Pentz, M. A., 228, 235, 237, 268, 318, 328
Perkins, R., 206, 207, 210, 250, 262
Perlick, D., 13, 14, 17, 58
Perry, C., 5, 14, 16, 33, 56, 103, 108, 109, 124, 126, 133, 142, 146, 232, 233, 235, 239, 243, 250, 264, 265, 284, 294, 301, 302, 328, 367, 376
Petersen, A., 13, 89, 408
Peterson, A., 266, 267, 268, 269
Peterson, K., 61, 197, 198, 250, 251, 259, 286, 288, 340, 364, 367, 397
Phelps, L., 53, 146, 191, 196, 202, 204, 207, 209, 213
Philliber, S., 95
Phillips, K. A., 55, 58, 59, 155, 242, 243, 262, 283, 291, 315, 324, 345
Phinney, J., 246
Piaget, J., 75
Pierce, J. P., 331
Pietrobelli, A., 60

Pike, K., 27, 28, 114, 116, 119
Pilawski, A., 365
Piran, N., 9, 16, 17, 29, 53, 54, 57, 60, 68, 77, 79, 80, 92, 94, 100, 105, 106, 108, 124, 125, 132, 133, 135, 141, 142, 145, 146, 147, 148, 150, 152, 157, 159, 162, 163, 164, 165, 167, 168, 169, 170, 171, 175, 179, 181, 191, 198, 200, 202, 205, 213, 221, 222, 239, 240, 241, 244, 246, 248, 260, 261, 262, 263, 269, 273, 276, 278, 285, 289, 290, 291, 298, 299, 300, 307, 308, 310, 311, 313, 318, 319, 320, 321, 333, 341, 342, 343, 352, 353, 361, 364, 369, 370, 371, 372, 373
Pirie, P. L., 235, 328
Pi-Sunyer, F. X., 38, 60
Polivy, J., 34, 35, 346
Pollard, J., 278
Pomeroy, C., 21, 285
Ponton, L. E., 136
Pope, H. G., Jr., 55, 58, 59, 155, 242, 243, 262, 283, 291, 308, 315, 324, 345
Porter, J., 182, 191
Posavac, E. J., 316
Posavac, H. D., 312, 316
Posavac, S. S., 312, 316
Power, C., 60
Powers, P. S., 57
Pratt, B. M., 179
Presnell, K., 223
Price, R. H., 4, 10, 15, 16
Prineas, R., 39
Prior, M., 48
Pryor, T., 398
Pryzbeck, T., 47
Puhl, R., 64, 65
Pung, M., 217
Pusztai, E. E., 338
Putnam, K., 49, 50

Q

Quinn, D., 174
Quinn, G. P., 331, 332

R

Rabak-Wagener, J., 318, 323
Raevuori, A., 47
Ragan, J., 217
Raj, A., 240
Rallo, J. S., 56
Ramey, S. L., 353
Ransley, J., 288, 293, 301
Raudenbush, S., 287
Reaman, J. A., 239, 244, 245, 247, 248
Reas, D, 189, 196, 197, 297, 300
Reed, D. L., 408
Reed, V., 200, 201
Reger, B., 328
Reiss, D., 16
Rende, R., 388
Renger, R., 26, 27, 131, 148, 408
Resnick, M., 55, 58, 65, 135–136, 246
Rex, J., 292, 368
Reynolds, K., 16, 126, 365
Ribisl, K. M., 237
Ricciardelli, L. A., 102, 242, 283, 289, 308, 344
Rice, C., 152, 158, 159, 171, 240, 246
Rice, R. E., 327, 328
Rich, T., 92, 189, 193, 199, 344, 366
Richards, A., 285
Richards, P. S., 12
Richman, R. D., 184, 187, 189, 194
Rieger, E., 24
Rietmeijer, C. A., 331
Ringwalt, C. L., 237
Ritchie, J., 185, 186, 188, 222
Ritter, P., 242
Roberto, N., 320, 331, 332
Roberts, S. R., 308
Roberts, T., 76, 152, 153, 155, 156, 157, 172, 175, 291
Robinson, A., 93
Robinson, T. N., 33, 40, 61, 67, 103, 408
Robison, J., 62
Rocco, P. L., 202, 204
Roche, A., 37
Rockett, H. R., 35, 349
Rodin, G. M., 216, 344
Rodin, J., 31, 66, 258
Rohrback, L., 237
Rohwer, J., 184, 185, 250
Roncolato, W., 185, 186, 188, 222
Roona, M. R., 79, 220, 228, 229, 231, 232, 233, 234, 239, 240, 243, 248, 250, 267, 284, 294, 338
Roosa, M. W., 244, 248
Rosen, J. C., 181, 201, 204
Rosen, K., 73
Rosenthal, R., 267
Rosenthal, S., 82
Rosenvinge, J. H., 16, 179, 222, 223, 290, 376
Rosner, B., 39, 349, 351
Rosnow, R. L., 267
Roth, J. L., 137–138, 386
Rothbaum, P. A., 140
Rothblum, E. D., 54, 64, 65, 110, 156
Rovera, G., 47
Rozin, P., 408
Rubin, K. H., 48
Ruble, A., 25, 78, 79, 102, 105, 336
Ruiz Lazaro, P. M., 399
Rush, A. J., 117, 119, 132
Russell, G. F. M., 387
Russell, V., 90, 152, 158, 159, 171, 240, 246
Ryan, J. A. M., 104
Rydall, A. C., 216, 344
Ryff, C. D., 408

S

Sacco, W. P., 408
Saelens, B. E., 37
Salimi, L., 353
Saltzberg, E., 181
Sameroff, A., 75
Sanders, M., 151
Sanderson, C. A., 207, 208, 222, 258, 259, 366
Sanson, A., 48
Santonastaso, P., 133, 201, 204, 205, 221, 250, 261, 341

Sapia, J., 53, 146, 191, 196, 202, 205, 207, 209, 213
Sargent, R., 151, 338
Sargiani, P., 13
Sartirana, M., 192, 196
Sasse, D. K., 58, 59
Saunders, S. E., 38, 60, 65
Sawrer, D., 154
Scales, P. C., 138, 141, 281
Schermer, F., 12, 32, 60, 87, 114, 133, 141, 148, 183, 184, 187, 222, 235, 249, 252, 255
Schmid, T., 287
Schmidt, L. A., 48
Schmidt, U., 338
Schneider-Rosen, K., 73
Schulenberg, J. E., 233
Schuman, M., 191, 196
Schupak-Neuberg, E., 308, 407
Schur, E., 151
Schutz, H. K., 114, 283, 290
Schuyler, T., 140
Schwitzer, A. M., 353
Scott, E., 272, 398
Seaver, A., 146, 193, 239, 294, 398
Secker-Walker, R. H., 235, 328
Severson, H. H., 230, 232, 258
Shaffer, D., 55, 56
Shafran, R., 116, 132
Sharma, A. R., 138
Sharpe, T., 26, 27, 206, 211, 408
Shatz, S., 353, 354
Shaw, B. F., 117, 119, 132, 146, 194, 300, 398
Shaw, H. E., 86, 136, 179, 205, 213, 220, 221, 222, 223, 233, 265, 267, 308, 335, 336, 338, 346, 351, 353, 357, 361, 389, 407
Shaw, J., 311
Sheffield, C., 155
Shepard, R. E., 201, 204
Sheridan, C., 320
Sherman, R., 403
Sherwood, N., 163, 164, 175, 181, 250, 260–261, 317, 318, 319, 336
Shields, S. A., 407
Shiltz, T. J., 272, 398
Shissiak, C., 11, 20, 25, 26, 27, 31, 78, 82, 102, 105, 131, 148, 174, 179, 202, 253, 336, 372, 408
Shore, R., 191, 202, 204
Shriver, T. P., 133, 141, 251, 376
Shukiban, L., 215
Shulenberg, J. E., 408
Shure, M. B., 353
Siegel, M., 403
Siegel-Gorelik, B., 242
Siervogel, R., 37
Silber, T., 21
Silberstein, L., 31, 258
Silverman, J. G., 240
Silverstein, B., 13, 14, 17, 58
Simmonds, B., 33, 40, 92, 103, 189, 193, 199, 344, 366, 408
Sivyer, R., 114
Sjostrom, L., 163, 164, 174, 175, 190, 194, 198
Slater, A., 156, 157
Smart, D., 48
Smith, J. E., 218
Smolak, L., 6, 9, 11, 12, 13, 14, 15, 16, 17, 21, 26, 31, 32, 34, 36, 45, 47, 48, 51, 52, 53, 54, 55, 59, 60, 67, 74, 76, 77, 78, 79, 80, 81, 82, 83, 83, 87, 90, 91, 92, 94, 97, 98, 99, 102, 103, 105, 105, 106, 110, 111, 113, 114, 116, 124, 132, 133, 135, 141, 145, 148, 150, 151, 152, 154, 155, 157, 158, 159, 161, 165, 171, 174, 175, 175, 179, 180, 183, 184, 186, 188, 197, 200, 213, 221, 222, 235, 240, 241, 242, 243, 245, 246, 247, 249, 250, 252, 253, 254, 255, 257, 258, 262, 277, 278, 279, 283, 291, 294, 306, 307, 308, 311, 330, 331, 345, 346, 349–350, 395, 408
Smolkowski, K., 236, 266, 268, 284, 384
Sobal, J., 38, 63, 64
Sobczak, C., 272, 398
Sobol, A. M., 61, 197, 250. 251, 259, 286, 288, 340, 367, 397
Sorter, R., 25

Specker, B., 26, 256, 346, 407
Speizer, F. E., 38
Spiller, B. B., 207, 210
Springer, E., 206, 207, 210, 211, 250, 262
Spurrell, E., 27
Srebnik, D., 181
Srikameswaran, S., 56, 105, 277, 291
Srinivasan, S., 37
Stackpole, K. M., 79, 220, 228, 229, 231, 232, 233, 234, 239, 240, 243, 248, 250, 267, 284, 294, 338
Stampfer, M. J., 38
Stanton, A. L., 123
Steen, S. N., 56
Stein, D., 56
Stein, N., 25, 99, 154, 162, 174, 189
Stein, R. I., 308, 407
Stein, S., 25
Steiner, H., 151
Steiner-Adair, C., 106, 159, 161, 163, 164, 171, 174, 175, 190, 194, 198, 255, 291, 311, 333
Stephens, J., 59
Stevenson, J. F., 386
Stewart, A., 95, 120, 127, 128, 129, 131, 145, 193, 364
Stewart, D. A., 127, 130, 132, 133, 189, 191, 194, 208, 222, 353
Stewart, T. M., 119, 122
Stice, E., 10, 11, 13, 15, 33, 34, 35, 40, 46, 47, 66, 86, 91, 92, 98, 101, 102, 105, 106, 107, 113, 114, 131, 134, 136, 157, 179, 205, 211, 213, 214, 214, 215, 217, 220, 221, 222, 223, 265, 266, 267, 282, 301, 306, 308, 321, 323, 335, 336, 337, 338, 341, 344, 345, 346, 349, 351, 353, 357, 361, 364, 368, 389, 407
Stoddard, C., 164, 307, 310, 311, 313, 318, 319, 320, 321, 338, 342, 361
Stone, E. J., 230, 232, 258
Stormer, S., 101, 211, 213, 214, 215, 312, 314, 315, 323, 364, 408
Story, M., 39, 55, 57, 58, 65, 67, 135–136, 138, 139, 240, 243, 246, 258, 270, 283, 292, 299, 368

Strachan, M. D., 214, 222, 223, 272
Strachowski, D., 33, 347
Strasburger, V. C., 334
Stratton, L., 146, 193, 239, 294, 398
Strauman, T. J., 122, 123
Streke, A. V., 79, 220, 228, 229, 231, 232, 233, 234, 239, 240, 243, 248, 250, 267, 284, 294, 338
Striegel-Moore, R. H., 17, 21, 27, 28, 31, 34, 77, 78, 80, 83, 92, 102, 106, 164, 245, 246, 247, 258, 272, 345, 349–350
Strober, M., 43, 44, 46, 47, 49, 50, 51, 78, 285
Strong, K. G., 114
Strong, K. O., 196, 311, 312
Sturgis, E. T., 207, 209
Sullivan, A. M., 160
Sullivan, P. F., 43, 44, 47
Sunday, S. R., 202, 204
Sussman, S., 230, 232, 258
Svrakic, D., 46
Swain, R., 24
Szymanski, M. L., 123

T

Tanofsky, M., 27
Tanofsky-Kraff, M., 60, 66
Tantleff-Dunn, S., 13, 14, 45, 51, 54, 67, 68, 101, 102, 114, 115, 116, 117, 119, 122, 123, 124, 152, 240, 241, 254, 283, 288, 290, 291, 306, 307, 308, 315, 345
Tarule, J. M., 150
Tavris, C., 149
Taylor, C. B., 26, 33, 35, 40, 55, 65, 66, 82, 89, 91, 92, 103, 106, 189, 193, 199, 203, 206, 207, 210, 211, 212, 217, 222, 242, 250, 258, 262, 301, 306, 308, 333, 340, 341, 344, 346, 347, 349, 351, 354, 355, 364, 408
Taylor, C. L., 346, 407
Taylor, J. M., 160
Taylor, M. J., 407

Taylor, S. E., 260
Terry, R., 151
Thaw, J., 189, 196, 197, 297, 300
Theander, S., 285
Thelen, M. H., 189, 194, 195, 340
Themba, M., 307, 329
Then, D., 308
Thom, A. S., 338
Thompson, B., 28, 77, 399
Thompson, J. K., 10, 11, 13, 14, 45, 51, 54, 59, 60, 67, 68, 86, 98, 101, 102, 114, 116, 117, 119, 122, 123, 124, 141, 152, 155, 157, 240, 241, 243, 254, 282, 283, 291, 306, 307, 308, 312, 314, 315, 323, 337, 345, 360, 408
Thompson, R. A., 403
Thompson, S., 54, 151, 185, 186, 188, 308
Thomsen, S. R., 308
Tiggemann, M., 156, 157, 170, 255, 292
Tilgner, L., 190, 195
Tobler, N. S., 79, 220, 228, 229, 231, 232, 233, 234, 239, 240, 243, 248, 250, 267, 284, 294, 338
Toledo, T., 372
Touyz, S., 24, 308
Tovèe, M., 151
Towell, T., 114
Treasure, J., 338
Treboux, D., 82
Troiano, R. P., 38, 61, 63, 64, 285
Trost, A., 215
Trotta, L., 332
Tucker, R., 163, 164, 174, 175, 190, 194, 198
Tweed, S., 146, 174, 190, 193, 194, 233, 250, 294, 295, 297, 300, 342, 398
Twenge, J., 174
Twigg, K., 190, 191, 195, 365

U

Ubriaco, M., 140
Utermohlen, V., 308
Utter, J., 258

V

Valdez, R., 287
Valoski, A., 66
van Hoeken, D, 6, 20, 21, 25, 52, 56, 87, 97, 259, 387
Van Strien, T., 92, 346, 407
Varady, A., 33, 40, 89, 92, 103, 193, 199, 344, 366, 408
Varnado-Sullivan, P. J., 189, 196, 197, 297, 300
Vigfusdottir, T. H., 243, 308, 356
Villapiano, M., 206, 211, 212, 213, 217, 262, 333, 340
Villena, J., 191
Vincent, M., 152, 156
Vincus, A. A., 237
Vitiello, B., 51
Vitousek, K., 116, 118, 119, 132
Vookles, J., 122, 123
Voorberg, N., 190, 193, 250, 275, 295, 342
Vorenberg, A. P., 241, 250, 259, 260, 261
Vukovic, N., 81, 202, 205, 247, 248, 399
Vulcano, B., 56

W

Wadden, T. A., 56
Wade, T. D., 43, 44, 181, 190, 205, 311, 318, 322, 323
Wall, M., 39, 258
Wallack, L., 307, 329
Waller, G., 311
Walsh, A. E. S., 49
Walsh, T., 55, 56
Walsh-Childers, K., 327
Wandersman, A., 147, 383, 386
Wang, E. Y., 235, 328
Wardrope, D., 190, 193, 250, 275, 295, 342
Warren, M., 40, 90
Waterhouse, D., 402
Waters, E., 82
Watt, N. F., 353
Weber, M. M., 308
Wechsler, H., 290
Weibel, D., 215, 341

Weigel, R. G., 312, 316
Weinberg, R. A., 138
Weiner, R., 292, 337
Weinshel, M., 403
Weiss, K. R., 200, 201, 222
Weissberg, R. P., 133, 134, 140, 141, 153, 251, 376
Weltzin, T. E., 47
Wenter, D. L., 237
Wertheim, E. H., 48, 114, 190, 191, 195, 202, 205, 290, 365
West, S. G., 353
Westjordet, M. Ø., 290
Whitaker, A., 55, 56
White, D., 407
White, M. A., 119, 122
Wichstrøm, L., 56, 89, 91, 106, 349, 351, 301
Wiecha, J., 61, 197, 198, 250, 251, 259, 286, 288, 340, 364, 367, 397
Wilfley, D., 25, 27, 28, 37, 60, 66, 151, 206–207, 210, 211, 217, 262
Willett, W. C., 38
Williams, Z., 308
Williams, C., 49
Williams, L. M., 83
Williamson, D., 25, 35, 36, 119, 122, 189, 196, 197, 287, 297, 300, 345
Williamson, I., 57
Wilson, D., 33, 40, 89, 92, 103, 189, 193, 199, 344, 347, 366, 408
Wilson, G. T., 26, 38, 66, 109, 127
Winett, R. A., 14, 17, 18
Wing, R. R., 66
Wing, Y., 24
Winzelberg, A., 203, 206, 207, 210, 211, 212, 217, 222, 250, 262, 333, 340, 341, 344, 351, 354, 355, 364

Wiseman, C. V., 202, 204
Withers, G. F., 190, 191, 195, 365
Wolf, N., 150, 321
Wolf, S. L., 58, 241, 324
Wolf-Bloom, M. S., 311, 312
Wolfe, B. L., 218
Wolitski, R. J., 331
Wonderlich, S., 44, 45, 46, 47, 48, 272
Wood, C., 141
Woodside, D., 87, 261, 287
Wooley, S. C., 38, 40, 66, 83, 99, 152, 159
Woolfenden, S. R., 179
Wootan, M. G., 328
Worden, J. K., 235, 328
Wright, A., 86, 205, 206, 208, 210, 353
Wroblewska, A.-M., 59

Y

Yanovski, S. Z., 38, 66
Yassouridis, A., 40
Yee, D., 213
Yesalis, C., 59
York-Crowe, E., 119, 122
Yuker, H. E., 40, 64

Z

Zabinski, M. F., 210, 217
Zaitsoff, S., 105, 277, 291
Zanetti, T., 132, 201, 204, 205, 221, 250, 261, 341
Zeckhausen, D., 266, 396, 397
Zlot, A., 287
Zoref, L., 58, 241, 324
Zucker, N., 189, 196, 197, 297, 300

Subject Index

A

Affective education, 229
Anorexia nervosa
    children, 285
    DSM–IV–TR definition of, 21–25
    Grand Ormand Street definition of, 30

B

Behavior genetics, 43–45
Behind Closed Doors (video), 320
Body image, 102
    media effects and, 308
    obesity, 67
    targeted prevention for, 213–217
        cognitive behavioral therapy, 213–214
        dissonance-based, 214–216
        psychoeducational, 216–217
Boys
    media effects, 308
    programs for, 242–243, 324–326
    role in prevention of eating problems in girls, 240–242
Bulimia nervosa
    children, 285
    DSM–IV–TR definition of, 25–27
    Grand Ormand Street definition of, 30

C

Cognitive-behavioral theory, 115–124
    basic concepts, 115–116
    body image, 116–121
    hypothesis testing and behavioral change, 120–121
    paralogical errors, 119–120
    research support, 121–124
    schema, 116–119
    Warneford Hospital Program, 127–130
Cognitive-behavioral therapy, 282
College students
    curriculum development, 261–262
    media literacy, 314–317, 323
    prevention programs, 205–213, 399
Comments to children and adolescents, 288–289
Computer-assisted prevention programs, 354–356, *see also* Cyber-prevention
Continuum of eating disorders, 31–36

464 SUBJECT INDEX

Control groups, 266–269
  contamination of, 267–268
  statistical power and, 267
CORE model of collaboration, 302–304
Curriculum development, 239–263
  developmental considerations, 252–262
  gender, 242–243
  race/ethnicity, 245–248
  themes, 248–252
Cyber-prevention, 331–333, *see also* Computer-assisted prevention programs

D

Developmental psychopathology, 73–94
  developmental contexts, 74–83
    implications for prevention, 77–83, 93
  developmental reciprocity, 81–83
  developmental trajectories, 83–87
  developmental transitions, 87–91
  methodological implications of, 91–92
Dieting
  prevention of, 217–219
    cognitive-behavioral psychoeducational approaches, 217–219
Disease-specific pathways, 130–131
Disembodiment (disrupted embodiment), 171–172
Dissonance reduction, 214–216, 365
Drive for muscularity, 58–60

E

Early adolescent transition, 84–85
Eating disorders
  anorexia nervosa
    DSM–IV–TR definition of, 21–25
    Grand Ormand Street definition of, 30
  bulimia nervosa
    DSM–IV–TR definition of, 25–27
    Grand Ormand Street definition of, 30
  continuum of, 31–36, 40, 97–98
  EDNOS
    children, 285
    DSM–IV–TR definition of, 28–29
    Grand Ormand Street definition of, 30
  food avoidance emotional disorder, 29–30
  gender and, 150–152
  males, 55–58
  neuropsychiatric approaches, 43–52
  prevalence, 11–12, 97
  signs and symptoms, 292–293
Ecological approaches to prevention
  assessing, 275–280, 383–387
  Bronfenbrenner's model, 75–77
    applied to prevention, 379–382
  collaboration, 302–304
  developmental psychopathology and, 74–83
  multiple settings, 297–305
  prevention and, 77–83
  school-based prevention of substance abuse and, 233–238
EDNOS
  DSM–IV–TR definition of, 28–29
  Grand Ormand Street definition of, 30
Elementary school
  curriculum development, 256
  eating disorders, 285
  media literacy, 317–319
  prevention programs, 184–188, 397
Ethnic minority groups
  eating disorders, 80–81
  prevention of eating disorders, 245–248
  resources for, 399
  substance abuse prevention programs, 243–245
Evaluation of prevention programs, 264–269, 383–387
  control groups, 266–269
  ecologically based programs, assessment of, 275–280

multiple settings, 298–302
program fidelity, 273–275

F

"Fat talk," 258, 290
Feminist-ecological-developmental (FED) model of prevention, 368–369, 377–387
Feminist-empowerment-relational model, 149–175, 363–365
  lived experience and proximal goals, 162–164
  program development and delivery, 158–164
  targeted prevention and, 340–343

G

Gender and eating disorders, 20–21, 80–81, 150–152
  curriculum development and, 240–243
  resources, 401

H

Health belief model, 365
Health promotion, 61–68
Health promoting schools, 370–376
High school
  curriculum development, 261
  media literacy programs, 314, 319–323
  prevention programs, 200–205, 398
    negative results, 200–204
    positive results, 204

I

Indicated (targeted) prevention defined, 9
Information-based programs, 229
Interactive delivery, 232–233

L

Life skills, 139–141
Life Skills Training Program, 231–232, 274
Lived experience, 162–164

M

Males, 52–60
  body dissatisfaction and drive for muscularity, 58–60
  cultural context participants, 53–55
  disordered eating and, 55–58
  media literacy, 314–315, 323–326
McKnight Risk Factor Screen, 347–348
Measures used in prevention studies, 407–408
Media activism, 307–309
  resources, 399–400
Media advocacy, 329–330
Media literacy, 309–327
  definition, 309–311
  goals and processes, 310–311
  resources, 399–400
Medicalization, 14
Middle school (junior high school)
  curriculum development, 257–261
  media literacy programs, 313–314, 317, 319
  prevention programs, 188–200, 397–398
    negative results, 193, 196–197
    positive results, 194–196

N

National Eating Disorders Association (NEDA), 329–330
Neurogenetic (neuropsychiatric) perspective on eating disorders, 43–52, 387–388
  behavior genetics, 43–45
  serotonin, 49–52
  temperament, 46–48

Non-Specific Vulnerability-Stressor model, 134–148, 363–365
 general model, 135–139
 prototypical elements of programs, 146
 proximal goals, 139–142
Normative developmental changes, 87–88
Nonnormative developmental changes, 88
Nutrition and exercise, 63, 285–288

O

Obesity, *see* Overweight and obesity
Objectification theory, 152–158
 reduction of objectification, 332
 self-objectification, 155–159
  effects of, 157–159
 sexual objectification, 153–155
Opportunities for non-appearance success, 291–292
Overweight and obesity
 definitions, 38–40
  adult, 38–39
  child, 39–40
 prevention of, 60–68, 367–368, 400–401
 relationship to eating disorders, 40, 367–368
 signs of, 292–294

P

Parents, 375–376
 parent education program, 295
 resources for, 402–404
Preschool
 curriculum development, 253–255
Prevention
 dangers of, 221–222, 389–390
 definitions, 6–10
 developmental psychopathology and, 77–83, 93
 effectiveness, 219–223, 366–367

feminist models, 149–175, 363–365, 368–369, 377–387
males
 role of, 53–55
 prevention for, 55–60
Non-Specific Vulnerability-Stressor model, 134–148
obesity, 60–68, 400–401
principles of, 13–18
proximal goals, 162–164
rationale for, 11–13
social cognitive approaches, 108–133
treatment, difference from, 361–363
Prevention programs, 397–399
 BodyWise, 372
 community-based programs, 235–238
  Communities That Care (substance abuse program), 237–238
  Project SixTeen (substance abuse program), 236–237
  Project Star (substance abuse program), 235–236
 feminist-empowerment-relational approach, 164–177
  The Ballet School Study, 165–170
  Full of Ourselves, 164, 198–199
  Just for Girls, 164–165, 174
 manuals, 272–273
 media literacy, 311–327
  ATLAS, 59, 324–326
  ATHENA, 59, 326–327
  Free to be Me, 317–319
  GO GIRLS!, 164, 174, 319–323, 343
 Non-Specific Vulnerability-Stressor approach, 142–148
  Everybody's Different, 142–145, 205
 psychoeducational programs, 216–219
  Body Traps, 210–211
  Eating Smart, Eating for Me, 183–184, 187, 274
  Every Body Is a Somebody, 193–194
  Five-Day Lesson Plan, 289–290
  Food, Mood, & Attitude, 211–212
  Freedom From Dieting, 219

SUBJECT INDEX 467

Healthy Body Images: Teaching Kids to Eat, and Love Their Bodies, Too!, 187–188
Student Bodies, 210–213, 220, 355–356
resource coordinator, 270–272, 371–372, 375
school-based programs, 294–297
Healthy Schools—Healthy Kids, 294–297
social cognitive approaches, 197–198
ATLAS, 324–326
ATHENA, 326–327
Planet Health, 197–198, 286
The Weigh to Eat!, 125–127
The Warneford Hospital curriculum, 127–130
Prevention resources, 393–406
advocacy and activism, 405–406
eating disorders organizations and websites, 393–394
ethnic minority resources, 399
fiction about body image and eating problems, 396
media literacy and activism, 399–400
prevention curricula and program guides, 397–399, *see also* Prevention programs
obesity, 400–401
Program delivery, 269–275
program fidelity, 273–275
Program participation effect (PPE), 193–194
Protective factors
definition of, 11, 104
types of, 104–106

R

Race, *see* Ethnic minority groups
Resilience, 11, 136–139
Resistance skills, 230–232
Risk factors, 33, 95–107
biological factors, 103–104
BMI, 102

body dissatisfaction, 102–103
definitions, 10, 95
problems with, 96–100
empirical support for, 101
identification of, 343–348
media, 307–308
Non-Specific Vulnerability-Stressor model and, 135–136
parent comments, 289
sociocultural factors, 36, 103
targeted prevention and, 344–345
weight concerns, 102–103
Role models, 289–291
educators as, 372–373

S

School-based programs, 228, 248–263, 294–297
developmental considerations, 252–262
ecological approaches, 233–235, 294–297
effectiveness of, 366–367
general themes, 248–252
Selective prevention, 9, 180, 336, 338
Serotonin, 49–51, 104
Sexual abuse, 98–99
experimental design and, 98–99
risk factor for eating disorders, 101
Sexual harassment, 76, 98–99, 289
experimental design and, 98–99
risk factor for eating disorders, 101
Slim Hopes (video), 313, 314, 316, 317, 323
Social cognitive/cognitive behavioral theory
the Big 3 paradigms, 363–365
social cognitive theory, 109–111
social learning theory, 111–115
direct experience, 111
observational learning, 111–112
research background, 113–115
symbolic communication, 112–113

SUBJECT INDEX

Social marketing and health promotion, 331
Social norm theory, 365
  correction of norm misperception, 208–209
Statistical power, 267
Steroid use, prevention of, 324–327
Substance use prevention, 227–239
  effective program components, 238
  ethnicity, 243–245
  lessons from, 228–233
  media campaigns and, 328–329

T

Targeted prevention, 213–223
  assessment of, 351–353
  body image, 213–217
  combined with universal prevention, 356–357
  chronic dieting and subclinical eating disorders, 217–219
  cost–benefits assessments, 348–351
  definition of, 9
  discussion groups, 340–343
  identification of participants, 343–348
    measures for, 345–348, 407–408
  programs, 213–223

Temperament, 46–48

U

Universal prevention, 181–213
  assessment of, 351–353
  combined with targeted, 353–356
  definition, 9
  effectiveness of, 220–223
  philosophy of, 339–340
  programs, 181–213
    elementary school, 184–188
    middle school, 188–200
    high school, 200–205
    college and young adult, 205–213

V

Voice, 159, 161–162

Y

Youth development programs, 137–139

Z

Zero indifference, 289